Global Health Security - Contemporary Considerations and Developments

Edited by Allincia Michaud, Stanislaw P. Stawicki and Ricardo Izurieta

Published in London, United Kingdom

Global Health Security - Contemporary Considerations and Developments
http://dx.doi.org/10.5772/intechopen.107822
Edited by Allincia Michaud, Stanislaw P. Stawicki and Ricardo Izurieta

Contributors
Allincia Michaud, Belay Desye, Belinda Hengel, Cheick Armand N. Palm, Ciprian M. Mihai Cirtiu, Elie Kabre, Hannah S. Jacobs-El, Ibrahim Khalil Dadari, Jeffrey S. Freed, Jibrailu L. Lot Maliyogbinda, Josep M. Ramon-Torrell, Julius Kenkoh Nkiese, Louise Causer, Marissa Smith, Mark Shephard, N. Stanislas Dimitri Meda, Nelly Sharpley, Ngozi Chioma Ewurum, Norayuni Ismail, Normand Fleury, Nur Ismah Izzati Ismail, Ram Roth, Rebecca Guy, Rudra Dahal, Samuel Oseloka Okafor, Sara Spowart, Sharifa Ezat Wan Puteh, Shona Hilton, Soo Y. Kwon, Stanislaw P. Stawicki, Stephanie Kininla Wirba, Susan Janet Matthews, Vincent Cirimele, Zachariah G. Goldsmith

First published in London, United Kingdom, 2024 by IntechOpen
IntechOpen is the global imprint of INTECHOPEN LIMITED, registered in England and Wales, registration number: 11086078, 167-169 Great Portland Street, London, W1W 5PF, United Kingdom

British Library Cataloguing-in-Publication Data
A catalogue record for this book is available from the British Library

Additional hard and PDF copies can be obtained from orders@intechopen.com

Global Health Security - Contemporary Considerations and Developments
Edited by Allincia Michaud, Stanislaw P. Stawicki and Ricardo Izurieta
p. cm.

This title is part of the Sustainable Development Book Series, Volume 17
Topic: Health and Wellbeing
Series Editor: Usha Iyer-Raniga
Topic Editor: Ann Hemingway

Print ISBN 978-1-83769-249-1
Online ISBN 978-1-83769-250-7
eBook (PDF) ISBN 978-1-83769-251-4
ISSN 2753-6580

IntechOpen Book Series

Sustainable Development

Volume 17

Aims and Scope of the Series

Transforming our World: the 2030 Agenda for Sustainable Development endorsed by United Nations and 193 Member States, came into effect on Jan 1, 2016, to guide decision making and actions to the year 2030 and beyond. Central to this Agenda are 17 Goals, 169 associated targets and over 230 indicators that are reviewed annually. The vision envisaged in the implementation of the SDGs is centered on the five Ps: People, Planet, Prosperity, Peace and Partnership. This call for renewed focused efforts ensure we have a safe and healthy planet for current and future generations.

This Series focuses on covering research and applied research involving the five Ps through the following topics:

1. Sustainable Economy and Fair Society that relates to SDG 1 on No Poverty, SDG 2 on Zero Hunger, SDG 8 on Decent Work and Economic Growth, SDG 10 on Reduced Inequalities, SDG 12 on Responsible Consumption and Production, and SDG 17 Partnership for the Goals

2. Health and Wellbeing focusing on SDG 3 on Good Health and Wellbeing and SDG 6 on Clean Water and Sanitation

3. Inclusivity and Social Equality involving SDG 4 on Quality Education, SDG 5 on Gender Equality, and SDG 16 on Peace, Justice and Strong Institutions

4. Climate Change and Environmental Sustainability comprising SDG 13 on Climate Action, SDG 14 on Life Below Water, and SDG 15 on Life on Land

5. Urban Planning and Environmental Management embracing SDG 7 on Affordable Clean Energy, SDG 9 on Industry, Innovation and Infrastructure, and SDG 11 on Sustainable Cities and Communities.

The series also seeks to support the use of cross cutting SDGs, as many of the goals listed above, targets and indicators are all interconnected to impact our lives and the decisions we make on a daily basis, making them impossible to tie to a single topic.

Meet the Series Editor

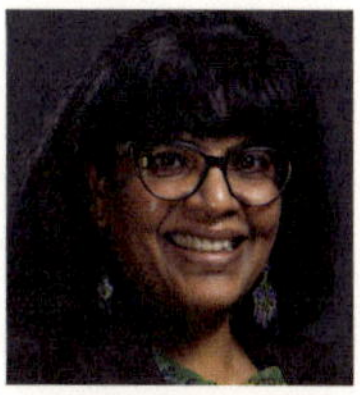

Usha Iyer-Raniga is a professor in the School of Property and Construction Management at RMIT University. Usha co-leads the One Planet Network's Sustainable Buildings and Construction Programme (SBC), a United Nations 10 Year Framework of Programmes on Sustainable Consumption and Production (UN 10FYP SCP) aligned with Sustainable Development Goal 12. The work also directly impacts SDG 11 on Sustainable Cities and Communities. She completed her undergraduate degree as an architect before obtaining her Masters degree from Canada and her Doctorate in Australia. Usha has been a keynote speaker as well as an invited speaker at national and international conferences, seminars and workshops. Her teaching experience includes teaching in Asian countries. She has advised Austrade, APEC, national, state and local governments. She serves as a reviewer and a member of the scientific committee for national and international refereed journals and refereed conferences. She is on the editorial board for refereed journals and has worked on Special Issues. Usha has served and continues to serve on the Boards of several not-for-profit organisations and she has also served as panel judge for a number of awards including the Premiers Sustainability Award in Victoria and the International Green Gown Awards. Usha has published over 100 publications, including research and consulting reports. Her publications cover a wide range of scientific and technical research publications that include edited books, book chapters, refereed journals, refereed conference papers and reports for local, state and federal government clients. She has also produced podcasts for various organisations and participated in media interviews. She has received state, national and international funding worth over USD $25 million. Usha has been awarded the Quarterly Franklin Membership by London Journals Press (UK). Her biography has been included in the Marquis Who's Who in the World® 2018, 2016 (33rd Edition), along with approximately 55,000 of the most accomplished men and women from around the world, including luminaries as U.N. Secretary-General Ban Ki-moon. In 2017, Usha was awarded the Marquis Who's Who Lifetime Achiever Award.

Meet the Volume Editors

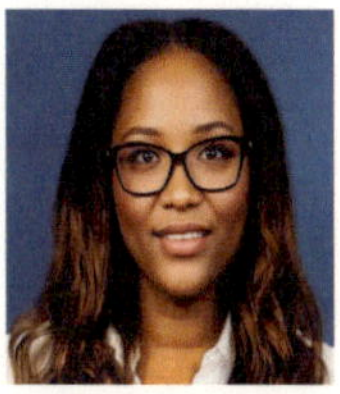

Allincia Michaud, MD, MPH, is a senior clinical postdoctoral research fellow at St. Luke's University Health Network, where she is engaged in various multidisciplinary research projects. Her research collaborations involve research protocol development, data evaluation, advanced analytics, and manuscript writing and editing. She's a proficient reviewer, editor, and author of several publications in reputed journals and has presented at various conferences. Additionally, she is also the managing editor of the *International Journal of Academic Medicine* (IJAM). She has a keen interest in international health, preventive medicine, the management of chronic diseases, health literacy, and the mitigation of health disparities.

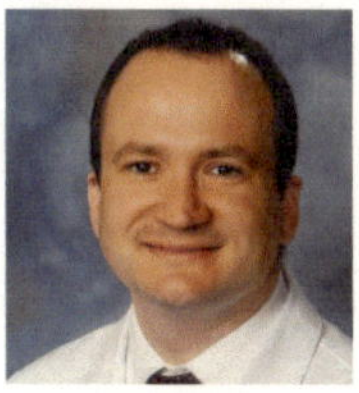

Stanislaw P. Stawicki, MD, MBA, is a professor of surgery and chair of the Department of Research & Innovation at St Luke's University Health Network. A specialist in general surgery and surgical critical care, he co-authored nearly 700 scholarly works, including more than 30 books. In addition to national and international medical leadership roles, he is a member of numerous editorial boards. His areas of expertise include academic international medicine, international health security, blockchain technology, patient safety, academic leadership, mentorship, trauma/critical care, and sonography.

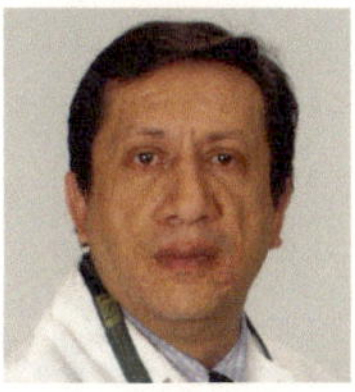

Ricardo Izurieta, MD, Dr. PH, MPH, is a professor and director of global communicable diseases at the College of Public Health and Director of the Public Health Scholar Concentration at Morsani College of Medicine, University of South Florida in Tampa. Dr. Izurieta received his MD from the Central University of Ecuador and, after graduation, carried out his postdoctoral training in public health and tropical infectious diseases at the University of Alabama at Birmingham (USA), Emory University (USA), and Universidad Cayetano Heredia (Peru). In 1991, he faced the cholera epidemic that spread through Latin American countries as national director of the Cholera Control Program in Ecuador's Ministry of Public Health. In 1997, he was appointed chief of the Department of Epidemiology and director of the Vaccine Center of the Armed Forces of Ecuador. During his studies, he has been a USAID Thomas Jefferson fellow, a PAHO Research fellow, an ORISE/CDC fellow, a Gorgas Memorial Institute fellow, and a FUNDACYT fellow. In 2003, Dr. Izurieta was elected vice president of the Gorgas Memorial Institute of Tropical and Preventive Medicine, and currently he is its Latin American liaison. He has been a panel reviewer for NIH, CDC, NSF, and the Wellcome Foundation, and additionally served on the ACAIM Taskforce on International Health Security and as a consultant for the United Nations Global Water Pathogens Project as well as for the United Kingdom and the Brazilian Academies of Sciences.

Contents

Preface XV

Section 1
Introduction 1

Chapter 1 3
Introductory Chapter: Contemporary Considerations and Developments in Global Health Security
by Allincia Michaud, Zachariah G. Goldsmith and Stanislaw P. Stawicki

Section 2
The Interconnected World: Preparedness and Management 15

Chapter 2 17
Perspective Chapter: Emerging Infectious Diseases as a Public Health Problem
by Josep M. Ramon-Torrell

Chapter 3 41
Perspective Chapter: The Pivotal Role of Vaccines and Interventional Equity and Appropriateness
by Ibrahim Khalil Dadari

Chapter 4 57
Perspective Chapter: Armed Conflict and Its Impact on Human Migration – The Healthcare Perspective
by Julius Kenkoh Nkiese and Stephanie Kininla Wirba

Chapter 5 85
Perspective Chapter: A Supposedly Developed Country's Response to a Healthcare Crisis – Lessons from the COVID-19 Pandemic for Future National Emergencies
by Jeffrey S. Freed, Hannah S. Jacobs-El, Soo Y. Kwon and Ram Roth

Section 3
The Power to Transform: Metrics and Leveraging Technology **101**

Chapter 6 **103**
Perspective Chapter: Application of Environmental Epidemiology for Exposure and Health Risk Assessment
by Belay Desye

Chapter 7 **115**
Contribution to the Management of Toxicological Risks in Burkina Faso: Design Process and Implementation Strategies for a Clinical Toxicology Laboratory
by N. Stanislas Dimitri Meda, Normand Fleury, Ciprian M. Cirtiu, Vincent Cirimele, Cheick Armand N. Palm and Elie Kabre

Chapter 8 **151**
Point-of-Care Testing in Rural and Remote Australia: An Emerging Technology to Address Global Health Challenges, Crises and Security
by Mark Shephard, Susan Matthews, Louise Causer, Belinda Hengel and Rebecca Guy

Section 4
Leadership, Workforce Development and Finance **175**

Chapter 9 **177**
Global Health Security: An Evaluation of Public Health Expenditure, Health Status and Economic Development in Nigeria
by Ngozi Chioma Ewurum and Samuel Oseloka Okafor

Chapter 10 **201**
Commodity Security: The Role of Drug Revolving Fund Scheme in Low- and Middle-Income Countries
by Jibrailu L. Maliyogbinda

Chapter 11 **229**
The Road to Universal Healthcare Coverage in the Face of COVID-19: South Africa's Struggles and Prospects
by Nelly Sharpley

Chapter 12 **243**
Perspective Chapter: Global Health Security through Psychoeducation and Microfinance with At-Need Groups
by Sara Spowart

Section 5
Cigarette Uses and Global Health **259**

Chapter 13 **261**
Regulatory and Policy-Making of E-Cigarettes Usage
by Sharifa Ezat Wan Puteh, Norayuni Ismail and Nur Ismah Izzati Ismail

Chapter 14 275
Global Regulatory Approaches towards E-Cigarettes, Key Arguments, and Approaches Pursued
by Marissa Smith and Shona Hilton

Chapter 15 301
The Electronic Cigarette Use in Canada – Local and Global Considerations
by Rudra Dahal

Preface

It is an undeniable fact that the global community remains largely unprepared to conduct early pandemic identification interception and to subsequently mount a reliable pandemic response. This is clearly evident from our experiences from the recent COVID-19 pandemic, with its global death toll of over 7 million people.[1] The pandemic has mercilessly exposed the frailty of communities around the globe, from local to national to international levels. However, as we delve into contemporary approaches and developments in global health security (GHS), we witness the global community's unwavering commitment to learn from these challenges and strengthen our collective response. This book offers a comprehensive analysis of the essentials of GHS and the strategies necessary to ensure robust leadership and systems-based approaches across nations. It examines the integrated efforts and developments by various governments, nongovernmental organizations, and other bodies, all working toward sustained investment to develop and implement rapid response mechanisms critical to ensuring a timely and effective response to mitigate the risks of future outbreaks or pandemics.

Global health (GH) security functions on a detect, prevent, respond, and recover[2] continuum. These four pillars are not isolated entities but rather a framework of interconnected systems, procedures, and policies that aim to minimize exposure and strengthen operations at key administrative and governmental levels. They operate independently and concurrently, with some functions overlapping from one pillar to the next during an outbreak. This intricate design creates a mutually supportive and reinforcing system, enabling a coordinated global response to health threats. This, in turn, ensures that countries are adequately prepared to respond to and contain outbreaks within their borders. These are critical components of GH governance and a testament to our shared responsibility and the need for continuous development to ensure the health and well-being of individuals worldwide. Identifying emerging and re-emerging infectious diseases and their impact on GHS is particularly relevant, especially with increasing outbreaks in under-developed and under-resourced areas, as well as the existing frailty even within relatively developed regions of the globe. Due to these factors, effective GHS actions often present a formidable challenge that not infrequently exceeds local capabilities. Within the current collection of book chapters, authors highlight some common emerging and re-emerging infectious disease threats and the dynamic relationships that exist between the associated factors and the occurrence of such diseases. This includes a discussion of various strategies to mitigate the impact of emerging and re-emerging infectious diseases. These insights are highly relevant and can be effectively utilized to anticipate and respond to the challenges posed by emerging infectious diseases. The book also emphasizes the

[1] World Health Organization. WHO Coronavirus (COVID-19) dashboard > Deaths [Dashboard]. World Health Organization 2023 data.who.int, https://data.who.int/dashboards/covid19/deaths

[2] Carlin EP, Moore MS, Shambaugh E, Karesh WB. 2021. Opportunities for Enhanced Defense, Military, and Security Sector Engagement in Global Health Security. EcoHealth Alliance.

critical role of vaccines in GHS, making a compelling case for vaccine interventional equity and appropriateness, advocating for a more secure global health landscape. Additionally, it provides essential insights into the public health attributes of armed conflict, its impact on individual and population health, and the spread of communicable diseases across various countries.

As the world grapples with the devastating impact of the COVID-19 pandemic, it becomes evident that the functions required to optimize GHS are beyond the capacity of any single government or sector. This also underscores the urgent need to re-establish a pandemic response committee around the globe, complete with international mechanisms for very close, joint, coordinated action. Therefore, we must not only renew our commitment to intercontinental and intergovernmental policies, programs, and engagement but also recognize the imperative of collective action. It is a shared responsibility to address the pillars of GHS—to detect, prevent, respond, and recover from health threats. With climate change, globalization, and various wars and conflicts, epidemics and pandemics are bound to occur more frequently. Consequently, the evolution of these pillars is not only critical but also a call to action for all of us to meet the ever-changing health landscape and ensure preparedness for future health crises.

Allincia Michaud MD, MPH and Stanislaw P. Stawicki MD, MBA, FACS, FAIM
Department of Research and Innovation,
St. Luke's University Health Network,
Bethlehem, Pennsylvania, USA

Ricardo Izurieta MD, DrPH, MPH
College of Public Health,
University of South Florida,
Tampa, Florida, USA

Section 1

Introduction

Chapter 1

Introductory Chapter: Contemporary Considerations and Developments in Global Health Security

Allincia Michaud, Zachariah G. Goldsmith and Stanislaw P. Stawicki

1. Introduction

The world has encountered a spectrum of global health threats, from several pandemics, bioterrorism, and antimicrobial resistance to natural disasters and, concurrently, changes in governance structures, policy frameworks, and legislation at both the national and international levels. The resulting loss of life, economic disruption, strain on healthcare systems, and social instability profoundly impacted countries' health security and threatened progress. As demonstrated repeatedly over the past several decades, countries around the globe are generally unprepared and ill-equipped to tackle the potential threats of epidemics, pandemics, and other public health emergencies [1, 2]. The fallout from the coronavirus disease (COVID-19) exposed the various deficiencies and vulnerabilities of health systems around the world, even among the most medically advanced nations [3, 4]. To further compound the already challenging global status quo, health equity issues adversely affect underserved communities and low-income countries, thus further contributing to the breakdown in global health security, especially in the era of rapid climate change, widespread medical misinformation, and increasing armed conflicts [5–8].

As we enter the post-pandemic era and reflect on the catastrophic impact and devastating rippling effects of the severe acute respiratory syndrome coronavirus 2 (SARS-CoV-2) on communities and nations, the need for a more robust, strategic, and systematic approach to health security has become more evident than ever before [3]. Global health security (GHS), according to the United States Agency for International Development (USAID), can be defined as "...the existence of strong and resilient public health systems that can prevent, detect, and respond to emerging infectious disease threats wherever they occur in the world" [2, 9–11] (**Figure 1**). Dramatic changes associated with globalization, population expansion, environmental degradation, armed conflicts, and chemical usage have advanced the spread of diseases, especially infectious agents, endangering the health of people and posing a grave threat to public health across geographical regions and international borders [1, 5]. These undeniable consequences led to the formation of the Global Health

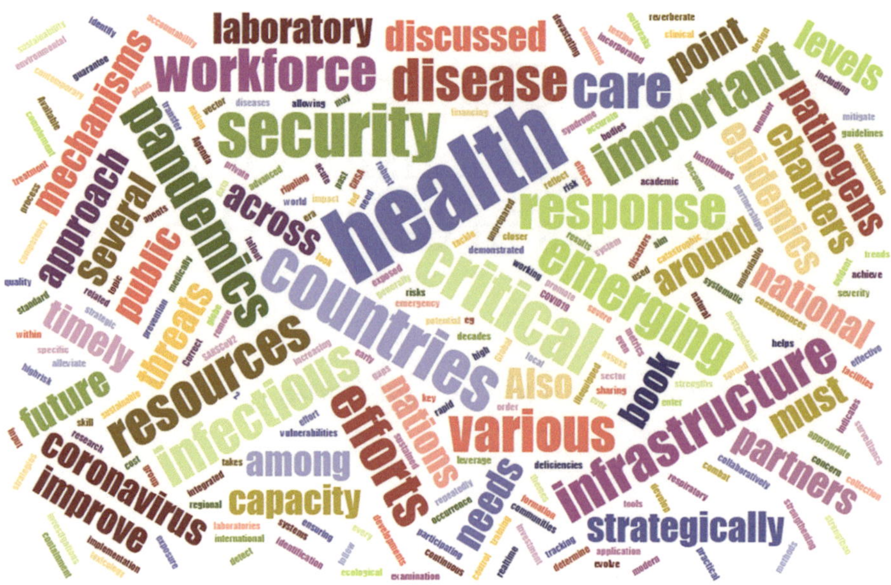

Figure 1.
Word cloud representing key concepts in global health security.

Security Agenda (GHSA). A committee of 70 countries, academic institutions, the private sector, and non-governmental organizations [2, 12–14], working strategically and collaboratively, these partnerships aim to leverage and complement the strengths and resources of their partners to develop sustainable financing mechanisms, improve information sharing and accountability across member countries to remove the needs and gaps, allowing for timely detection, response, and prevention, in an effort to alleviate the increasing occurrence and severity of epidemics, pandemics, and other emerging infectious disease threats [14–16]. Additionally, recognizing that emerging diseases are two times more likely to be caused by zoonotic pathogens [17], the implication and influence of the 'One Health Approach,' a term coined during the 2003 severe acute respiratory disease (SARS) avian influenza H5N1 outbreak is vital in addressing global health security threats. This concept emphasizes the interconnectedness of animal, human, and environmental health [18]. Consequently, a robust GHS framework is essential for safeguarding population health, while investing in GHS is critical to promoting sustainable development (**Figure 2**).

With the evolving landscape of global health threats, above all, it is increasingly imperative to integrate efforts from various governments and non-governmental organizations, leveraging existing partnerships to address underlying determinants of health and misinformation during health emergencies to foster effective public health responses, achieve sustained investment and rapid response mechanisms that are critical to ensuring a timely and effective mitigating response to prevent future outbreaks or pandemics.

Thus, the GHSA member partners' 2024 strategic framework and some of the core areas the Centers for Disease Control and Prevention (CDC) determined essential to reducing global health security risk's themes focus on preparedness, leadership development, technical knowledge, and health data information, initiates to achieve universal health care, and collaborative foundation [18–22].

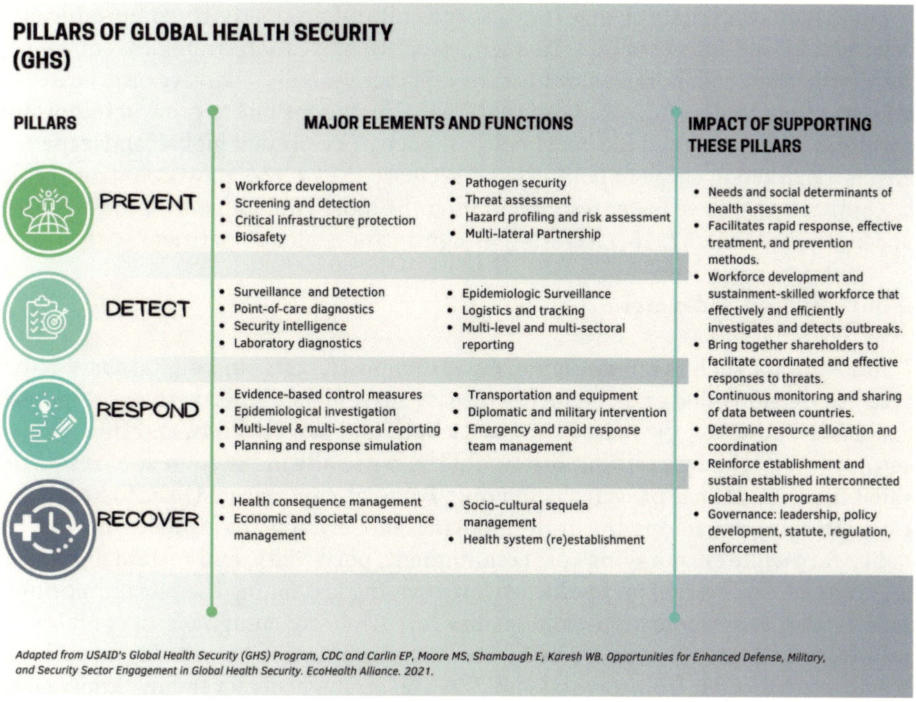

Figure 2.
The global health security framework consists of four pillars of interconnected systems, procedures, and policies that aim to mitigate health risks, minimize exposure, and strengthen countries' operations for sustainable health security.

1.1 Preparedness and management

Preparedness is crucial to handling any emergency or emerging situation. Preparedness, as stipulated by the World Health Organization (WHO) and The United Nations, is a comprehensive approach that involves the acquisition of knowledge and the development of skills by governments, response and recovery organizations, communities, and individuals to effectively anticipate, respond to, and recover from the effects of foreseeable, imminent, or current disasters or threat [2, 23, 24]. A country's ability to effectively identify and respond to health security threats depends on several factors, such as its surveillance systems, preparedness response, infrastructure, and established preventive measures [24, 25]. Consequently, a lack of preparedness cripples the country's economy and causes a significant loss of human life. As such, preparedness is fundamental to any country's health security and management. The average country's Global Health Security Index (GHS) score in 2021 was 38.9 out of 100, with no country scoring within the top tier 5, suggesting weaknesses in the global healthcare systems and an urgent need for preparedness actions [2]. The growing importance of preparedness management is also underscored by the impact of climate change on global health security. Rising temperatures and altered habitats for disease vectors have been shown to increase the spread of infectious diseases like malaria, dengue fever, and cholera [26]. Extreme weather events, such as hurricanes and floods, have led to displacement, food shortages, and damage to health infrastructure, heightening vulnerability to disease outbreaks and emergencies [27].

Furthermore, climate change impacts agricultural productivity, compromising food security and nutrition [28]. As such, effective mitigation strategies requiring interdisciplinary collaboration, robust surveillance systems, adaptive healthcare infrastructure, and coordinated international efforts continue to grow in importance to address both direct and indirect health impacts. The present global landscape reflects a marked upsurge in political and security risks across most countries, with the countries that have fewer resources being the most vulnerable with the biggest gaps in preparedness [2, 16], resulting in significant health disparities.

1.2 Surveillance and metrics

Innovations, such as telemedicine, rapid diagnostic tests, and digital surveillance tools, are transforming and enhancing disease surveillance and countries' response capabilities; however, the need for capacity building, partnerships, and finance at multiple levels while preserving sustainability, especially in the context of resource availability [29–31] has proven challenging. Point-of-care testing (POCT) and point-of-care imaging are among the most important modern tools to promote high-yield quality care while encouraging cost containment, portability, and sustainability [32–35]. Point-of-care testing and point-of-care imaging are among the most important modern tools to promote high-yield quality care while encouraging cost containment, portability, and sustainability [32–35]. However, as point-of-care strategies evolve, it's evident that input from key stakeholders and strategically leveraging knowledge and skills in existing programs across regions, countries, and continents are of critical importance to the long-term success of point-of-care imaging and laboratory programs. Periodic gap analyses are mandatory to ensure that overall progress is being accurately measured and any emerging issues are promptly addressed [32, 36, 37].

One of the barriers to progress in GHS is the relative paucity of shared published evidence-based approaches, interventions, outcome measurements, and lessons learned among countries [38–40]. It is critical for every nation to assess its health systems (e.g., facilities, laboratories, and related critical infrastructure) and other security metrics and needs in order to guarantee that participating stakeholders and partners follow standard guidelines, accurate knowledge and skill dissemination, training and competency, and continuous data monitoring [41–43]. Correct identification, early detection of specific pathogens, real-time tracking, and the transfer of information at the local, regional, national, and international levels are approaches used to combat and control the spread of infectious agents and determine appropriate treatment plans [41–43]. Available research indicates that strengthening disease surveillance helps identify high-risk infectious diseases' pathogens of national concern, detect emerging trends, and strengthen vector monitoring capacity [44, 45]. Also of great importance, pharmaceutical quality surveillance systems prevent antimicrobial resistance transmission in healthcare facilities [46–48]. Overall, this reinforces countries' and partners' relationships and inevitably enhances GHS optimally within a self-improving paradigm. The success of these systems typically requires scientific and expert partnerships, health ministries, and organizations working in concert at various levels (local and global) [49, 50].

1.3 Workforce development, finance and equity

Another fundamental theme and element in maintaining GHS is a country's workforce. Workforce and capacity development requires the mobilization of multi-sectoral efforts, coordination of public health resources on lessons learned, and collaboration of governments at various levels to reinforce their health security infrastructure and train future and current workforce based on evidence-based resources [51, 52]. With billions of dollars in economic losses and increasing frequency of public and global health emergencies, workforce and capacity development are vital facets of health security [53, 54]. Central to sustainable global workforce development is the importance of the support and collaboration of various leaders and partners in health security, especially so in the context of diversity, equity, and inclusion [55–57]. Significant gaps and challenges regarding women's leadership in GHS have been identified over the years and are increasingly and more effectively being addressed at this time [58–60]. As previously mentioned, one of the central premises of GHS is sustainability, and investments from various partners and stakeholders are crucial to facilitating GHSA's strategic objectives. Often under-recognized, the contributions of sustainable financing tend to be overlooked as contributors to GHS. But the ability to provide adequate resources often equates to empowerment, manifesting over a number of critical domains, such as one's independence, authority, status, agency, and living standards. This, in turn, directly and indirectly impacts population health and, inevitably, health security [61–63].

2. Synthesis and conclusion

In conclusion, the discourse on global health security underscores the urgent need for coordinated action to address the myriad challenges posed by infectious diseases, pandemics, natural disasters, and health inequities. The COVID-19 pandemic has starkly exposed the vulnerabilities of health systems worldwide, compelling a reevaluation of preparedness, response mechanisms, and the broader infrastructure supporting global health security. As we navigate the post-pandemic landscape, it is evident that a robust and strategic approach to health security is paramount. The Global Health Security Agenda (GHSA) exemplifies the collaborative efforts required to bolster health security across nations. Through partnerships and sustainable financing mechanisms, GHSA endeavors to strengthen disease surveillance, response capabilities, and workforce development, thereby enhancing the resilience of public health systems.

Key themes essential to advancing global health security include preparedness and management, surveillance, metrics, workforce development, and finance. Addressing these themes necessitates a multifaceted approach, encompassing the integration of evidence-based interventions, capacity-building initiatives, and equitable resource allocation. In essence, investing in global health security is not only a matter of safeguarding individual well-being but also a critical component of promoting sustainable development and fostering resilience in the face of future health threats. By embracing a collaborative, holistic approach, we can strive towards a safer, more equitable world for all.

Acronyms and abbreviations

CDC	Centers for Disease Control and Prevention
COVID-19	coronavirus disease of 19
GHS	global health security

GHSA	Global Health Security Agenda
POCT	point-of-care testing
SARS	severe acute respiratory disease
SARS-CoV-2	severe acute respiratory syndrome coronavirus 2
USAID	United States Agency for International Development
WHO	World Health Organization

Author details

Allincia Michaud[1], Zachariah G. Goldsmith[2] and Stanislaw P. Stawicki[1*]

1 Department of Research and Innovation, St. Luke's University Health Network, Bethlehem, PA, USA

2 Department of Urology, St. Luke's University Health Network, Easton, PA, USA

*Address all correspondence to: stawicki.ace@gmail.com

References

[1] Le NK, Garg M, Izurieta R, Garg SM, Papadimos TJ, Arquilla B, et al. International health security: A summative assessment by ACAIM consensus group. In: Contemporary Developments and Perspectives in International Health Security. Vol. 1. London, UK: IntechOpen; 2020

[2] Bell JA, Nuzzo JB. Global Health Security Index: Advancing Collective Action and Accountability amid Global Crisis: GHS Index. 2021. Available from: https://www.GHSIndex.org

[3] Papadimos TJ, Soghoian SE, Nanayakkara P, Singh S, Miller AC, Saddikuti V, et al. COVID-19 blind spots: A consensus statement on the importance of competent political leadership and the need for public health cognizance. Journal of Global Infectious Diseases. 2020;**12**(4):167

[4] Stawicki SP, Jeanmonod R, Miller AC, Paladino L, Gaieski DF, Yaffee AQ, et al. The 2019-2020 novel coronavirus (severe acute respiratory syndrome coronavirus 2) pandemic: A joint American college of academic international medicine-world academic council of emergency medicine multidisciplinary COVID-19 working group consensus paper. Journal of Global Infectious Diseases. 2020;**12**(2):47

[5] Yellapu V, Malan S, Merkert B, Kharecha H, Alam A, Stawicki SP. Impact of climate change on international health security: An intersection of complexity, interdependence, and urgency. In: Contemporary Developments and Perspectives in International Health Security. Vol. 3. London, UK: IntechOpen; 2021

[6] Hoffman SJ. The evolution, etiology and eventualities of the global health security regime. Health Policy and Planning. 2010;**25**(6):510-522

[7] Kelle A. Securitization of international public health: Implications for global health governance and the biological weapons prohibition regime. Global Governance: A Review of Multilateralism and International Organizations. 2007;**13**(2):217-235

[8] Conti K, Desai S, Stawicki SP, Papadimos TJ. The evolving interplay between social media and international health security: A point of view. In: Contemporary Developments and Perspectives in International Health Security. Vol. 1. London, UK: IntechOpen; 2020

[9] Bianchi KM. Global health security: A blueprint for the future. Emerging Infectious Diseases. 2022;**28**(12):352

[10] Binder S, Levitt AM, Aguilar JR. Preventing emerging infectious diseases: A strategy for the 21st century: US Department of Health and Human Services. Centers for Disease Control and Prevention. 1998;**1**:17-24

[11] Quinn SC, Kumar S. Health inequalities and infectious disease epidemics: A challenge for global health security. Biosecurity and Bioterrorism: Biodefense Strategy, Practice, and Science. 2014;**12**(5):263-273

[12] Dokubo EK, Shang JD, N'Dir A, Ndongmo CB, Okpu G, Fadil YM, et al. Building on capacity established through US Centers for Disease Control and Prevention global health programs to respond to COVID-19, Cameroon. Emerging Infectious Diseases. 2022;**28**(Suppl. 1):S181

[13] Armstrong-Mensah EA, Ndiaye SM. Global health security agenda implementation: A case for community engagement. Health Security. 2018;**16**(4):217-223

[14] Morgan J, Kennedy ED, Pesik N, Angulo FJ, Craig AS, Knight NW, et al. Building global health security capacity: The role for implementation science. Health Security. 2018;**16**(S1):S-5-S-7

[15] Paranjape SM, Franz DR. Implementing the global health security agenda: Lessons from global health and security programs. Health Security. 2015;**13**(1):9-19

[16] Fitzmaurice AG, Mahar M, Moriarty LF, Bartee M, Hirai M, Li W, et al. Contributions of the US Centers for Disease Control and Prevention in implementing the Global Health security agenda in 17 partner countries. Emerging Infectious Diseases. 2017;**23**(Suppl. 1):S15

[17] Taylor LH, Latham SM, Woolhouse ME. Risk factors for human disease emergence. Philosophical Transactions of the Royal Society of London. Series B, Biological Sciences. 2001;**356**(1411):983-989

[18] Carlin EP, Moore MS, Shambaugh E, Karesh WB. Opportunities for Enhanced Defense, Military, and Security Sector Engagement in Global Health Security. New York, USA: EcoHealth Alliance; 2021

[19] Herrera CA, Báscolo E, Villar-Uribe M, Houghton N, Massuda A, Bennett S. The World Bank–PAHO lancet regional health Americas commission on primary health care and resilience in Latin America and the Caribbean. The Lancet Regional Health–Americas. 2023;**28**

[20] Daszak P, Keusch GT, Phelan AL, Johnson CK, Osterholm MT. Infectious disease threats: A rebound to resilience: Commentary reviews the US approach to pandemic preparedness, its impact on the response to COVID-19, and offers policy options to strengthen US pandemic resilience. Health Affairs (Washington, DC, USA). 2021;**40**(2):204-211

[21] Gresham L, Alemu W, Divi N, Alhusseini N, Awoniyi O, Bashir A, et al. Modernizing Public Health Surveillance. Modernizing Global Health Security to Prevent, Detect, and Respond. Massachusetts, USA: Elsevier; 2024. pp. 307-327

[22] Greiner A, Stehling-Ariza T, Hoffman A. Guidance for US Centers for Disease Control and Prevention Staff for the Establishment and Management of Public Health Rapid Response Teams for Disease Outbreaks. Georgia, USA: Centers for Disease Control and Prevention; 2020

[23] Chiossi S, Tsolova S, Ciotti M. Assessing public health emergency preparedness: A scoping review on recent tools and methods. International Journal of Disaster Risk Reduction. 2021;**56**:102104

[24] Kandel N, Chungong S, Omaar A, Xing J. Health security capacities in the context of COVID-19 outbreak: An analysis of international health regulations annual report data from 182 countries. The Lancet. 2020;**395**(10229):1047-1053

[25] Heymann DL, Rodier G. Global surveillance, national surveillance, and SARS. Emerging Infectious Diseases. 2004;**10**(2):173

[26] Watts N, Amann M, Arnell N, Ayeb-Karlsson S, Belesova K, Boykoff M, et al. The 2019 report of the lancet countdown on health and climate change: Ensuring that the health

of a child born today is not defined by a changing climate. The Lancet (Amsterdam, Netherlands). 2019;**394**(10211):1836-1878

[27] Haines A, Ebi KL, Smith KR, Woodward A. Health risks of climate change: Act now or pay later. The Lancet. 2014;**384**(9948):1073-1075

[28] Patz JA, Frumkin H, Holloway T, Vimont DJ, Haines A. Climate change: Challenges and opportunities for global health. Journal of the American Medical Association. 2014;**312**(15):1565-1580

[29] Dodd R, Lane C. Improving the long-term sustainability of health aid: Are Global Health partnerships leading the way? Health Policy and Planning. 2010;**25**(5):363-371

[30] Sikka V, Chattu VK, Popli RK, Galwankar SC, Kelkar D, Sawicki SG, et al. The emergence of zika virus as a global health security threat: A review and a consensus statement of the INDUSEM joint working group (JWG). Journal of Global Infectious Diseases. 2016;**8**(1):3

[31] Dana E, Nour AM, Kpa'Hanba GA, Khan JS. Point-of-care ultrasound (PoCUS) and its potential to advance patient Care in low-Resource Settings and Conflict Zones. Disaster Medicine and Public Health Preparedness. 2023;**17**:e417

[32] Yager P, Domingo GJ, Gerdes J. Point-of-care diagnostics for global health. Annual Review of Biomedical Engineering. 2008;**10**:107-144

[33] Nayak S, Blumenfeld NR, Laksanasopin T, Sia SK. Point-of-care diagnostics: Recent developments in a connected age. Analytical Chemistry. 2017;**89**(1):102-123

[34] Luppa P, Junker R. Point-of-Care Testing: Principles and Clinical Applications. New York, USA: Springer; 2018

[35] Dhawan AP, Heetderks WJ, Pavel M, Acharya S, Akay M, Mairal A, et al. Current and future challenges in point-of-care technologies: A paradigm-shift in affordable global healthcare with personalized and preventive medicine. IEEE Journal of Translational Engineering in Health and Medicine. 2015;**3**:1-10

[36] Parsons LM, Somoskövi Á, Gutierrez C, Lee E, Paramasivan C, Al A, et al. Laboratory diagnosis of tuberculosis in resource-poor countries: Challenges and opportunities. Clinical Microbiology Reviews. 2011;**24**(2):314-350

[37] Greaves RF, Bernardini S, Ferrari M, Fortina P, Gouget B, Gruson D, et al. Key questions about the future of laboratory medicine in the next decade of the 21st century: A report from the IFCC-emerging technologies division. Clinica Chimica Acta. 2019;**495**:570-589

[38] Kennedy ED, Morgan J, Knight NW. Global health security implementation: Expanding the evidence base. Health Security. 2018;**16**(S1):S-1-S-4

[39] Worsley-Tonks KE, Bender JB, Deem SL, Ferguson AW, Fèvre EM, Martins DJ, et al. Strengthening global health security by improving disease surveillance in remote rural areas of low-income and middle-income countries. The Lancet Global Health. 2022;**10**(4):e579-ee84

[40] Ravi SJ, Meyer D, Cameron E, Nalabandian M, Pervaiz B, Nuzzo JB. Establishing a theoretical foundation for measuring global health security: A scoping review. BMC Public Health. 2019;**19**:1-9

[41] Berkeley AR, Wallace M, Coo C. A framework for establishing critical infrastructure resilience goals. In: Final Report and Recommendations by the Council, National Infrastructure Advisory Council. Washington D.C., USA: Department of Homeland Security; 2010. pp. 18-21

[42] World Health Organization. Monitoring the Building Blocks of Health Systems: A Handbook of Indicators and their Measurement Strategies. Geneva: World Health Organization; 2010

[43] Jovanović A, Klimek P, Renn O, Schneider R, Øien K, Brown J, et al. Assessing resilience of healthcare infrastructure exposed to COVID-19: Emerging risks, resilience indicators, interdependencies and international standards. Environment Systems and Decisions. 2020;**40**:252-286

[44] Zhang X-X, Jin Y-Z, Lu Y-H, Huang L-L, Wu C-X, Lv S, et al. Infectious disease control: From health security strengthening to health systems improvement at global level. Global Health Research and Policy. 2023;**8**(1):38

[45] Hitchcock P, Chamberlain A, Van Wagoner M, Inglesby TV, O'Toole T. Challenges to global surveillance and response to infectious disease outbreaks of international importance. Biosecurity and Bioterrorism: Biodefense Strategy, Practice, and Science. 2007;**5**(3):206-227

[46] World Health Organization. Global Antimicrobial Resistance Surveillance System (GLASS) Report: Early Implementation 2020. Geneva: World Health Organization; 2020

[47] Endale H, Mathewos M, Abdeta D. Potential causes of spread of antimicrobial resistance and preventive measures in one health perspective-a review. Infection and Drug Resistance. 2023;**16**:7515-7545

[48] Ferri M, Ranucci E, Romagnoli P, Giaccone V. Antimicrobial resistance: A global emerging threat to public health systems. Critical Reviews in Food Science and Nutrition. 2017;**57**(13):2857-2876

[49] Harman S. Global Health Governance. London, United Kingdom: Routledge; 2012

[50] Organization WH. Delivering Quality Health Services: A Global Imperative. Paris, France: OECD Publishing; 2018

[51] Doble A, Sheridan Z, Razavi A, Wilson A, Okereke E. The role of international support programmes in global health security capacity building: A scoping review. PLOS Global Public Health. 2023;**3**(4):e0001763

[52] World Health Organization. Advanced Global Health Security: From Commitments to Actions. Geneva: World Health Organization; 2016

[53] Kalra S, Kelkar D, Galwankar SC, Papadimos TJ, Stawicki SP, Arquilla B, et al. The emergence of Ebola as a global health security threat: From 'lessons learned' to coordinated multilateral containment efforts. Journal of Global Infectious Diseases. 2014;**6**(4):164

[54] Stawicki SP, Firstenberg MS, Galwankar SC, Izurieta R, Papadimos T. Contemporary Developments and Perspectives in International Health Security. Vol. 1. London, United Kingdom: BoD–Books on Demand; 2021

[55] World Health Organization. Global Strategy on Human Resources for Health: Workforce 2030. Geneva: World Health Organization; 2016

[56] Organization WH. Working Together for Equity and Healthier Populations: Sustainable Multisectoral Collaboration Based on Health in all Policies Approaches. World Health Organization; 2023

[57] Organization WH. Essential Public Health Functions, Health Systems and Health Security: Developing Conceptual Clarity and a WHO Roadmap for Action. 2018

[58] Smith SG, Sinkford JC. Gender equality in the 21st century: Overcoming barriers to women's leadership in global health. Journal of Dental Education. 2022;**86**(9):1144-1173

[59] Ingle E, Rencken C, Seide J, Badshah A. Women's leadership in global health. Gates Open Research. 2023;**7**(16):16

[60] Ayaz B, Martimianakis MA, Muntaner C, Nelson S. Participation of women in the health workforce in the fragile and conflict-affected countries: A scoping review. Human Resources for Health. 2021;**19**:1-14

[61] Gough I, McGregor JA. Wellbeing in Developing Countries: From Theory to Research. New York, USA: Cambridge University Press; 2007

[62] Missoni E, Pacileo G, Tediosi F. Global Health Governance and Policy: An Introduction. London, United Kingdom: Routledge; 2019

[63] Alla F, Ahmed TI. Understanding the Influence of Income Generating Activities on Women's Empowerment: A Case Study of JASMAR Human Security Organization's Project for Female Sex Workers in the Republic of the Sudan. Ohio, USA: Ohio University; 2021

Section 2

The Interconnected World: Preparedness and Management

Chapter 2

Perspective Chapter: Emerging Infectious Diseases as a Public Health Problem

Josep M. Ramon-Torrell

Abstract

Emerging infectious diseases (EIDs) can be defined as diseases that have recently appeared in a population or are rapidly increasing in incidence or geographic range. An "emerging infection" refers to either a new infection that has never appeared before or a known infection that has experienced a recent increase in prevalence. The Human Immunodeficiency Virus (HIV) pandemic and Severe Acute Respiratory Syndrome Coronavirus (SARS-CoV) outbreaks are prototypical examples of emerging infectious diseases that were not prevalent before the 1980s and 2003, respectively. On the other hand, a "re-emerging infection" is a familiar infection that resurfaces. The influenza A virus pandemics of 1918, 1957, and 1968 serve as prototypical examples of re-emerging infections. This chapter aims to define the concepts of emerging and re-emerging infectious diseases and explore their main causes, the microorganisms involved, and why they can become significant global public health problems.

Keywords: emerging infectious diseases, re-emerging infectious diseases, climate change, public health impact, impact on human health, associated factors

1. Introduction

Emerging infectious diseases (EIDs) had been a public health problem for decades and continue to pose a challenge to global health. Throughout history, there have been numerous infectious diseases that were once considered emerging and had a significant impact on human health and society as a whole. The frequency of EIDs has notably increased in the past 30 years, and it is expected to further rise in the near future.

Some examples of historically emerging infections include the 1918 Spanish flu pandemic that claimed millions of lives worldwide [1]. Another example is the emergence of Human Immunodeficiency Virus/Acquired Immunodeficiency Syndrome (HIV/AIDS) in the 1980s, which has caused millions of deaths since its onset and remains a significant public health issue today [2]. In the past decade, we have witnessed the emergence of new infectious diseases, such as the Ebola virus in West Africa in 2014, the Zika virus in South America in 2015, and the Coronavirus 2019 (COVID-19) pandemic, worldwide in 2019.

Emerging infectious diseases can be broadly defined as infections that have recently appeared in a population or have existed but have experienced an increase in incidence or geographic range [3]. They can manifest as rapidly spreading diseases that pose a significant threat to public health and the global economy.

The difference between an emerging infection and a re-emerging infection lies in the temporal and epidemiological context in which they occur. Emerging infections are those that appear for the first time in a population or experience a significant increase in incidence. On the other hand, re-emerging infections are those that have existed previously but have resurfaced or experienced an increase in incidence after a period of decline or apparent control.

Emerging infections are often associated with various factors, including the emergence of new pathogens through genetic mutation, pathogen transfer from one species to another, or the introduction of a pathogen into a susceptible population. Additionally, they can result from diverse and complex factors such as environmental and climatic changes, ecosystem disruptions, human migration, globalization, and intensive agricultural practices [4].

On the other hand, re-emerging infections are diseases that have been present in a population in the past but have experienced a resurgence in their incidence. This can be due to various factors, including the weakening of control measures, the emergence of drug-resistant strains, a decrease in population immunity, or changes in human behavior that increase exposure to the pathogen [5].

In summary, the definition of EIDs can include various categories: [6].

a. True new diseases that arise in humans from zoonotic sources.

b. Previously identified diseases that may have been unknown or prevalent but are now being evaluated.

c. Widely known re-emerging diseases that increase in frequency and may emerge as coinfections that facilitate their spread (such as HIV).

Over 60% of these new EIDs are associated with zoonoses, where 23% are vector-borne diseases (VBDs) and 72% originate from wildlife [7]. EIDs can arise from different sources, such as changes in the environment, pathogen evolution, drug resistance, and globalization. Early identification and rapid response are crucial in preventing the spread of emerging diseases.

The factors associated with the emergence of diseases include a variety of biological, environmental, social, and cultural elements. Some of these factors include:

- Climate change and destruction of natural habitats, along with changes and geographic expansion of vector habitats.
- Globalization and increased international trade and travel.
- Increased population density and urbanization.
- Changes in agriculture and animal farming.
- Drug resistance and antimicrobial therapy.

- Evolution and mutation of pathogens.
- Emergence of new technologies and their impact on public health.
- International travel.

These factors can interact and often unpredictable ways, leading to the emergence of new infectious diseases.

Emerging infectious diseases have historically represented the most feared plagues for humans, and new infections continue to arise today, giving rise to new significant epidemics and pandemics. In fact, the emergence of the new coronavirus "COVID-19" in December 2019 is a clear example of what these emerging diseases represent, and we will delve further into this chapter. Let us examine some of the diseases that, due to their characteristics, have great potential to become a global problem in the short or medium term.

First, the influenza virus, which has caused historic pandemics throughout the centuries. In the last 100 years, there have been four influenza pandemics: H_1N_1 (Spanish flu) in 1918 with 50 million deaths, H_2N_2 (Asian flu) in 1957, H_3N_2 (Hong Kong flu) in 1968, and the new H_1N_1 (swine flu) in 2009. Influenza type A virus has the highest potentiality to become a new pandemic in the future due to its ability to undergo significant genetic modifications through mutations and recombination, resulting in the emergence of new viral variants with novel characteristics. One crucial aspect of influenza type A virus that makes it more concerning is its capacity to infect both humans and animals, including aquatic birds and mammals, known as zoonotic hosts. This creates an environment conducive to interspecies transmission and the possibility of genetic recombination between human and animal strains of the virus. A specific subtype of influenza A virus that has been a cause for concern in recent decades is H_5N_1, known as highly pathogenic avian influenza. This subtype has been responsible for outbreaks in poultry and wild birds and has occasionally transmitted the virus to humans, resulting in severe infections and mortality, though its mutations have not yet been allowed for sustained human-to-human transmission. Other subtypes, such as H_7N_9 and H_9N_2, have also shown the ability to infect humans and have been under surveillance due to their pandemic potential.

Second, the Ebola virus can cause hemorrhagic fever. It is essential to highlight that the Ebola virus has certain characteristics that give it a high potential to become a new global health problem. Although the outbreaks that have occurred so far have been regional, it is crucial to consider some factors that make this virus a concern. The Ebola virus is highly lethal, with mortality rates reaching up to 90%. This characteristic is worrying since, in the event of broader transmission, it could cause a significant number of deaths and overwhelm healthcare systems. The virus is a zoonosis originating in fruit bats and occasionally transmitted to humans through contact with wild animals. The major concern would be if the virus jumps to new species and adopts a more efficient form of human-to-human transmission. Transmission from an infected person to a healthy one occurs through direct contact with infected blood and fluids. If a variant with higher human-to-human transmission capability were to appear, it could trigger a faster and broader spread.

Finally, the dengue virus is a mosquito-borne disease endemic in more than 100 countries, mainly in tropical and subtropical regions. In recent years, outbreaks have been reported in various European countries, indicating a potential spread beyond its usual territories. The widespread distribution of the *Aedes aegypti* mosquito, the main vector of dengue, coupled with increased trade, international travel, and climate change—which can influence the distribution and activity of mosquito vectors, expanding their geographic range—increase the likelihood of its introduction to new areas, potentially triggering outbreaks and rapid global spread.

There are four distinct serotypes of the dengue virus (DEN-1, DEN-2, DEN-3, and DEN-4), and a previous infection with one serotype provides lifelong immunity only against that specific serotype. However, subsequent infection with another serotype increases the risk of developing severe dengue, a more severe form of the disease. Thus, the coexistence of multiple serotypes in a region increases the possibility of outbreaks and clinical complications. Although there are dengue vaccines available, a universal vaccine providing complete protection against all serotypes has not been developed yet, making control and prevention more challenging.

In this chapter, we will analyze the current state of knowledge about emerging infectious diseases, describe some characteristics of the microorganisms causing these diseases, and detail the factors contributing to their emergence. We will also review their global impact on public health.

2. Factors associated with emerging infectious diseases

Although, as we have seen previously, there are various factors associated with the increase in EIDs, we can summarize them as: social and behavioral changes, environmental changes, and changes in the causative microorganisms. These factors would act synergistically, increasing the emergence of certain pathogens, affecting transmission mechanisms, and leading to greater host susceptibility [8].

Table 1 provides a more detailed classification of the factors that, either individually or in combination, enhance the occurrence of EIDs.

2.1 Demographic factors

Demographic factors play a significant role in the emergence and spread of emerging infectious diseases. Factors, such as rapid population growth, uncontrolled urbanization, and changes in population distribution, are key elements that affect the dynamics of infectious diseases. These demographic factors interact with other socioeconomic and environmental aspects to influence the emergence and spread of diseases.

Environmental factors	Anthropological factors	Pathogenetic balance	Virulence
Temperature Humidity Drought	Socioeconomic factors Globalization Land use	Host immunity Geographical redistribution of the pathogen Exposure to a new species Recombination and adaptation	Increased cytotoxicity Increased susceptibility Antimicrobial resistance Emergence of a pathogen in a new host

Table 1.
Factors that enhance the appearance of emerging infectious diseases (EIDs).

First, rapid population growth can increase population density in urban areas, facilitating disease transmission. A study by Smith et al. [9] pointed out that urban growth creates conducive conditions for the spread of infectious diseases, as proximity among individuals facilitates transmission.

Second, changes in population distribution can also play a role in EIDs. Human mobility, including international travel, can lead to the rapid global spread of diseases. In 2019, 1.5 billion tourists traveled outside their borders worldwide, facilitating the spread of these infectious diseases within days or weeks, as demonstrated by the Severe Acute Respiratory Syndrome Coronavirus 2 (SARS-CoV-2) pandemic. Tatem et al. [10] demonstrated that patterns of human mobility can predict the spread of infectious diseases, such as influenza, across different geographic regions. Demographic changes in population size and density through urbanization can also affect infection dynamics. For example, influenza tends to have more persistent outbreaks in densely populated urban regions, with a similar pattern observed in the early COVID-19 pandemic [11].

If demographic change has significantly altered the context of infectious diseases in recent years, an even greater effect can be attributed to changes in the emergence of immunomodulatory infections, which, in turn, can affect other infections. For instance, the emergence of HIV has amplified the burden of tuberculosis [12].

On the other hand, demographic changes such as population aging also have a significant influence on the emergence of EIDs. Older individuals tend to have a weakened immune system, making them more susceptible to infections. Additionally, the presence of comorbidities in the elderly population can complicate the body's response to infections.

These demographic factors have a significant impact on the emergence and spread of EIDs. Rapid population growth, uncontrolled urbanization, changes in population distribution, and population aging are key demographic elements that influence the dynamics of infectious diseases. Understanding and addressing these demographic factors is crucial for effectively preventing and controlling emerging infectious diseases.

2.2 Social factors

Transformations in human behavioral patterns, cultural practices, and social interactions can significantly influence the dynamics and spread of diseases. One social factor that can contribute to the emergence of EIDs is the increase in mobility and international travel. Mass movements of people facilitate the rapid spread of pathogens across different geographical regions. Furthermore, the globalization of trade and tourism has increased interconnectivity between communities, allowing for the introduction and dissemination of diseases in new areas [13].

Changes in food production and consumption practices can also have a significant impact. Intensive agriculture and overcrowded animal farming increase the risk of zoonotic disease transmission, facilitating the transmission of diseases from animals to humans. The mass production of food, particularly animal protein, often incorporates the use of antibiotics to enhance the growth and productivity of livestock such as chickens, pigs, and cattle. Additionally, the distribution of food to markets can introduce new pathogens into the food chain through food handlers, even distal to the markets where they are sold.

On the other hand, changes in behaviors and social interactions can also influence the spread of emerging infectious diseases. Risky sexual practices, such as unprotected sex and promiscuity, can increase the transmission of sexually transmitted diseases (STDs) such as HIV/AIDS and syphilis. Likewise, changes in personal hygiene behaviors and healthcare practices can affect the transmission of respiratory, gastrointestinal, and contact diseases.

2.3 Climate change

The negative impact of infectious diseases on health and well-being is intrinsically related, as we have seen before, to a combination of multiple stressful or driving factors, to which we should add poor sanitation, access to clean water and food, the quality of public health services, political instability and conflicts, drug resistance, and movements of animal and/or human populations. Changes in climate patterns, environmental degradation, and ecosystem disruption can trigger the emergence and expansion of infectious diseases, creating a conducive environment for their transmission.

How we shape and adapt to the environment, through our impact on land use (deforestation/reforestation and agricultural activities), the construction of artificial water bodies or dams, and measures taken to control infectious diseases, such as the development of vaccines and drugs, insecticide spraying, distribution of insecticide-treated bed nets, and the development of rapid diagnostic tests, are also critical factors affecting the transmission of infectious diseases [14]. Climate has a direct impact on the dynamics of a subset of infectious diseases, including vector-borne diseases (VBDs), some waterborne diseases such as cholera, and other pathogens transmitted through soil and food. The climate also has multiple indirect effects through socio-economic factors; for example, floods can hinder ongoing disease control measures, including vector control [15].

Infectious VBDs are primarily transmitted by arthropod vectors, which are particularly sensitive to climate changes for several reasons. Arthropods are ectothermic, with their internal temperature regulated by external environmental conditions [16]. Their larval developmental stage usually requires the presence of water bodies and/or specific humidity conditions. Vector biting rates tend to increase with temperature up to an upper threshold, after which they decrease. The development and replication of vector-transmitted pathogens (the extrinsic incubation period or EIP) or in the environment also occur faster at higher temperatures [17]. Additionally, the development and survival of vectors are significantly affected by seasonal conditions [18].

Many transmission-related life cycle traits of the mosquito (biting rate, adult lifespan, population size, and distribution) and the pathogen (extrinsic incubation rate) are temperature sensitive, and oviposition patterns depend on water availability [19]. Consequently, the geographical range for dengue, malaria, and other vector-borne diseases [20–23] is affected by the local climate, and there is substantial effort to understand how these ranges may change with climate change [24–26]. For certain vector-borne diseases such as Zika virus disease, climate change may lead to an expanded range [27]. However, for other diseases, such as malaria, climate change may shift the spatial range of the infection to higher latitudes. As ever, the footprint of human interventions may loom larger than these changes in local conditions.

One of the main effects of climate change is the increase in global temperature. Global warming has led to the expansion of areas conducive to the proliferation of vectors, such as mosquitoes, which transmit diseases such as dengue, malaria, and the Zika virus. A study conducted by Caminade et al. [28] found a significant relationship between temperature increase and the geographical expansion of disease-transmitting vectors.

Furthermore, climate change can alter rainfall patterns and season distribution, impacting the spread of waterborne diseases such as cholera. Heavy rains and floods can contaminate sources of drinking water and facilitate pathogen spread, while prolonged droughts can increase water scarcity and inadequate hygiene conditions. Ecological change, such as deforestation and ecosystem degradation, can also contribute to the emergence of emerging infectious diseases. Destruction of natural habitats and loss of biodiversity can lead to increased contact between humans and disease-carrying animals. This increases the risk of zoonotic disease transmission, such as West Nile virus and Ebola virus [29]. Additionally, changes in migratory patterns of animal species due to climate change can alter disease dynamics. For example, the displacement of disease-carrying animals to new geographic areas can introduce pathogens into susceptible human populations, leading to outbreaks and epidemics [30].

Addressing climate and ecological change is crucial as part of the global strategy to prevent and control emerging infectious diseases. Implementation of climate change adaptation and mitigation measures can reduce the spread of vector-borne and waterborne diseases. Furthermore, the protection of ecosystems and conservation of biodiversity are essential to avoid disruption of natural disease cycles. Rising temperatures, changes in precipitation patterns, and biodiversity loss can alter natural habitats, favoring the proliferation and spread of disease-causing microorganism. Furthermore, deforestation, urbanization, and ecosystem destruction can lead to closer contact between humans and animals, thus increasing the risk of emerging infectious disease transmission.

Climate and ecological change are closely linked to the emergence and spread of emerging infectious diseases. Changes in climate patterns, environmental degradation, and ecosystem disruption promote disease transmission and increase the risk of outbreaks. Addressing these challenges requires climate change adaptation and mitigation measures, as well as biodiversity conservation and public awareness. Interdisciplinary research and collaboration are key to understanding and tackling this complex issue.

2.4 Antimicrobial resistance

The ability of disease-causing microorganisms to develop resistance to existing antimicrobial drugs represents a serious challenge to public health. Drug resistance is a natural phenomenon that occurs when microorganisms such as bacteria, viruses, fungi, and parasites develop the ability to survive and multiply in the presence of antimicrobial agents that were originally effective in combating them. Continuous exposure and inappropriate use of antimicrobial drugs in humans, animals, and agriculture have accelerated the emergence and spread of drug resistance [31]. This resistance compromises the effectiveness of treatments and increases the burden of infectious diseases worldwide.

The relationship between drug resistance and emerging infectious diseases is complex and multifaceted. Antimicrobial resistance can increase the emergence of new diseases or the re-emergence of previously controlled diseases. When antimicrobial drugs are ineffective in treating an infection, the microorganism can spread and cause severe and difficult-to-treat illnesses. Additionally, resistance can lead to an increase in the duration of the disease, the burden of morbidity, and mortality [32]. A prominent example is antibiotic resistance, one of the most pressing issues in public health. Bacteria resistant to multiple antibiotics, known as multidrug-resistant bacteria or superbugs, have emerged and spread worldwide.

Antibiotic resistance has become a threat to global public health. It is estimated that each year, 2.8 million deaths occur due to infections resistant to antibiotics, and this figure is expected to rise to 10 million deaths by 2050. The countries reporting the highest number of cases of antibiotic-resistant bacteria are India, China, Brazil, Russia, and the United States of America. It is estimated that approximately 70% of Gram-negative bacteria and 30% of Gram-positive bacteria have developed some degree of antibiotic resistance. On the other hand, drugs with the highest antibiotic resistance are carbapenems, macrolides, and fluoroquinolones, which are used in the treatment of severe infections as meningitis, pneumonia, or tuberculosis.

Pathogens, such as methicillin-resistant *Staphylococcus aureus* (MRSA) and carbapenem-resistant Enterobacteriaceae (CRE), pose a significant threat to human health due to the limited availability of effective treatment options [33]. The enzyme NDM-1 (New Delhi metallo-beta-lactamase-1) causes resistance to nearly all antibiotics and initially emerged in India, from where it has spread to more than 120 countries. It took its name from the city (New Delhi) where the first infected patient is believed to have been, and from where it rapidly disseminated. It was found in drinking water in Delhi and in the upper reaches of the Ganges River. The resistance of *Klebsiella pneumoniae* to carbapenems increased from 2–52% in just 5 years. From 2008 to 2013, *Escherichia coli* became resistant in 83% to cephalosporins, broad-spectrum antibiotics, and in 85% to fluoroquinolones, a synthetic drug. For example, these bacteria, *E. coli*, present a 92% resistance to aminopenicillins (a group to which amoxicillin belongs) in India.

Natural selection plays a significant role in resistance development, as microorganisms with genetic traits that confer resistance have a survival advantage in an environment exposed to antimicrobial drugs [34]. The transmission of resistance genes can also occur between different species of microorganisms, further amplifying resistance spread.

Moreover, inappropriate use of antimicrobial drugs is a key factor in resistance development. Self-medication, unnecessary prescription, incorrect dosing, and premature treatment discontinuation can promote drug resistance. Additionally, the use of antimicrobials in agriculture, such as the use of antibiotics in intensive animal farming, also contributes to the emergence and spread of resistance [35, 36].

The issue of drug resistance and antimicrobial therapy has implications not only for human health but also for animal health and food safety. Drug resistance can be transmitted between humans and animals, leading to an increase in zoonotic diseases and greater difficulty in treating infections in both humans and animals. Furthermore, the presence of resistant microorganisms in food can pose a risk to public health if adequate control and prevention measures are not taken.

The emergence of emerging infectious diseases is also related to climate change and environmental degradation. Rising temperatures, changes in precipitation patterns, and biodiversity loss can alter natural habitats, favoring the proliferation and spread of disease-causing microorganisms. Additionally, deforestation, urbanization, and ecosystem destruction can lead to closer contact between humans and animals, thereby increasing the risk of emerging infectious disease transmission [13, 37].

Addressing the challenge of drug resistance and emerging infectious diseases requires concerted global action. It is necessary to strengthen epidemiological surveillance to monitor drug resistance and detect outbreaks of emerging diseases. Additionally, measures should be implemented to promote responsible use of antimicrobial drugs, including education and awareness regarding their proper use in both clinical and agricultural settings.

Research and development of new antimicrobial drugs are also crucial to tackle resistance. Investments in research and development are needed to discover new molecules and therapeutic approaches, as well as to foster innovation in the field of rapid and accurate diagnostics [38]. Furthermore, promoting international collaboration and cooperation among the human, animal, and environmental health sectors is necessary to comprehensively address the issue of drug resistance.

Drug resistance and antimicrobial therapy pose a significant threat to public health and are closely related to emerging infectious diseases. The emergence and spread of resistance compromise the effectiveness of treatments and increase the burden of infectious diseases worldwide. It is necessary to adopt a comprehensive approach that addresses drug resistance, including measures to promote responsible use of antimicrobial drugs, strengthen epidemiological surveillance, invest in research and development of new drugs, and foster international collaboration. Only through a multidisciplinary approach and coordinated action can we tackle this challenge and ensure the effectiveness of antimicrobial treatments in the future.

3. Characteristics of microorganisms causing emerging infectious diseases

Recent research highlights the importance of understanding the characteristics of microorganisms associated with emerging infectious diseases. Pathogenic microorganisms, such as bacteria, viruses, parasites, and fungi, can cause emerging infectious diseases with a significant impact on global public health and socioeconomic stability.

The microorganisms that cause emerging infectious diseases have several characteristics in common. Some of the characteristics of microorganisms include their ability to mutate and adapt, their capacity for quick replication, and their ability to overcome host defenses. Another important characteristic of microorganisms associated with emerging infectious diseases is their ability to efficiently transmit from one host to another.

Many of these microorganisms have a high capacity for propagation between human and animal populations. This means that they are capable of being transmitted from animals to humans, which we know as zoonotic diseases. Factors that favor this transmission would include environmental factors—degradation of the environment—close contact between humans and animals, the consumption of wild animals, and the expansion of intensive agriculture [39]. Recent decades have seen repeated pathogen emergence from wild or domestic animal reservoirs into human populations, from HIV-1 and HIV-2, to the 1918 influenza virus, to Middle East Respiratory Syndrome Coronavirus, to SARS-CoV-2 (Refs. [2–4]). For a novel pathogen to become a threat to human populations, first, contact between humans and the animal reservoir must occur; the pathogen must either have or evolve the capacity for human-to-human transmission and finally, this human-to-human transmission must enable expansion of the pathogen's geographical range beyond the zone of spillover [40].

Unlike diseases such as HIV or highly transmissible coronaviruses, microorganisms that jump from animals to humans often have limited or no ability to transmit from person to person. In these cases, transmission occurs when humans come into direct contact with infected animals or their products, such as meat, milk, or excrement. This form of transmission is considered a "dead-end transmission" because there is no sustained spread of the microorganism within the human population. Importantly, although "dead-end" transmission of these microorganisms does not usually lead to epidemic outbreaks or pandemics, their individual and local consequences should not be underestimated. These zoonotic transmission events can cause severe and even lethal disease in cases where infection occurs in humans.

Throughout history, we have witnessed the emergence of various microorganisms that have posed a significant threat to global public health. These emerging microorganisms, including viruses, bacteria, fungi, and other pathogens, have emerged from different sources and have demonstrated their ability to cause severe diseases and spread rapidly. As we move further into the twenty-first century, it is crucial to be prepared to identify and respond to potential emerging microorganisms that may arise in the coming years.

One of the microorganisms that has generated significant concern in recent years is the Rift Valley Fever Virus (RVFV). This mosquito-borne virus primarily affects animals such as livestock and sheep but has shown the ability to infect humans and cause severe diseases, including fever, hemorrhage, and neurological problems. Although person-to-person transmission is still limited, RVFV outbreaks have caused high mortality and morbidity in regions of Africa and are considered a potential threat to global public health [41]. Another microorganism deserving attention is the avian influenza virus H_7N_9. This virus, primarily transmitted from birds to humans, has caused sporadic outbreaks in China since 2013. While sustained human-to-human transmission has not been observed thus far, human cases of H_7N_9 infection have been severe with a high mortality rate. We must remain vigilant about the possibility of this virus acquiring mutations that enable more efficient spread among humans, which would pose a significant threat to global public health. Additionally, we should also be attentive to Nipah viruses, such as the Nipah virus (NiV) and the Hendra virus (HeV). These zoonotic viruses have caused outbreaks in Southeast Asia and Australia, respectively. NiV has demonstrated the ability to spread from person to person in certain outbreaks, increasing concerns about its potential to trigger a large-scale epidemic. Nipah virus infections have been associated with a high mortality rate and severe symptoms such as encephalitis and pneumonia [42].

Furthermore, some bacteria also pose an emerging threat to public health. Carbapenem-resistant *Klebsiella pneumoniae* (KPC) and methicillin-resistant *Staphylococcus aur*eus (MRSA) are prominent examples of multidrug-resistant bacteria. The resistance to antibiotics limits treatment options and presents a significant challenge for controlling infections caused by these bacteria [43]. When considering possible emerging microorganisms that could pose a threat to global public health in the coming years, it is essential to mention the Marburg virus. This virus belongs to the same family as the Ebola virus and has caused sporadic outbreaks in Central Africa since its discovery in 1967. Although Marburg fever outbreaks have been less frequent than Ebola, the high mortality rate associated with this disease (up to 90%) and the lack of specific treatments make it a significant global threat [44]. Another microorganism that has garnered attention is the Middle East Respiratory Syndrome Coronavirus (MERS-CoV) and various variants of coronaviruses. MERS-CoV was first identified in Saudi Arabia in 2012 and has caused sporadic outbreaks since then. Although person-to-person transmission is limited, cases of MERS-CoV infection have been severe, with high mortality rates. The concern lies in the possibility that this virus may undergo mutations that allow more efficient transmission among humans, potentially leading to a large-scale epidemic [45].

4. Impact of emerging infectious diseases on populations, public health, and the global economy

Emerging infectious diseases represent a constant challenge and danger to public health and the global economy. These diseases, caused by new pathogens or the emergence of resistant strains, have a high potential for transmission with significant impacts on populations and healthcare systems. The recent outbreak of SARS-CoV-2 has highlighted the threat posed by these emerging diseases to public health and the global economy. We must assess what the emergence of these new germs and diseases means for populations, global public health, and the economy at both regional and global levels. **Table 2** shows the human and economic impact of major emerging diseases.

The rapid spread of these diseases can result in epidemics or pandemics that affect entire communities. In addition to direct deaths caused by these diseases, there are serious consequences in terms of long-term morbidity and disability. Furthermore, these diseases can disproportionately impact vulnerable populations, such as children, the elderly, and people with chronic illnesses. According to a study conducted by Johnson et al. [54], it was found that the impact of emerging infectious diseases on the population can be particularly severe in areas with fragile healthcare systems and limited resources. Additionally, infectious diseases can negatively affect people's quality of life, causing stress, anxiety, and an increase in disease burden.

4.1 Examples of the impact produced by EIDs

At the end of the late 1970s of the last century, the general perception was that the era of major epidemics had come to an end; we had made progress in treating bacterial diseases with the advent of antibiotics and vaccines, which offered broad protection against multiple viral diseases. However, the Human Immunodeficiency Virus (HIV) emerged and changed everything, along with the Acquired Immunodeficiency Syndrome (AIDS) associated with its infection. A zoonosis that encountered the perfect environment: mutations that made its transmission among humans more

Year	Event	Estimated mortality and morbidity	Economic cost
1981	AIDS/HIV	70 million infections. 37 million deaths [46]	3–4% of GDP in Africa [47]
2003	SARS	8100 cases and 744 deaths [48]	US $3 billions in China US $6 billions in Canada US $5 billions in Singapore [49]
2013	Ebola	20,646 cases 11,323 deaths [50]	US$2 billion loss in Guinea, Liberia, and Sierra Leone [51]
2020	COVID	767.984.989 cases* 6.943.390 deaths* [52]	4,3% del GPD worldwide [53]

*June 2023.

Table 2.
Impact of various emerging diseases on morbidity and mortality and their economic cost.

efficient, social changes associated with new sexual behaviors, and the emergence of parenteral heroin use. These factors amplified and facilitated its expansion.

Human Immunodeficiency Virus is a spherical retrovirus, equipped with an envelope and a protein capsid. Its genome is a single-stranded RNA chain that is temporarily copied to DNA in order to replicate and integrate into the genome of the infected cell. The protein antigens on the outer envelope specifically assemble with membrane proteins of susceptible cells, especially cluster of differentiation 4 (CD4) T cells. The process of converting RNA to DNA is a key feature of retroviruses and is carried out through enzymatic actions of reverse transcriptase. The Human Immunodeficiency Virus Type 1 (HIV-1), responsible for the current pandemic, has been closely related to Simian Immunodeficiency Virus (SIVcpz), which infects populations of the Central African subspecies of the common chimpanzee, while Human Immunodeficiency Virus Type 2 (HIV-2), on the other hand, originates from Simian Immunodeficiency Virus (SIVsm), which is found in the mangabey monkeys inhabiting the coastal forests from Senegal to Ivory Coast.

As a result, the emergence of HIV and its associated AIDS pandemic demonstrates how an EID can significantly impact global health. It highlights the importance of understanding the factors that contribute to the spread and adaptation of these pathogens to human populations. Furthermore, it serves as a reminder of the ongoing need for research, surveillance, and preparedness to effectively respond to the ever-changing landscape of infectious diseases.

It is estimated that 38.4 million people are living with HIV worldwide, and the annual number of deaths from HIV-related illnesses, which has decreased to below one million since 2017, still stands at around 700,000 deaths as of 2021. The accumulated incidence since the beginning of the pandemic is 85.6 million cases, with nearly 41 million infected individuals having died worldwide. The cost of HIV, both in terms of population and economics, has been enormous, particularly in African countries.

Until 2022, AIDS (Acquired Immunodeficiency Syndrome) has had a profound macroeconomic impact worldwide. This impact has been especially notable in regions with high rates of HIV infection, such as some parts of sub-Saharan Africa, but it has also affected both developed and developing economies. One of the primary aspects, though not the only one, of the economic cost of the infection's impact has been the significant increase in healthcare expenses in affected countries. The costs associated with prevention, diagnosis, and treatment, including antiretroviral drugs and other medications, have been enormous. Additionally, treating HIV/AIDS-related complications has required considerable resources in terms of medical personnel, hospitals, and medical equipment. Moreover, the loss of human capital due to the death of productive-age individuals, particularly in sub-Saharan countries, has been devastating. AIDS has disproportionately affected young and working-age people, leading to imbalances in the population and depriving economies of valuable human resources for socioeconomic development.

On the other hand, AIDS has placed a significant burden on affected families and communities. The disease has led to the orphanhood of children, creating a need for more resources for the care and education of these orphans. It has also increased the caregiving burden for family members who have to attend to people with HIV/AIDS. The socioeconomic consequences of HIV/AIDS have been far-reaching, affecting not only individuals but also societies and economies as a whole.

Addressing the economic impact of HIV/AIDS requires a comprehensive approach, including continued investment in prevention, treatment, and support services. Ensuring access to antiretroviral therapy and other essential healthcare services for all those living with HIV is crucial to reducing the economic burden of the disease. Additionally, efforts to promote education and awareness about HIV transmission and prevention can help to reduce new infections and the associated economic costs. Supporting affected families and communities through social programs and initiatives is also vital to alleviate the broader socioeconomic consequences of HIV/AIDS. Only through concerted and sustained efforts can we effectively address the economic challenges posed by HIV/AIDS and work toward a future free from this devastating disease. It is estimated that by 2025, 29 billion US dollars (in US dollars of 2019) will be needed for the HIV response in low- and middle-income countries, including countries that were previously considered high-income countries, in order to end AIDS as a threat to global public health.

Coronaviruses are an extensive group of RNA viruses that can cause various conditions, ranging from the common cold to more severe diseases such as bronchitis, bronchiolitis, pneumonia, Middle East Respiratory Syndrome Coronavirus (MERS-CoV), or Severe Acute Respiratory Syndrome (SARS-CoV), among others. Toward the end of 2019, Chinese authorities reported an outbreak of a new coronavirus (SARS-CoV-2) in the city of Wuhan, originating from a zoonosis. To contain the SARS-CoV-2 outbreak, China imposed lockdowns and restricted population movements in several cities to prevent the virus's spread, as the Chinese New Year triggers the world's largest annual migration. By January 24, 2020, some sources indicated over 1300 identified cases, primarily in China, but also in the United States of America, France, Thailand, Japan, Nepal, and South Korea. On March 11, 2020, the World Health Organization (WHO) declared the SARS-CoV-2 outbreak a pandemic.

The SARS (Severe Acute Respiratory Syndrome) outbreak in 2002 and 2003 had a significant impact on the global economy. While the spread of SARS was quickly controlled and did not escalate into a large-scale pandemic like the current one, the macroeconomic cost of this outbreak was considerable (**Table 2**). During the SARS outbreak, there was a significant decrease in tourism, hospitality, and international travel in the affected regions. Countries and cities with SARS cases experienced a drastic reduction in foreign visitors and an increase in travel cancelations, resulting in revenue loss for the tourism industry and related services. The SARS outbreak created uncertainty among consumers and investors. Consumer confidence declined due to fear of the disease, leading to reduced spending and commercial activities. Investors also became cautious and hesitant to invest in the regions affected by the outbreak. Despite the relatively quick containment of the SARS outbreak compared to other emerging viruses, its macroeconomic consequences were notable. Global estimates of direct and indirect economic losses due to SARS vary in different reports, but the total cost is estimated to have ranged from several billions to tens of billions of dollars.

The MERS coronavirus, previously known as "novel coronaviru" "(nCoV), is a single-stranded RNA virus. It causes Middle East Respiratory Syndrome Coronavirus (MERS-CoV), first detected in Saudi Arabia in 2012. The origin of this virus is currently unknown but is believed to have likely originated from an animal source. The virus is now spreading to South Korea, raising concerns as coronaviruses can often mutate, potentially leading to a pandemic. All known cases have been linked to the Arabian Peninsula, either occurring there or in nearby countries. There are many uncertainties regarding the origin and transmission of MERS-CoV, which is typical of an emerging disease. Various possibilities, including environmental factors, animal sources, and human exposures, are being considered. As a result, the precise modes of transmission of the MERS coronavirus remain to be well defined.

Middle East Respiratory Syndrome outbreaks have resulted in temporary closures of medical facilities, hotels, and other businesses, leading to income loss in these sectors. Additionally, the implementation of control and prevention measures has resulted in restrictions on commercial activities, negatively affecting the local economy and companies operating in those regions.

The emergence of HIV in the last century, the Ebola virus disease epidemic in West Africa, the rise of antimicrobial-resistant pathogens, and the COVID-19 pandemic have reinforced the concept of Global Health. In addition to the impact these diseases have on population health, we must consider their far-reaching economic implications. Broader economic evaluations can provide a multisectoral translational perspective on the costs of the disease beyond approaches focused solely on human health, which consider disease cases, direct medical expenses, and public health functions and interventions [55]. In a study published by Fan et al. [56], it was estimated that the COVID-19 outbreak could have a significant impact on the global economy, with estimated economic losses in trillions of dollars. Additionally, the most affected countries may experience a decline in their gross domestic product (GDP) and an increase in public debt burden. These economic impacts can have long-lasting effects on communities and hinder long-term recovery.

The traditional approach to assessing the economic impact on health focuses on evaluating the direct costs of the disease burden (care, diagnosis, and treatment of the disease) and indirect costs (wages, productivity losses, etc.). However, this approach does not provide a comprehensive view of the economic impact of these diseases, such as the implementation of contagion control measures, lockdowns, trade closures, travel restrictions, etc., as we have seen during the early months of the SARS-CoV-2 pandemic, along with the collapse of healthcare systems leading to diagnostic delays and premature deaths associated with this fact [55]. The World Health Organization (WHO) has proposed a framework to calculate a broader economic impact of diseases [57] that allows for analyzing the economic consequences of biological threats by examining wider impacts, including human behavior, resilience speed, and the "fear factor."

Let us take a look at some examples of the multisectoral economic impact of emerging infectious diseases (EIDs). As we mentioned earlier in this chapter, over 60% of EIDs have a zoonotic origin, which can result in significant economic impacts on the agricultural and livestock sectors. According to data provided by the World Organization for Animal Health [58], zoonotic diseases lead to a significant percentage of livestock culling as part of control strategies, along with a decline in livestock exports.

If we analyze the impact of COVID-19 on global agriculture, it has been significant and has affected various aspects of the food chain and agricultural production. First, there has been a major disruption in the food supply chain due to the pandemic, resulting in varying degrees of food supply disruptions depending on the country or region. This includes movement restrictions, logistical disruptions in distribution, and border closures. These factors have hindered the timely delivery of seeds, fertilizers, and pesticides, as well as the harvesting and distribution of agricultural products [59].

Second, movement restrictions and social distancing measures have limited the availability of agricultural labor, especially in countries that rely on migrant agricultural workers. This has affected the capacity for planting, harvesting, and crop maintenance, resulting in production losses and increased labor costs. Furthermore, the economic crisis associated with the pandemic, coupled with rising prices, has led to a decrease in demand and changes in consumption patterns, particularly in sectors such as horticulture and perishable products. Changes in consumption patterns, such as the closure of restaurants and a preference for nonperishable products, have also affected the marketing and prices of certain agricultural products, leading to a decline in demand.

During the SARS outbreak in 2003, tourism in Hong Kong dropped by 60%, and in Singapore by over 70%, with similar impacts observed in Mexico during the swine flu outbreak. However, possibly the greatest impact has been witnessed during the recent COVID-19 pandemic, which has had a significant impact on the tourism and airline industry. The measures implemented to contain the spread of the virus led to a massive decrease in travel and tourism demand. Airlines, hotels, tour operators, and other industry stakeholders experienced a drastic reduction in occupancy and revenue. The closure of tourism-related businesses and the decrease in travel demand have resulted in a substantial loss of jobs in the sector. Additionally, we should consider the significant decline in tourism revenues, which have had a significant impact on local and national economies, particularly in destinations heavily reliant on tourism [60, 61].

Furthermore, we should not underestimate the environmental impact that follows the emergence of EIDs. The damage to natural resources, loss of wildlife populations, and environmental pollution are often overlooked in economic assessments related to these diseases [55]. These pathogens, including viruses, bacteria, and other microorganisms, have the potential to cause outbreaks and pandemics resulting in considerable morbidity, mortality, and negative economic impact, with a potentially devastating effect on population health. Emerging infectious diseases pose a constant threat to healthcare systems worldwide. These pathogens can cause outbreaks and pandemics that test the responsiveness and resources of healthcare systems. One of the most feared consequences is the increased healthcare burden due to these diseases, which generate a rapid surge in demand for care and services, often within a short period of time. This will require a quick and effective response from healthcare systems, involving an increase in the number of consultations, hospitalizations, and intensive care. This additional burden can put pressure on available resources, resulting in a shortage of beds, medical personnel, and necessary supplies, to provide quality care. Moreover, control measures will be necessary to minimize the impact of these diseases, including contact tracing, case isolation, and other measures, which will require a rapid and effective mobilization of professional and material resources. All of this should be considered alongside the stress, fatigue from increased healthcare workload, and fear of contagion among healthcare personnel.

5. Strategies to address the impact of emerging infectious diseases

Emerging infectious diseases pose a significant threat to human, animal, and environmental health globally. Outbreaks of diseases, such as SARS-CoV-2, Ebola virus, avian flu, and Zika virus, among many others, have highlighted the need for a comprehensive and multidisciplinary approach to address these public health crises. Prevention and control of these diseases are crucial to reducing their impact on populations, public health, and the economy. Some key strategies include:

- Strengthenicnd resilient healthcare systems is essential, with the capacity to rapidly detect and respond to outbreaks of emerging infectious diseases. This involves improving healthcare infrastructure, training healthcare personnel, and strengthening epidemiological surveillance.

- The fight against antibiotic resistance must incorporate some important measures. It is essential to educate healthcare professionals, patients, and the general public about the proper use of antibiotics. Clear guidelines should be provided on when to prescribe them and when not to, as well as the importance of completing the treatment cycle. Prudent use of antibiotics is crucial. Antibiotics should be used only when necessary and for the treatment of bacterial infections. Additionally, it is crucial to establish surveillance systems to monitor antibiotic resistance and track usage patterns in different regions and populations. This will help identify emerging issues and take preventive measures (Centers for Disease Control and Prevention (CDC) and European Centre for Disease Prevention and Control (ECDC) programs) along with data exchange between countries to track drug resistance patterns. A prominent example of this is the Global Antimicrobial Resistance Surveillance System (GLASS). GLASS is an initiative led by the World Health Organization (WHO) that aims to collect, analyze, and share data on antimicrobial resistance worldwide. Through GLASS, countries can provide data on antibiotic resistance and antimicrobial use in humans and animals. These data are collected and analyzed globally to identify emerging resistance patterns, areas of concern, and trends over time.

- Research and development of vaccines and treatments: Investments in research and development are needed to accelerate the creation of effective vaccines and antiviral or antibiotic treatments. This includes supporting international collaboration and the exchange of data and samples.

- Enhancing surveillance and early detection: Strengthening epidemiological surveillance systems is necessary to quickly identify outbreaks of emerging infectious diseases and monitor their evolution. This involves implementing technology-based surveillance systems, improving healthcare staff training, and promoting collaboration between countries.

- Education and public communication: Promoting education and public awareness about emerging infectious diseases is essential. This includes providing accurate and timely information about these diseases, their modes of transmission, and preventive measures. Additionally, clear and transparent communication by health authorities is needed to build trust in prevention and control strategies.

- International cooperation: Cooperation and collaboration between countries are critical to addressing emerging infectious diseases globally. This includes sharing information, resources, and best practices, as well as coordinating efforts to prevent the spread of cross-border diseases. This concept is known as Global Health.

- Addressing associated factors: Effectively preventing emerging infectious diseases requires addressing underlying factors contributing to their emergence and spread. These factors include deforestation, environmental degradation, climate change, rapid urbanization, and antimicrobial resistance. Policies and measures must be implemented to tackle these challenges, including promoting sustainable agricultural practices, conserving natural ecosystems, and properly regulating the use of antimicrobials.

An outstanding example of the effective adaptation of specific policies in a strategy to minimize the impact of an emerging infection is the global response to the HIV/AIDS pandemic. Through collaboration among governments, international organizations, and civil society, prevention and treatment programs, access to antiretroviral drugs, and educational campaigns have been implemented, significantly reducing the impact of HIV/AIDS in many parts of the world. The fight against this disease has demonstrated that a coordinated and evidence-based response can make a difference in mitigating the impact of emerging infections.

Several countries and communities have demonstrated resilience and effective adaptation strategies against emerging infections. Let us look at some prominent examples.

During the COVID-19 pandemic, Taiwan implemented a rapid and efficient response to contain the virus spread. Their approach focused on early detection, contact tracing, isolating positive cases, and extensive use of information and communication technologies for monitoring and communication. This response has been widely praised for its effectiveness in containing the virus and minimizing its impact on the community. Singapore was another example of a country that has shown a quick and effective response to emerging infections. During the SARS pandemic in 2003 and the COVID-19 pandemic, Singapore implemented strict control measures, including contact tracing, quarantine, and social distancing. Clear and transparent communication with the public has also been a key component of their strategy. Uganda, on the other hand, has developed a comprehensive approach to address HIV/AIDS, which includes prevention, treatment, and healthcare programs for affected individuals. Additionally, they have worked to reduce the stigma and discrimination associated with the disease, which has contributed to improved access to care and support services. Finally, Brazil demonstrated an effective response to outbreaks of yellow fever and other infectious diseases. The country has carried out massive vaccination campaigns, improved epidemiological surveillance, and strengthened its healthcare system to address outbreaks promptly and in a coordinated manner.

These examples highlight the importance of a timely, coordinated, and evidence-based response to address emerging infections. Resilience and effective adaptation in these communities and countries have been crucial in minimizing the impact of infectious diseases and protecting public health.

5.1 The "One Health" approach and emerging infectious diseases

As mentioned earlier, emerging infectious diseases (EIDs) constitute a significant threat to global human health. The "One Health" approach is based on the recognition that human, animal, and environmental health are intrinsically interconnected. It proposes a holistic perspective that encompasses the interaction between humans, animals, plants, and the environment, acknowledging that public health challenges cannot be effectively addressed without close collaboration and integration of knowledge and efforts across disciplines.

The concept of "One Health" is not new and dates back at least 200 years [62]. The most commonly used definition shared by the Centers for Disease Control and Prevention (CDC) in the United States of America and the One Health Commission is: "One Health is defined as a collaborative, multisectoral, and transdisciplinary approach that works at the local, regional, national, and global levels to achieve optimal health outcomes by recognizing the interconnection between people, animals, plants, and their shared environment." A simpler version of this definition is provided by the One Health Institute at the University of California, Davis: "One Health is an approach to ensure the well-being of people, animals, and the environment through collaborative problem-solving at the local, national, and global levels" [63].

In the context of EIDs, the "One Health" approach focuses on understanding the factors contributing to the emergence and spread of these diseases. This involves evaluating the links between human and animal health, monitoring diseases in animals and their potential transmission to humans, as well as assessing environmental factors that may influence disease spread. The "One Health" approach is crucial in understanding emerging infectious diseases due to several key factors.

Many of these diseases originate in animals and are transmitted to humans. Disease surveillance in animals, such as respiratory viruses in birds or rodent-borne viruses, is essential to identify potential transmission to humans. The "One Health" approach promotes collaboration between human and animal health professionals to monitor and prevent the spread of these diseases [64]. Furthermore, climate change and environmental degradation can influence the spread of emerging infectious diseases. Rising temperatures, deforestation, and urbanization can disrupt ecosystems and lead to increased contact between humans, animals, and pathogens. The "One Health" approach emphasizes the importance of assessing environmental impacts and climate change in the emergence and spread of emerging infectious diseases. It recognizes the need to understand the effects of climate change and environmental degradation on human and animal health and advocates for integrated management of these issues.

Antimicrobial resistance is becoming an increasing concern in the context of EIDs. Overuse and inappropriate use of antibiotics in humans and animals contribute to the development of resistance, making treatment more difficult. This approach promotes the implementation of policies and practices for responsible use of antimicrobials in both human and animal health. Lastly, early detection and rapid response are crucial in controlling EIDs. The "One Health" approach emphasizes the importance of establishing integrated surveillance systems that enable early detection of outbreaks in humans and animals, facilitating a rapid and effective response to contain the spread.

6. Conclusions

We can conclude by stating that emerging infectious diseases represent a significant threat to public health and global stability. As the world faces the emergence of new pathogens and unexpected outbreaks, it is crucial that we are prepared to respond quickly and effectively. These diseases have the potential to cause high morbidity and mortality, as well as trigger health and socioeconomic crises. We have witnessed how COVID-19 has affected millions of people worldwide, overwhelming healthcare systems, imposing mobility restrictions, and having a significant impact on the global economy.

Early detection, epidemiological surveillance, strengthening healthcare systems, and implementing preventive measures are key elements in responding to emerging infectious diseases. Scientific research, development of effective vaccines and treatments, as well as public education and awareness, also play a fundamental role in mitigating these outbreaks. Furthermore, it is essential to strengthen international cooperation and collaboration to jointly address these threats. Governments, international organizations, healthcare professionals, and society as a whole must come together to share information, resources, and best practices. Additionally, it is crucial that healthcare systems are prepared and flexible enough to meet the challenges posed by emerging infectious diseases. Addressing inequalities in access to healthcare and strengthening health systems in low-resource countries are also necessary, as emerging infectious diseases can have a particularly devastating impact in these regions. Learning from lessons of past outbreaks such as Ebola and SARS is crucial to improve our preparedness and response to future emerging infectious diseases. Cooperation between the public and private sectors, collaboration among countries, and global coordination are essential to effectively confront these challenges and protect the health of populations worldwide.

In summary, emerging infectious diseases constantly pose a threat to public health and global stability. Their impact on the population and the economy is significant, and a strong and coordinated global response is required. Investment in research, international cooperation, preparedness, and strengthening of healthcare systems, as well as public education and awareness, are key elements to address and mitigate the effects of these diseases. Only through a joint and collaborative approach can we be prepared to face the challenges presented by emerging infectious diseases. The "One Health" approach promotes multidisciplinary collaboration among professionals in human health, veterinary medicine, ecology, epidemiology, and other related disciplines. This collaboration allows for a better understanding of the factors contributing to the emergence and spread of emerging infectious diseases, as well as the development of more effective preventive and control strategies.

Conflict of interest

The author declares no conflict of interest.

Author details

Josep M. Ramon-Torrell
Clinical Science Department, School of Medicine and Health Sciences, University of Barcelona, Spain

*Address all correspondence to: jmramon@ub.edu

References

[1] Taubenberger JK, Morens DM. 1918 influenza: The mother of all pandemics. Emerging Infectious Diseases. 2006;**12**(1):15-22. DOI: 10.3201/eid1201.050979

[2] Fauci AS, Folkers GK. Emerging infectious diseases: A 10-year perspective from the National Institute of Allergy and Infectious Diseases. Emerging Infectious Diseases. 2012;**18**(2):207-214. DOI: 10.3201/eid1802.110312

[3] McCloskey B, Dar O, Zumla A, Heymann DL. Emerging infectious diseases and pandemic potential: Status quo and reducing risk of global spread. The Lancet Infectious Diseases. 2014;**14**:1001-1010. DOI: 10.1016/S1473-3099(14)70846-1

[4] Morens DM, Folkers GK, Fauci AS. The challenge of emerging and re-emerging infectious diseases. Nature. 2014;**430**(6996):242-249. DOI: 10.1038/nature02759

[5] Morse SS, Mazet JA, Woolhouse M, Parrish CR, Carroll D, Karesh WB, et al. Prediction and prevention of the next pandemic zoonosis. The Lancet. 2012;**380**(9857):1956-1965. DOI: 10.1016/S0140-6736(12)61684-5

[6] Jones BA, Grace D, Kock R, Alonso S, Rushton J, Said MY, et al. Zoonosis emergence linked to agricultural intensification and environmental change. Proceedings of the National Academy of Sciences of the United States of America. 2013;**110**(21):8399-8404. DOI: 10.1073/pnas.1208059110

[7] Dantas-Torres F. Climate change, biodiversity, ticks and tick-borne diseases: The butterfly effect. International Journal for Parasitology: Parasites and Wildlife. 2015;**4**:452-461. DOI: 10.1016/j.ijppaw.2015.07.001

[8] Kobayashi N. Impact of emerging, re-emerging and zoonotic viral infectious diseases in a virologist's perspective. Open. Virology Journal. 2018;**12**(Suppl-2):131-133. DOI: 10.2174/1874357901

[9] Smith KF, Goldberg M, Rosenthal S, Carlson L, Chen J, Chen C, et al. Global rise in infectious diseases associated with urbanization. National Academy of Sciences of the United States of America. 2014;**111**(52):18513-18517. DOI: 10.1098/rsif.2014.0950

[10] Tatem AJ, Rogers DJ, Hay SI. Global transport networks and infectious disease spread. Advances in Parasitology. 2006;**62**:293-343. DOI: 10.1016/S0065-308X(05)62009-X

[11] Rader B, Scarpino SV, Nande A, Hill AL, et al. Crowding and the shape of COVID-19 epidemics. Nature Medicine. 2020;**26**:1829-1834. DOI: 10.1038/s41591-020-1104-0

[12] Kwan CK, Ernst JD. HIV and tuberculosis: A deadly human syndemic. Clinical Microbiology Reviews. 2011;**24**:351-376. DOI: 10.1128/CMR.00042-10

[13] Jones KE, Patel NG, Levy MA, Storeygard A, Balk D, Gittleman JL, et al. Global trends in emerging infectious diseases. Nature. 2008;**451**(7181):990-993. DOI: 10.1038/nature06536

[14] Kibret S, Wilson GG, Ryder D, et al. The influence of dams on malaria transmission in sub-Saharan Africa. EcoHealth. 2017;**14**:408-419. DOI: 10.1007/s10393-015-1029-0

[15] Boyce R, Reyes R, Matte M, et al. Severe flooding and malaria transmission in the western Ugandan highlands: Implications for disease control in an era of global climate change. The Journal of Infectious Diseases. 2016;**214**:1403-1410. DOI: 10.1093/infdis/jiw363

[16] Scott TW, Amerasinghe PH, Morrison AC, et al. Longitudinal studies of Aedes aegypti (Diptera: Culicidae) in Thailand and Puerto Rico: Blood feeding frequency. Journal of Medical Entomology. 2000;**37**:89-101. DOI: 10.1603/0022-2585-37.1.89

[17] Reisen WK, Fang Y, Martinez VM. Effects of temperature on the transmission of West Nile virus by Culex tarsalis (Diptera: Culicidae). Journal of Medical Entomology. 2006;**43**:309-317. DOI: 10.1603/0022-2585(2006)043[0309:EOTOTT]2.0.CO;2

[18] Brady OJ, Johansson MA, Guerra CA, et al. Modelling adult Aedes aegypti and Aedes albopictus survival at different temperatures in laboratory and field settings. Parasites & Vectors. 2013;**6**:351. DOI: 10.1186/1756-3305-6-351

[19] Mordecai EA, Cohen JM, Evans MV, et al. Detecting the impact of temperature on transmission of Zika, dengue, and chikungunya using mechanistic models. PLoS Neglected Tropical Diseases. 2017;**11**:e0005568. DOI: 10.1371/journal.pntd.0005568

[20] Rocklöv J, Dubrow R. Author correction: Climate change: An enduring challenge for vector-borne disease prevention and control. Nature Immunology. 2020;**21**:695. DOI: 10.1038/s41590-020-0648-y

[21] Brady OJ, Golding N, Pigott DM, Kraemer MU, Messina JP, Reiner RC Jr, et al. Global temperature constraints on Aedes aegypti and ae. Albopictus persistence and competence for dengue virus transmission. Parasites & Vectors. 2014;**7**:338. DOI: 10.1186/1756-3305-7-338

[22] Kraemer MUG, Sinka ME, Duda KA, et al. The global distribution of the arbovirus vectors Aedes aegypti and ae. Albopictus. eLife. 2015;**4**:e08347. DOI: 10.7554/eLife.08347

[23] Hales S, de Wet N, Maindonald J, Woodward A. Potential effect of population and climate changes on global distribution of dengue fever: An empirical model. Lancet. 2002;**360**:830-834. DOI: 10.1016/S0140-6736(02)09964-6

[24] Wagner CE, Hooshyar M, Baker RE, Yang W, Arinaminpathy N, Vecchi G, et al. Climatological, virological and sociological drivers of current and projected dengue fever outbreak dynamics in Sri Lanka. Journal of the Royal Society Interface. 2020;**17**:20200075. DOI: 10.1098/rsif.2020.0075

[25] Couper LI, MacDonald AJ, Mordecai EA. Impact of prior and projected climate change on US Lyme disease incidence. Global Change Biology. 2021;**27**:738-754. DOI: 10.1111/gcb.15435

[26] Ryan SJ, Carlson CJ, Tesla B, Bonds MH, Ngonghala CN, Mordecai EA, et al. Warming temperatures could expose more than 1.3 billion new people to Zika virus risk by 2050. Global Change Biology. 2021;**27**:84-93. DOI: 10.1111/gcb.15384

[27] Ryan SJ, Lippi CA, Zermoglio F. Shifting transmission risk for malaria in Africa with climate change: A framework for planning and intervention. Malaria Journal. 2020;**19**:170. DOI: 10.1186/s12936-020-03224-6

[28] Caminade C, McIntyre KM, Jones AE, Morse AP. Mapping recent and future climate suitability for dengue transmission in Europe. National Academy of Sciences of the United States of America. 2018;**114**(9):1941-1946. DOI: 10.1111/nyas.13950

[29] Keesing F, Belden LK, Daszak P, Dobson A, Harvell CD, Holt RD, et al. Impacts of biodiversity on the emergence and transmission of infectious diseases. Nature. 2010;**468**(7324):647-652. DOI: 10.1038/nature09575

[30] Altizer S, Ostfeld RS, Johnson PT, Kutz S, Harvell CD. Climate change and infectious diseases: From evidence to a predictive framework. Science. 2013;**341**(6145):514-519. DOI: 10.1126/science.1239401

[31] Laxminarayan R, Duse A, Wattal C, Zaidi AK, Wertheim HF, Sumpradit N, et al. Antibiotic resistance—The need for global solutions. The Lancet Infectious Diseases. 2013;**13**(12):1057-1098. DOI: 10.1016/S1473-3099(13)70318-9

[32] Alanis AJ. Resistance to antibiotics: Are we in the post-antibiotic era? Archives of Medical Research. 2005;**36**(6):697-705. DOI: 10.1016/j.arcmed.2005.06.009

[33] Tacconelli E, Carrara E, Savoldi A, Harbarth S, Mendelson M, Monnet DL, et al. Discovery, research, and development of new antibiotics: The WHO priority list of antibiotic-resistant bacteria and tuberculosis. The Lancet Infectious Diseases. 2018;**18**(3):318-327. DOI: 10.1016/S1473-3099(17)30753-3

[34] Gould IM, Bal AM, Newell DG. Antibiotic resistance: A global response. Frontiers in Public Health. 2018;**6**:209. DOI: 10.2147/IDR.S173867

[35] Ventola CL. The antibiotic resistance crisis: Part 1: Causes and threats. Pharmacy and Therapeutics. 2015;**40**(4):277-283

[36] Landers TF, Cohen B, Wittum TE, Larson EL. A review of antibiotic use in food animals: Perspective, policy, and potential. Public Health Reports. 2012;**127**(1):4-22. DOI: 10.1177/003335491212700103

[37] Haines A, Kovats RS, Campbell-Lendrum D, Corvalán C. Climate change and human health: Impacts, vulnerability, and mitigation. The Lancet. 2014;**383**(9928):2105-2118. DOI: 10.1016/S0140-6736(06)68933-2

[38] Goff DA, Kullar R, Goldstein EJ, Gilchrist M, Nathwani D, Cheng AC, et al. A global call from five countries to collaborate in antibiotic stewardship: United we succeed, divided we might fail. The Lancet Infectious Diseases. 2017;**17**(2):e56-e63. DOI: 10.1016/S1473-3099(16)30386-3

[39] Woolhouse ME, Gowtage-Sequeria S. Host range and emerging and reemerging pathogens. Emerging Infectious Diseases. 2005;**11**(12):1842-1847. DOI: 10.3201/eid1112.050997

[40] Baker RE, Mahmud AS, Miller IF, et al. Infectious disease in an era of global change. Nature Reviews. 2022;**20**:193-205. DOI: doi. 10.1038/s41579-021-00639-z

[41] Mohammed M, Lorenzo G, Busquets N, Brunl A. Rift Valley fever virus: Insights into pathogenesis, recent outbreaks, and countermeasures. Viruses. 2021;**13**(5):893. DOI: 10.1128/JVI.02641-10

[42] Satterfield BA, Lim T, Wang L. Nipah virus infection: Current outbreak and future directions. Clinical Infectious Diseases. 2018;**66**(5):748-755. DOI: 10.1128/JCM.01875-17

[43] Mathers AJ, Stoesser N, Sheppard AE, et al. Klebsiella pneumoniae carbapenemase (KPC)-producing K. Pneumoniae: A review of epidemiology, treatment, and outcomes. Infectious Diseases and Therapy. 2019;**8**(1):1-12. DOI: 10.1128/AAC.04292-14

[44] Kortepeter MG, Dierberg K, Shenoy ES, Cieslak TJ. Marburg virus disease: A summary for clinicians. International Journal of Infectious Diseases. 2020;**99**:233-242. DOI: 10.1016/j.ijid.2020.07.042

[45] Memish ZA, Perlman S, Van Kerkhove MD, Zumla A. Middle East respiratory syndrome. The Lancet. 2019;**395**(10229):1063-1077. DOI: 10.1016/S0140-6736(19)33221-0

[46] WHO Global Health Observatory data. Available from: http://www.who.int/gho/hiv/en [Accessed: May, 2023]

[47] Dixon S, McDonald S, Roberts J. AIDS and economic growth in Africa: A panel data analysis. Journal of International Development. 2001;**13**(4):411-426. DOI: 10.1002/jid.795

[48] Wang M-D, Jolly AM. Changing virulence of the SARS virus: The epidemiological evidence. Bulletin of the World Health Organization. 2004;**82**(7):547-548

[49] Keogh-Brown MR, Smith RD. The economic impact of SARS: How does the reality match the predictions? Health Policy. 2008;**88**(1):110-120. DOI: 10.1016/j.healthpol.2008.03.003

[50] Ebola Situation Report. Weekly data report, April 15. Available from: http://www.who.int/mediacentre/ [Accessed: May, 2023]

[51] World Bank. The Economic Impact of the 2014 Ebola Epidemic: Short- and Medium-Term Estimates for Guinea, Liberia, and Sierra Leone", Working Paper 90748. Washington, DC: World Bank; 2014

[52] Available from: https://covid19.who.int [Accessed: June, 2023]

[53] (FMI). World Economic Outlook: Managing Divergent Recoveries. Available from: https://www.imf.org/en/Publications/WEO/Issues/2021/03/23/world-economic-outlook-april-2021 [Accessed: June, 2023]

[54] Johnson NF, Mueller JL, Jones RG. Potential trade-offs between the health, economic, and equity impacts of an influenza pandemic. Bulletin of Mathematical Biology. 2020;**82**(1):1-31. DOI: 10.1007/s11538-020-00717-y

[55] Smith KM, Machalabaa CC, Seifmanc R, Feferholtza Y, Karesha DWB. Infectious disease and economics: The case for considering multi-sectoral T impacts. One Health. 2019;**7**:100080. DOI: 10.1016/j.onehlt.2018.100080

[56] Fan VY, Jamison DT, Summers LH. The economic consequences of a pandemic. The World Bank Research Observer. 2020;**35**(1):1-33

[57] World Health Organization. WHO Guide to Identifying the Economic Consequences of Disease and Injury. World Health Organization; 2009. Available from: https://apps.who.int/iris/handle/10665/137037 [Accessed: June, 2023]

[58] World Bank. People, Pathogens and our Planet: The Economics of One Health. Washington, DC: World Bank; 2012

[59] Swinnen J, McDermott J. Impact of COVID-19 on agriculture, food systems,

and rural livelihoods. IFPRI Policy Brief 15. 2020. Available from: https://www.ifpri.org/publication/impact-covid-19-agriculture-food-systems-and-rural-livelihoods [Accessed: June, 2023]

[60] UNWTO. 2020. Tourism and COVID-19: UNWTO Briefing Note. 2020. Available from: https://www.unwto.org/tourism-covid-19 [Accessed: March, 2023]

[61] WTTC. Economic Impact Reports. 2021. Available from: https://wttc.org/Research/Economic-Impact. [Accessed: March, 2023]

[62] Atlas RM. One health: Its origins and future. Current Topics in Microbiology and Immunology. 2013;**365**:1-13. DOI: 10.1007/82_2012_223

[63] Mackenzie JS, Jeggo M. The one health approach—Why is it so important? Tropical Medicine and Infectious Disease. 2019;**4**:88. DOI: 10.3390/tropicalmed4020088

[64] Morens DM, Fauci AS. Emerging infectious diseases: Threats to human health and global stability. PLoS Pathogens. 2013;**9**(7):e1003467. DOI: 10.1371/journal.ppat.1003467

Chapter 3

Perspective Chapter: The Pivotal Role of Vaccines and Interventional Equity and Appropriateness

Ibrahim Khalil Dadari

Abstract

The current COVID-19 pandemic saw the world deploying the latest technology as fast as it could to tackle the situation hurriedly. The world saw vaccine "grabbing" of immense magnitude from the most powerful nations which some defined as vaccine apartheid. This deprived less powerful nations of timely access to the vaccine meant to interrupt the pandemic. Moreso, countries were faced with a generalized approach to the response which may have exacerbated existing inequities and further entrenched deprivations not just at the subnational levels but between nations as well. Once the stronger nations have had enough of their hoarded vaccines, these were then dumped on these weaker nations with additional consequences. This chapter explores the dynamics at play and what could be done better going further.

Keywords: equity, appropriate interventions, vaccine apartheid, vaccine diplomacy, global health

1. Introduction

The world needs to be better prepared to adequately mitigate and respond to global health emergencies. With the unprecedented response mounted to control the COVID-19 pandemic of recent, lessons are still being learned on how best the response should have been handled. This is despite human's perceived intellectual prowess and current advancement in medical technology and innovation. Vaccines became the centerpiece of the global response to control the pandemic, as was the case with several previous outbreaks. In the process, various factors, actions, and inactions had consequences on the overall and local outcomes of the pandemic including the emergence of new concepts which will have long-lasting effects on the future of pandemic response and global health security. Dissecting the interplay of these factors will be beneficial to future pandemic mitigation and response efforts.

Between 1996 and 2022, over 2200 disease outbreaks were reported across 233 countries and territories, with diseases among those with the highest number of outbreaks being COVID-19, Influenza, Cholera, and Meningitis [1]. The top five countries with the highest number of outbreaks included the Democratic Republic of Congo, Nigeria, the United States of America, Sudan, and Brazil. Sub-Saharan Africa has the highest frequency of disease outbreaks as reported. As of August 2023,

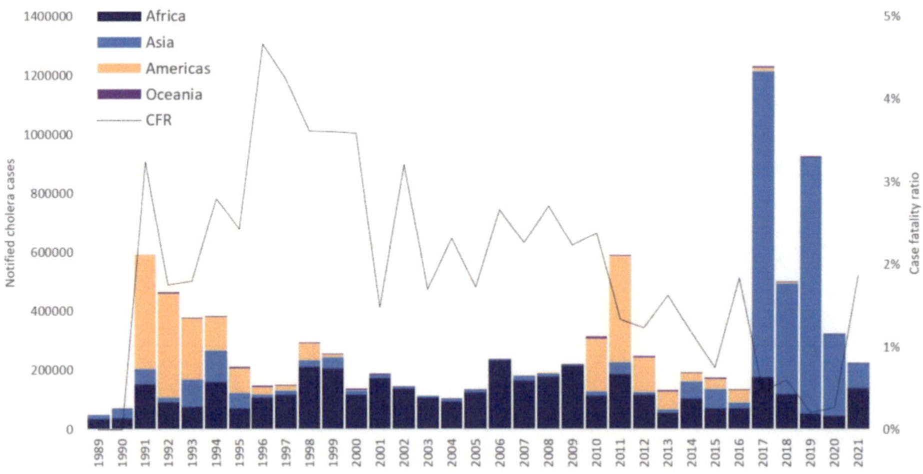

Figure 1.
Cholera cases reported to WHO by year and continent between 1989 and 2021. (Source: WHO Cholera – Global situation [3].)

over 760 million COVID-19 cases have been reported with about 7 million deaths [2]. Similarly, there has been a surge of cholera cases globally with about 30 countries reporting cases as of the end of 2022 most of which have prolonged cases [3]. **Figure 1** shows the annual case distribution of Cholera over the past several decades. Thousands of cases of Measles and other diseases have also been reported over the years.

Most of these diseases can be controlled through vaccination. Vaccines are one of the most cost-effective public health interventions with a net high return on investment greater than 20 for each dollar spent [4, 5]. It is stated that the full value of vaccinations is not fully quantified through a lot of these economic evaluations, for example, the impact of reduced resources consumed by the hospital from a future antimicrobial resistance or management of secondary diseases that may emanate from non-control of the primary vaccine-preventable disease (VPD) entity [6]. The value of vaccines cannot be overemphasized with the crucial role it continues to play in the control and eradication of diseases such as smallpox and the polio virus [7, 8]. Several new vaccines have been made available recently targeting both subsisting and (re)emerging diseases [8–10]. Unlike medicines that treat an existing infection, vaccines improve population immunity against the disease by making people resistant to the infection or its severe form [8]. This was the case with the COVID-19 pandemic where vaccines contributed substantially to controlling the disease: potentiating the effect of nonpharmaceutical interventions (NPI) [11]. It is pertinent to always correct the notion that vaccines are not cure but prevention, which is a misconception often seen in people with limited understanding of the role and mechanism of action of vaccines.

Vaccines remain the most complex medical products to develop, from conceptualization to pre-approval when sufficient evidence of quality, safety, and efficacy have been obtained and scrutinized to ensure they are much more beneficial relative to any risks they may portend associated with their use [12]. In emergencies, vaccines having satisfied all the standards get pre-approved as emergency use listing (EUL) to allow for rapid deployment to save lives as seen in the case of the COVID-19 pandemic. Even while they are deployed, robust surveillance is instituted to ensure tracking and reporting of any untoward effects which are referred to as adverse events following immunization

(AEFI), some of which are directly related to the vaccine products with others being coincidental events [13]. Like many medications and even foods, these untoward events are bound to happen in quite a few numbers but that does not take away from the extremely high safety standards accorded these products – nothing like a perfect vaccine, medicine or even food product exists! But people should note the rigorous process of vaccines approval at the national, regional, and global levels where the World Health Organization (WHO) and even national regulatory agencies (NRA) institute very stringent screening and approval processes to ensure the safety of the product being ingested, most especially as these are administered to healthy individuals whose tolerance threshold for reactions will be quite low as against someone who is already sick.

It is one thing to have the vaccine manufactured and approved; available for use and another to ensure the most in need get these vaccines without social, economic, cultural, or even ethnic barriers – the concept of equity in vaccine access and utilization. Health and in effect, vaccine equity ensures each nation or individual gets the opportunity to access quality vaccines unhindered by any personal or individual attributes or associations, including geography or location, gender, wealth, or other socioeconomic variables [14]. The Immunization Agenda 2030 (IA2030) emphasizes equity as one of its three goals (Goal 2: Promoting equity) to highlight its importance in ensuring universal vaccination coverage [15]. There exist inequities across regions, countries, states, or people, in access to and utilization of health services with the world making considerable progress towards reducing these disparities. Emergencies bring out the worst of humanity – greed, as was seen during the COVID-19 pandemic where nations were grabbing vaccines in surplus of their needs without any concern for fellow humans who may not have the quantum of resources to compete and grab as well. This phenomenon has been described by many as vaccine apartheid where over 90% of vaccines were grabbed by rich countries with no iota of concern for the not-so-rich nations [16]. The concepts of vaccine diplomacy or empathy became even more pertinent in the pandemic response [17]. While vaccine empathy described the nation or individual's capability to show sympathy to other nations or individual's needs for vaccines, vaccine diplomacy described the actual effort made by stronger nations and individuals to build mutually beneficial relationships to address the other individual or nation's vaccine needs [17]. We discuss the interplay of these factors vis-a-vis the global health security epidemiology, and what these portend for the future.

2. Nature of global health security

Many nations who hitherto were thought to have built a formidable health system capable of withstanding any threat were seen to falter when confronted with the reality of the pandemic of COVID-19 proportion; you could imagine what would happen if we had something worse. The United States Centers for disease control and Prevention (CDC) [18] describes today's top global health security threats to include:

- Emergence and spread of new infectious diseases.
- Ever-increasing globalization of travel and trade enables disease to spread.
- Rise of drug-resistant, disease-causing pathogens
- Potential for accidental release, theft, or illicit use of dangerous pathogens

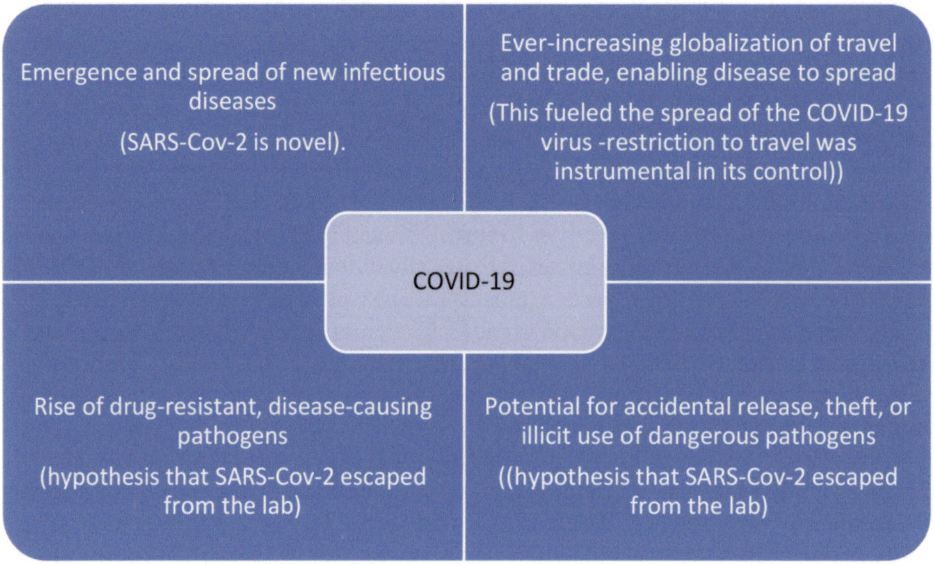

Figure 2.
Triggers and sustainers of global health emergencies.

One or more of the above, or even their mix could lead to a catastrophic and unimaginable global health crisis that needs to be prepared for. Benchmarking these top threats against the COVID-19 pandemic shows an interplay of each of the components to directly or indirectly trigger and sustain the pandemic as shown in **Figure 2**.

Although not all cases of emerging infectious diseases result in crisis, some do lead to large-scale morbidity and mortality. For instance, the COVID-19 pandemic has affected over 700 million persons as reported and resulted in about 7 million deaths; the 2009 H1N1 (swine flu) resulted in more than 284,000 deaths worldwide [2].

2.1 Emergence and spread of new infectious diseases

New and re-emerging infectious diseases are continually seen every day due to predominantly overt or covert human activity which could be intentional or accidental in nature. The US National Institute of Allergy and infectious diseases (NIAD) defines emerging infectious diseases as outbreaks of previously unknown diseases or known diseases that are rapidly increasing in incidence or geographic coverage in the last 2 decades or even persistent infectious diseases that failed to be controlled [19]. Re-emerging diseases are those that reappear after control or significant decline has been achieved and this could be due to human behaviors such as poor antimicrobial usage resulting in antimicrobial resistance (AMR) or even disruption in public health measures. Infectious diseases are (re)emerging quite fast with about 40 infectious diseases discovered since 1970 [18]. Some of these diseases of note include the severe acute respiratory syndrome viruses (SARS), the middle east respiratory syndrome virus (MERS), the Ebola virus, the Chikungunya virus, the Avian flu, the Swine flu virus, The Zika virus and most recently COVID-19, caused by a new coronavirus, SARS-CoV-2. The spread of these diseases is facilitated by globalization making them a global threat that could or have resulted in a pandemic which is a globalized spread of a health threat.

2.2 Ever-increasing globalization of travel and trade enables disease to spread

We live in an increasingly globalized world with travel, trade, and other human endeavors bringing people closer to each other physically or otherwise. Most infectious diseases are spread by contact or near contact through aerosols, airborne, body fluids, etc. The more people mingle and connect the easier it is to spread these diseases. It is challenging to restrict travel and human contact in an increasingly globalized world. Of most concern is international travel and the challenge thereof in limiting potentially deadly infectious diseases within borders [20]. A potent way to provide immunity against such diseases in these contexts will be prior exposure to the pathogen which carries potential for severe morbidity or mortality, or to use vaccines or immune products.

2.3 Rise of drug-resistant, disease-causing pathogens

More and more pathogens are becoming drug-resistant resulting in the re-emergence of previously controlled diseases spiking into outbreaks and epidemics. Antimicrobial resistance (AMR) is therefore a pandemic serving as a precursor for more pandemics in a chain-like reaction. Data suggests an estimated 4·95 million deaths associated with bacterial AMR in 2019 with the highest all-age death rate attributable to resistance seen in western sub-Saharan Africa put at 27·3 deaths per 100,000 [21]. While rich countries do face this serious menace, the data clearly shows a more daring situation in poorer countries of sub-Saharan Africa. Some of the top threats from AMR include *Escherichia coli*, *Staphylococcus aureus*, *Klebsiella pneumonia*, and *Streptococcus pneumoniae.*

2.4 Potential for accidental release, theft, or illicit use of dangerous pathogens

Several incidents of accidental or purposeful exposure to, or infection by, a highly infectious pathogenic agent have been reported and documented. Some of the causes of these include pathogen mix-ups where two or more pathogens are mixed up in the lab, laboratory accidents as seen in the Anthrax case of 2003 at the University of New Mexico, state bioweapon program accidents as seen in the 1979 Sverdlovsk Anthrax Leak, bioterrorism as seen in the 2001 anthrax mailing incidents [22]. These incidences have been one of the theories depicting the introduction and spread of some notable emerging infectious agents. Evidence on these may be hard to find particularly when the consequences of these actions are large and entities or nations responsible fear the 'punishments' that could arise from such which may come with heavy economic implications for the concerned entities.

According to Tom Inglesby, the director of the Center for Health Security at the Johns Hopkins Bloomberg School of Public Health (JHSPH), "*threats to U.S. health, safety, and security include not only major global and regional epidemics of emerging infectious diseases such as Ebola and Zika, but changes to the ways that known diseases, including dengue, chikungunya, yellow fever, and Middle Eastern respiratory syndrome coronavirus (MERS-CoV), are spreading throughout the world.*" [23].

Although many rich nations including the US, were thought to be well prepared to respond to massive epidemics or pandemics, the COVID-19 pandemic did reveal otherwise and showed the reality of unpreparedness of most countries in the world. Some poorer nations fared better than the wealthier ones. Understanding the nature of global health security threat and potential mitigation or control measures which includes both non-medical and medical measures such as vaccines, and making adequate provisions for equitable access and utilization globally will be pivotal in defeating future global health threats.

3. Approaches to addressing pandemics and epidemics: the role of vaccines

Health system preparedness to mitigate and assist in effectively curbing the future pandemic or global health emergencies should they occur, should be the mainstay of addressing global health emergencies. Some of the preparedness efforts include establishing and sustaining early warning systems, developing a preparedness and response plan including relevant protocols to monitor and mitigate global health emergencies, having a standby governance or command and control center to manage global health emergencies, identifying, and maintaining surge human and material resource capacity, among others.

Response on the other hand relates to the management and mitigation activities following the declaration of a global health event and are often adapted to the events epidemiology which describes the distribution, determinants, and deterrents of the global health emergency. The response often includes curative services meant to treat or cure those who have been afflicted with the condition, and preventive services meant to mitigate the spread of the condition and limit transmission of the disease within the population. The International Health Regulations (IHR) 2005 which is a legally-binding instrument of international law on 196 countries has an overarching legal framework that defines the countries' rights and obligations in handling public health events and emergencies with the potential to cross borders [24]. The IHR has criteria that help the global health community and countries define whether a public health event such as a disease outbreak or epidemic could be classified or need to be declared as a public health emergency of international concern (PHEIC). It also designates steps countries need to take to ensure public health preparedness and response including designating an IHR focal point, improving country disease surveillance capabilities, and safeguards to protect individuals and communities during travels in the event of a public health emergency. To ascertain the applicability of the IHR during pandemics, a panel of about 20 experts reviewed and ascertained the usefulness and appropriateness of the IHR tool [25]. It was noted that many countries did not deploy the full capabilities of the IHR tool as such the deficiencies noted were not those inherently within the tool but from limited application by countries during the COVID-19 pandemic. It is therefore crucial for countries to be sensitized and mechanisms to be put in place such that the full benefits of the IHR tool are harnessed in the event of any future public health event.

3.1 Vaccines deployed in public health emergencies

With most of the global health events being infectious diseases, vaccines have been and will continue to play a central role in both the preparedness and response for these emergencies. During the recent COVID-19 pandemic, many response initiatives were instituted to adapt existing global structures for pandemic preparedness and response and included proposals for a pandemic treaty, a pandemic fund, and mechanisms for ensuring equitable access to medical countermeasures such as the Access to COVID-19 Tools (ACT) Accelerator which includes COVAX which is the vaccines pillar of the ACT accelerator [26]. These interventions signify the agility of the global pandemic preparedness and response mechanisms, being tweaked to manage the prevailing public health emergency. A lot of lessons were learned which informed some reforms or reorganization of the global health pandemic preparedness and response architecture. Some of these reforms included setting up the COVID-19 vaccine delivery partnership (CoVDP) launched in December 2021 which has supported countries administering over 13 billion doses of COVID-19 vaccines to the most vulnerable and most-at-risk populations including the elderly, those with chronic underlying conditions and health workers. The COVAX mechanism was not without criticisms including the fact that COVAX could not reach half of its goal to distribute 2 billion doses to participating countries which were mostly from the global south by December 2021 [27].

MenAfriVac is another vaccine that has been very effective in controlling and eliminating the devastating epidemics of Meningitis caused by *Neisseria meningitides* type A, which happen over a cycle of a few years across countries in the Meningitis belt of Africa. Before the development of the MenAfriVac vaccine, several epidemics of the disease happened with one of the most severe one's ever recorded happened around 1996 to 1997 with over 250,000 cases and about 10% case fatality [28]. The incidence of cases has dropped significantly over the years with several of the countries not recording any cases in many years. Thanks to the Bill and Melinda Gates Foundation (BMGF) funded Meningitis Vaccine Project (MVP), several million susceptible people in sub-Saharan Africa were protected with the vaccine which resulted in population immunity. An impact analysis documented about a 57% decline in cases across several countries [28]. Furthermore, the appropriateness of the vaccine characteristics including being licensed for use at room temperature as a controlled temperature chain (CTC) vaccine has contributed immensely to achieving very high coverage and effectiveness [29]. This highlights the value of not only developing vaccines to combat epidemics and pandemics but also ensuring the use of the most appropriate technology in doing so.

Cholera is one of the oldest pandemic-prone diseases with several pandemics recorded over the last two centuries. It is a feco-oral disease which is characterized by watery diarrhea which may result in death without proper fluid and electrolyte replacements or management. The disease outbreak showed a spike in 2022 with more than 29 countries reporting outbreaks. Over 73 million doses of oral cholera vaccines (OCV) were shipped to several countries by the International Coordinating Group (ICG) – a body that coordinates and manages the stockpiles and supply of these vaccines during emergencies, since the stockpile was established. The vaccine is given as a two-dose regimen over 6 months. Due to global shortages, the ICG was able to recommend a single-dose regimen which was shown to be quite effective in an epidemic. The key point of note here is the flexibility of the dosing regimen to adapt to the emerging needs of the public health emergency.

While several epidemic and pandemic-prone diseases have vaccines developed, however, a key challenge for most of the global health events is the non-availability of vaccines at the onset as was the case more recently with Ebola viral disease (EVD), Zika, and the COVID-19 pandemic. Normally vaccines can take 5 to 10 years from conceptualization to pre-approval or approval ready for use. The bulk of the capacity, which goes with funding as well, for vaccine development and commercialization is mostly in the global north – Europe and the US, with some capacity seen in India and China. This lopsided resource positioning creates an unequal race to access vaccines which was typified by one of the worst vaccine-grabbing histories ever known to man manifested during the COVID-19 pandemic seen. This depicts the extant market failure that public goods could face if left in the open market for the strongest buyer to take. While rich countries accumulated so many vaccines, they ended up donating near-expiry vaccines to many poorer countries who already were grappling with numerous other challenges and were now being faced with the need to race vaccination of expiring vaccines with the limited resources they have. The case of EVD is different since the disease mostly affected countries with limited resources, such as racing to develop and license vaccines within about 6 months was not strongly demonstrated.

Nonetheless, vaccines have shown extraordinary effectiveness in the control of some of these pandemics and epidemics. Several infectious diseases outbreaks such as meningitis, measles, and cholera have in numerous instances been controlled with massive vaccination efforts. COVID-19 was no exception in getting the benefits of being controlled by vaccines. The rapidity of the vaccine development and pre-approval seen during the COVID-19 pandemic was unprecedented and worthy of commendation. However, the process of getting vaccines available within months as against the usual 5 or more years was rather hijacked and used as a weapon by the antivaccination conspiracy theorists to propagate misinformation with the sole aim of festering vaccination rejection and an overall decline in vaccine confidence, which occurred in part across countries. This misinformation propaganda was aided by the globalized world and easy access to information both verified and unverified. The challenge of declining vaccine confidence or hesitancy may keep growing ahead of the next pandemic, as such it is therefore important to keep this in mind and strategize as part of preparedness for the next epidemic or pandemic. It is thus very important to highlight that the whole required processes and steps from vaccine conceptualization to approval were observed but with speed, which made the vaccine products available at a much shorter time duration than usual.

3.2 Innovations

Newer technologies are being deployed in vaccine development to address public health emergencies such as the use of messenger Ribonucleic Acid (mRNA) deployed by pharmaceutical companies during the COVID-19 pandemic. The Meningitis Vaccine Project in the 2000s also developed a conjugate vaccine that was thermostable at room temperature for a few days facilitating seamless vaccine deployment to the remotest of areas in the Meningitis belt. At each moment, the global health community makes efforts to utilize the latest technology including innovating where necessary to develop and deploy effective vaccines for the epidemic or pandemic. mRNA vaccines could have applications beyond infectious diseases to include chronic illnesses like cancer. There is potential for vaccines developed as nasal sprays that will make pandemic prevention and response easier and more widespread. A huge obstacle for many vaccine deployments has been and continues to be the requirement for cold chain storage which if addressed could ease vaccination by improving vaccine reach and decreasing costs [29]. Investing in innovations and more appropriate technology for vaccines portends great benefits for the future of vaccine development with the same or even faster rapidity in the development and deployment of vaccines for public health emergencies as a scale.

4. What did we learn from the vaccination during public health emergencies?

Several vaccines have been and continue to be used during emergencies for either preventive or reactive campaigns including but not limited to COVID-19, meningitis,

Cholera, Ebola, and Measles. Over the years lessons have been learned that highlight the successes and challenges encountered as well as opportunities for improvements. These lessons have guided improvements in vaccination during emergencies and vaccinations overall for an improved outcome. Prior to the COVID-19 pandemic, millions of doses of OCV have been deployed through the ICG from the global stockpile of cholera vaccines set up since 2013 both proactively and reactively. Measles remains an epidemic-prone disease in several low- and middle-income countries, and often large-scale preventive and response vaccination campaigns are conducted with millions of doses every year. The Meningitis burden particularly across the meningitis belt has significantly declined thanks to the Meningitis vaccination campaigns which has been included as part of the routine immunization schedule of some countries. And finally, the Ebola viral diseases outbreak of 2014 to 2016 saw support countries and partners accelerating vaccine development and deployment to contain the disease [30].

Over 13 billion doses of the COVID-19 vaccine were deployed globally as of June 2023 using several vaccine types. These were delivered through the CoVDP or as direct purchases by High-Income Countries (HIC). Due to the priority of the pandemic as a public health emergency of international concern (PHEIC) coupled with the urgency and speed required to deliver the vaccines, nations used a variety of approaches including creating novel platforms often associated which very high political offices to using the routine immunization delivery platforms. This vaccine delivery came at a cost to the primary health care and routine immunization systems. Existing human and material resources for routine immunization and PHC systems were repurposed to not only deliver COVID-19 vaccines but to plan and implement the broader COVID-19 pandemic response. In some instances, parallel systems were established solely for the COVID-19 vaccination and will need to integrate the delivery into existing PHC and RI systems to have a more sustainable platform to continue the control of the virus. Guidelines have been developed to support country integration of COVID-19 initiatives [31].

4.1 Successes recorded

Through the various initiatives by governments, and bilateral and multilateral partners, there were numerous efforts to guarantee supply for low- and middle-income countries (LMIC). To effectively assess the situation is to look at the counterfactual of the non-existence of such initiatives such as the COVAX in aiding country access to COVID-19 vaccines in a timely and affordable manner; the OCV stockpile in containing cholera outbreaks through the ICG or even the traditional measles vaccines to prevent and respond to outbreaks. While the targets and aspirations of the initiatives may not have been fully achieved, credit should be given to the different initiatives and the additional lives that were saved by the little gesture. The Meningitis Vaccine Project funded by the BMGF supported the development and rollout of MenAfriVac which has resulted in the near elimination of Neisseria meningitis in some countries with a significant decline in outbreak frequency and disease mortality across the meningitis belt [28]. The International Coordinating Group (ICG) was established to manage the stockpiles of Oral Cholera Vaccines during emergencies and has been successful in rationing the OCV stockpile, especially during cholera epidemics or pandemics [30]. The pandemic treaty is an intergovernmental negotiating body created by a special session of the World health assembly in late 2021 with the core of it being the equitable sharing of lifesaving medical resources to support health emergency preparedness, response, and resilience [27]. Furthermore, the COVAX humanitarian buffer is an initiative that provides a safety net for the most vulnerable populations including displaced and conflict-affected persons.

There was enhanced global, regional, and even national coordination for improved vaccination delivery across the different vaccines. Several inter and intra-agency working groups were set up at all levels where governments and partners came together to strategize, prepare, and discuss an equitable model of vaccine allocation and delivery. This often brings a heightened awareness and involvement of the top political leadership on vaccination, more seen during the COVID-19 pandemic. This is an opportunity that could be leveraged for strengthening routine immunization and PHC.

Acceleration of the pace of vaccine development was leveraged during the EVD and even enhanced during the COVID-19 pandemic. With the precedence set, vaccines for responding to public health emergencies could be developed within weeks and deployed to help in controlling the situation. Furthermore, innovations seen during the MenAfriVac, Ebola, and even COVID-19 vaccines have shown a progressive advancement in vaccine technology. But we also learn from measles vaccines that traditional vaccines do have a role to play in epidemic and pandemic disease management.

COVID-19 vaccination brought to foe several issues. The concepts of vaccine empathy and vaccine diplomacy became more pronounced recently. While vaccine empathy refers to an individual or a nation's capability to sympathize with other individuals or nations' vaccine wants and needs, vaccine diplomacy is a nation's vaccine efforts that aim to build mutually beneficial relationships with other nations [17]. Several LMIC countries receive donations of vaccines from high-income countries in an attempt to bridge the widened gap in access and utilization of COVID-19 vaccines which persists to date. **Figure 3** shows the COVID-19 immunity gaps from lower vaccination access and utilization in developing countries.

Some of the vaccines had a very short shelf life resulting in mass expiry of vaccines in the hands of poorer nations who now had to grapple with a double jeopardy scenario of scarcity amid plenty. Another attempt was the struggle with the transfer of vaccine manufacturing technology from Big Pharma in the richer countries to the developing economies. Several issues of intellectual property right came up. There is no way we can achieve an equitable and appropriate global health emergency control when tools

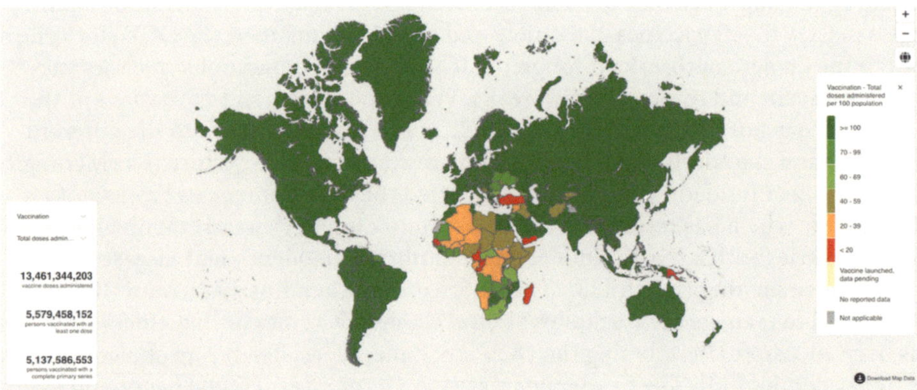

Figure 3.
COVID-19 vaccination coverage globally shows developing countries still lagging. This stark difference is driven largely by vaccine inequity. (Source: WHO COVID-19 dashboard.)

needed for effective preparedness and response are left solely to market forces without meaningful interventions. Some waivers of intellectual property rights and mutually beneficial technology transfer are needed to effectively manage any future emergency.

4.2 Challenges encountered

For most of the vaccines deployed for epidemic or pandemic mitigation and response, shortages were universal. This results in coordinating bodies reorganizing themselves to ensure vaccines are widely distributed as possible while providing the desired effectiveness. Vaccine shortages have been seen with cholera vaccines which resulted in a revision of the dosing regimen from 2 to 1 dose during an outbreak response to accommodate as many susceptible persons as possible. The shortages seen in the COVID-19 era were phenomenal where richer nations were seen to use their wealth and power in securing excess vaccines for their people with little or no consideration for the poorer countries until much later in the response.

The African Union set up a 10-member team in August 2020 known as the African Vaccine Acquisition Task Team (AVATT) chaired by The President of South Africa Cyril Ramaphosa. The AVATT's key aim was to ensure the continent secured sufficient COVID-19 vaccines to protect its close to a billion population. Cyril Ramaphosa is one of the notable persons from the continent who have been vocal on the COVID-19 vaccine allocation and manufacturing disparity. Using the terrible experiences from South Africa's long dark history of racial injustice, he refers to the vaccination injustice as a vaccine apartheid that must be ended.

"*Although the advent of coronavirus vaccines has broadened the frontiers of hope for a sustainable global recovery, the inequitable distribution of these vaccines means that the recovery will be uneven and, potentially, short-lived. If the world is to overcome the pandemic in 2022, it needs to end vaccine apartheid.*" – President Cyril Ramaphosa [32]. His words are loaded with wisdom and carry a strong but reassuring message to the world that for any global health security to be properly managed, equity and social justice in preparedness and response efforts are pivotal. Several discussions and negotiations ensued with many actors including the World Trade Organization, the WHO, and World Intellectual Property Organization finally securing a Trade-Related Aspects of Intellectual Property Rights (TRIPS) COVID-19 vaccines waiver in July 2022 to potentially cover COVID-19 diagnostics and therapeutics.

Recently in his remarks at the summit for a New Global Financial Pact in Paris, President Ramaphosa stated that there persists resentment towards the West due to the treatment meted on African and poorer nations during the pandemic response and he stated that African nations "felt like we were beggars when we needed access to vaccines.".

These are the consequences of one of the most historic vaccine grabbing ever witnessed by mankind where rich countries secured pre-manufactured vaccines in multiples of their population needs and requirements and dolled off the leftover with mostly short shelf life to poorer nations when these countries have achieved a certain level of control of the pandemic already. We must implement and not just vocalize concrete steps towards this vaccine equity and interventional appropriateness hearing the voices of all concerned before pushing the bitter pills down the throats of the marginalized.

Some of the key challenges summarized by Lal et al. included an over-reliance on global health security interventions at the expense of broader universal health coverage (UHC), gaps in mitigating socioeconomic factors and wider determinants of health, and the lack of inclusive and equitable engagement mechanisms in public health decision making [26].

5. Future approaches (recommendations and conclusions)

To better achieve vaccines and interventional equity and appropriateness for global health security, certain fundamental steps will need to be taken particularly with the many learnings from the COVID-19 pandemic response.

5.1 Governance, one and equal voices

The global health landscape was awash with numerous coordinating bodies and structures striving hard to make a difference building on experiences from previous public health events. No doubt this provided a platform, which some may argue as unequal, to allow for some meaningful engagements and discussions. The different initiatives set up including the COVAX, the pandemic fund, etc. were borne from these coordinating bodies where key issues related to ensuring an overall framework for global health security. At the global, regional, and national levels, some form of governance was instituted and played a key role in the pandemic response. It is important to leverage these structures and reposition them for preparedness starting now and not wait till the next global health threat. Progress is being made with setting up hubs such as the WHO Hub for Pandemic and Epidemic Intelligence. Are these bodies equitable in their decision-making arms? While LMICs should work on strengthening their institutional weaknesses to have more resilient systems, they must be given a seat and be heard during preparedness and response to ensure a healthier world for all. Keeping poorer nations as mere recipients of crumbs will not in any way better global health security but result in protracted crises.

5.2 Development and manufacturing of vaccines

The TRIPS waiver secured for the COVID-19 vaccines was a welcome development but came albeit late to transform the COVID-19 pandemic response, but will be a valuable tool for future public health threats. A clear framework and process to fasten the transfer of technology and waivers for intellectual property rights should be available and should be pre-approved at the inception of vaccine trials. LMICs should be carried along in the development stride for vaccines and tools for mitigating or managing global health threats. Equal participation in pre-clinical and clinical trials to ensure the appropriateness of an intervention finally certified for use. The Big pharma and rich nations who often invest in the Research & Development (R&D) of the pharmaceutical companies should take deliberate positive steps to fully transfer technology and support vaccine manufacture in LMICs. AstraZeneca was one company that made great progress in that area, and we can build on the successes so far. But also, LMICs must promote national policies and investments to support local R&D and be ready to share technology with rich countries as well. This is towards a mutually beneficial model which will see effective vaccine diplomacy for the overall global good.

5.3 Pre-approval and licensing

One of the weaknesses of LMICs is in the regulation and approval of medicinal products through their respective national regulatory authorities (NRA). Deliberate collaborations should be established between countries with well-developed NRAs and LMICs to ramp up capacity and support preparedness and response for future emergencies. The pre-approval and licensing of vaccines are managed through a robust process by the WHO. A means to socialize better the process and refining to mitigate issues related to countries pushing for vaccines to be released ahead of WHO pre-approval.

5.4 Procurement and distribution

Several developing countries do not have the resources or mechanisms for cost-effective procurement and distribution of vaccines. Mechanisms for supporting the pooling and procurement of vaccines for LMICs, a much-improved version of the COVAX and similar tools will be beneficial.

5.5 Sustainable initiatives

Responding to global health emergencies often requires extraordinary measures which may mean creating separate coordination structures and systems to battle the emergency and restore normalcy. Efforts should be made to leverage and strengthen existing systems by incorporating resilience in preparedness and response plans including conducting sustainability assessments where feasible. Scenario analysis and drills to prepare adequately for global health emergencies will be quite useful.

6. Conclusion

This chapter discussed the pivotal role of vaccines and interventional equity and appropriateness citing sources from the several vaccines deployed during public health emergencies including Oral cholera, Ebola, Meningitis, Measles, and the COVID-19 pandemic. Drivers of inequity in vaccine development, procurement, distribution, and use were discussed and suggestions were made. Several initiatives were discussed including the Meningitis Vaccine Project, the ICG for Cholera vaccines, the COVAX humanitarian buffer, vaccine apartheid, grabbing, etc. Finally, future approaches to guarantee global health security were summarized.

Conflict of interest

The authors declare no conflict of interest.

Author details

Ibrahim Khalil Dadari
United Nations Children's Fund, New York, USA

*Address all correspondence to: ibrahimddr@gmail.com

References

[1] Torres Munguía JA et al. A global dataset of pandemic-and epidemic-prone disease outbreaks. Scientific Data. 2022;**9**(1):683

[2] World Health Organization (WHO). WHO Coronavirus (COVID-19) Dashboard. n.d. Available from: https://covid19.who.int/ [Accessed: Feb 2023]

[3] WHO. Cholera – Global situation. 2022. Available from: https://www.who.int/emergencies/disease-outbreak-news/item/2022-DON426

[4] Sim SY et al. Return on investment from immunization against 10 pathogens in 94 low- and middle-income countries, 2011-30. Health Affairs (Millwood). 2020;**39**(8):1343-1353

[5] Ozawa S et al. Return on investment from childhood immunization In low- and middle-income countries, 2011-20. Health Affairs (Millwood). 2016;**35**(2):199-207

[6] Bonanni P, Picazo JJ, Rémy V. The intangible benefits of vaccination – What is the true economic value of vaccination? Journal of Market Access & Health Policy. 2015;**3**(1):26964

[7] Okwo-Bele J-M, Cherian T. The expanded programme on immunization: A lasting legacy of smallpox eradication. Vaccine. 2011;**29**:D74-D79

[8] Whitney CG et al. Benefits from immunization during the vaccines for children program era - United States, 1994-2013. Morbidity and Mortality Weekly Report. 2014;**63**(16):352-355

[9] Sinnis P, Fidock DA. The RTS, S vaccine—A chance to regain the upper hand against malaria? Cell. 2022;**185**(5):750-754

[10] Woolsey C, Geisbert TW. Current state of Ebola virus vaccines: A snapshot. PLoS Pathogens. 2021;**17**(12):e1010078

[11] Doroshenko A. The combined effect of vaccination and nonpharmaceutical public health interventions—Ending the COVID-19 pandemic. JAMA Network Open. 2021;**4**(6):e2111675-e2111675

[12] World Health Organization (WHO). Regulation and Prequalification. 2023. Available from: https://www.who.int/teams/regulation-prequalification/eul/covid-19

[13] World Health Organization (WHO). Adverse Events Following Immunization (AEFI). n.d. Available from: https://www.who.int/teams/regulation-prequalification/regulation-and-safety/pharmacovigilance/guidance/aefi

[14] World Health Organization. Social Determinants of Health: Key Concepts. 2013. Available from: https://www.who.int/news-room/q-a-detail/social-determinants-of-health-key-concepts [Accessed: November 2021]

[15] World Health Organization. Implementing the Immunization Agenda 2030. 2021. Available from: https://www.who.int/publications/m/item/implementing-the-immunization-agenda-2030 [Accessed: January 7, 2021]

[16] Zajączkowski K. European Union initiatives supporting Sub-Saharan Countries in combating the covid-19 pandemic. In: The EU Towards the Global South During the COVID-19 Pandemic. Bern: Peter Lang International Academic Publishers; 2022. p. 55

[17] Su Z et al. COVID-19 vaccine donations—Vaccine empathy or vaccine

diplomacy? A narrative literature review. Vaccine. 2021;**9**(9):1024

[18] Centers for Disease Control and Prevention [CDC]. What is Global Health Security? 2022

[19] National Institute of Allergy and Infectious Diseases (NIAID). NIAID Emerging Infectious Diseases/ Pathogens. 26 July 2018. Available from: https://www.niaid.nih.gov/research/ emerging-infectious-diseases-pathogens

[20] Oshitani H. Globalization and emerging infectious diseases. Nihon Rinsho. Japanese Journal of Clinical Medicine. 2016;**74**(12):1956-1961

[21] Murray CJ et al. Global burden of bacterial antimicrobial resistance in 2019: A systematic analysis. The Lancet. 2022;**399**(10325):629-655

[22] Manheim D, Lewis G. High-risk human-caused pathogen exposure events from 1975-2016. F1000Research. 2021;**10**:752. DOI: 10.12688/ f1000research.55114.2

[23] National Academies of Sciences, Engineering, and Medicine. Examining Challenges and Possible Strategies to Strengthen U.S. Health Security: Proceedings of a Workshop. Washington, DC: The National Academies Press; 2018. DOI: 10.17226/24856

[24] World Health Organization (WHO). International Health Regulations (2005). 3rd ed. Geneva: WHO; 2016

[25] Aavitsland P et al. Functioning of the international health regulations during the COVID-19 pandemic. Lancet. 2021;**398**(10308):1283-1287

[26] Lal A et al. Pandemic preparedness and response: Exploring the role of universal health coverage within the global health security architecture. The Lancet Global Health. 2022;**10**(11):e1675-e1683

[27] Gostin LO. A new architecture for Global Health emergency preparedness and response—The imperative of equity. JAMA Health Forum. 2022;**3**(6):e222197-e222197

[28] Trotter CL et al. Impact of MenAfriVac in nine countries of the African meningitis belt, 2010-15: An analysis of surveillance data. The Lancet Infectious Diseases. 2017;**17**(8):867-872

[29] Dadari IK, Zgibor JC. How the use of vaccines outside the cold chain or in controlled temperature chain contributes to improving immunization coverage in low- and middle-income countries (LMICs): A scoping review of the literature. Journal of Global Health. 2021;**11**:04004

[30] Walldorf JA et al. Lessons learned from emergency response vaccination efforts for cholera, typhoid, yellow fever, and Ebola. Emerging Infectious Diseases. 2017;**23**(13):S210-S216

[31] WHO-UNICEF. Considerations for Integrating COVID-19 Vaccination into Immunization Programmes and Primary Health Care for 2022 and Beyond. Geneva: WHO; 2022. Available from: https://www.who.int/publications/i/ item/9789240064454

[32] The Econonomist. Cyril Ramaphosa Says the World Must End Vaccine Apartheid. New York: The Economist Newspaper Limited; 2021

Chapter 4

Perspective Chapter: Armed Conflict and Its Impact on Human Migration – The Healthcare Perspective

Julius Kenkoh Nkiese and Stephanie Kininla Wirba

Abstract

Armed conflict can result in loss of human life, displace people, and violate human rights. While human migration often results from various causes like the search for food and shelter, armed conflicts also cause migration. Most armed conflicts stem from bad governance and religious radicalism. With bad governance, revendication from the marginalised often results in severe opposite repression from the state instead of dialogue. Migration from armed conflict imposes a disproportionate distribution of the population with the displaced lodged in camps thanks to some United Nations (UN) agencies like the High Commissioner for Refugees (UNHCR), the World Food Program (WFP), the UN Population Fund (UNFPA), and the United Nation Children's Emergency Fund (UNICEF), in the areas of food provision, shelter, and medical care to the displaced and affected populations. Refugee camps can become an epicentre for diseases outbreaks like Tuberculosis, childhood diarrhoea, cholera, and HIV. Health workers are caught in the web, being attacked by armed groups, taking care of the wounded, while caring for themselves as well. It is important to address the major causes of armed conflict if we truly want to attain Universal Health Coverage, maintain a peaceful world, and achieve the Sustainable Development Goals by 2030.

Keywords: armed conflict, refugee, human migration, sustainable development goals, universal health coverage

1. Introduction

Armed conflicts have become preponderant in the world today. Almost every continent of the world has an epicentre of armed conflicts. Over 110 armed conflicts exist in the world over, with some having lasted as much as 50 years [1]. While some continents may have multicentric armed conflict zones, others have just occasional clashes that may occur sporadically between groups of varying opinion and ethnicity. Some of the armed conflict areas around the world include, but are not limited to Ukraine, Iran, Yemen, Ethiopia, Democratic Republic of Congo (DRC), The Sahel Region

(Islamic Insurgencies), Haiti, Pakistan, and a probable armed conflict in Taiwan if care is not taken [2]. North Africa and the Middle East appear to be the most affected of all the world continents, while Australia appears to be the most peaceful. **Figure 1** below illustrates the conflict hotspots on the globe.

From **Figure 1**, we observe a preponderance of armed conflicts in Northern Africa, the Middle East, South-East Asia, and the Northern part of South America. Of note is especially conflicts that claim more than 10,000 lives in conflict-related deaths. The question remains: why is there such a rapid proliferation of armed conflicts in these areas? This is probably attributable to the persistent susceptibility to armed conflicts in these areas due to governance failures in most Arab countries, the still unfolding consequences of the 2003 US-led Iraq invasion, and the complex relations and rivalries among regional powers [3].

The real impact of armed conflicts on each continent is diverse and depends on a couple of factors. One of the latest conflicts, which is affecting almost the entire globe is the Russo-Ukrainian war, whose impact on each region varies. The impact of this war on the African continent is derailing its slow recovery from the COVID-19, bringing diverse effects on the economy [4]. Armed conflicts in Africa have moved from focusing on the autonomy of the states (pre-independence) to that of the struggle to control political power post-independence [5], thus practically stagnating, and in some cases, pushing the economy to like 10 to 15 years pre-conflict.

In Asia, especially Southeast Asia, and Europe, the Russo-Ukrainian war threatens the balance of power and peace in the European Union (EU), thus endangering the peace in Europe that has reigned post World War II [6], with resultant rises in prices in the global south, and destabilising their economic and fiscal conditions. Most countries are struggling to meet their energy requirements. Ghimire, underscores the

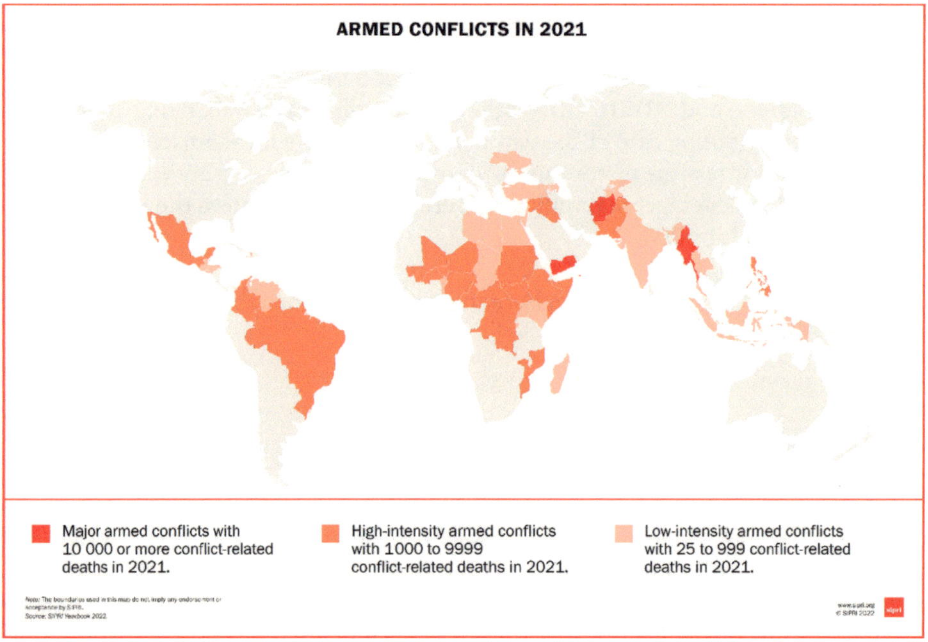

Figure 1.
Armed Conflict Hotspots, 2021. Source; SIPRI Year Book 2022.

prediction from the world bank that 60% of the poorest countries were already in debt distress or at high risk because of the global pandemic, and the Russo-Ukrainian war has compounded the distress due their dependence on 3F imports (Food, Fuel and Fertilisers). Therefore, armed conflicts have a detrimental effect on the economic and social wellbeing of people [7], indicating that the economy proves to be a more decisive factor than others in predicting the incidence and demonstrating the aftermath of armed conflicts.

2. Definition of terms

2.1 Armed conflicts

Armed conflicts are defined as political conflicts where the use of armed force by two parties of which at least one is the Government of a State results in at least 25 battle-related deaths [8]. A 'major armed conflict' is a contested incompatibility concerning government and/or territory over which the use of armed forces between the military forces of two parties of which at least one is the government of a state results in at least 1000 deaths in the course of the conflict in a single calendar year [9].

Two categories of armed conflict are identified: international armed conflicts (IAC) occurring between two or more States; and non-international armed conflicts (NIAC) which occur between State and non-governmental armed groups, or only between armed groups [8].

Summarily, according to the International Committee of the Red Cross [10] the following must apply for a situation to be considered and "armed conflict" under humanitarian low:

1. The armed groups have a level of organisation that enables them to carry out military operations (i.e., conduct hostilities).

2. Those groups have the capacity to maintain protracted operations.

3. The armed clashes are of a military nature.

4. The armed clashes are between the government's armed forces and organised armed groups, or between organised armed groups.

5. The armed clashes occur within the territory of a State.

The above definition does not take into consideration armed conflicts that arise between ethnic groups within a country, though the causes may be similar to those of armed conflicts as defined above. Besides, the death tool used above to define armed conflicts ignores deaths less than 25. To determine the exact death toll during conflict is rendered complex by the fact that a qualified medical practitioner seldom certifies death [11]. One limitation, however, to the above definition, is that the actual conflict-related death toll could be much more different, especially in areas where the nature of the conflict makes it difficult to determine such figures, like burial in mass graves. No matter the number of deaths registered, every human life is valuable, and must be protected. Any conflict that results in death violates the fundamental human right to life [12] and by extension, deprives the affected from food, education, work, health, and liberty.

2.2 Refugees

Refugees are people who have fled war, violence, conflict, or persecution, and have crossed international boundaries to find safety in another country [13]. Internally Displaced Persons (IDPs), on the other hand refers to people who have been forced to flee their home or places of habitual residence, as a result of, or in order to avoid the effects of armed conflicts, situations of generalised violence, violations of human rights, or natural home-made disasters, and who have not crossed an internationally recognised border [14].

2.3 Human migration

The Encyclopaedia Britannica defines Human Migration as the permanent change of residence by an individual or group; it excludes such movements as nomadism, migrant labour, commuting, and tourism, all of which are transitory in nature [15]. According to National Geographic, on the other hand, Migration is defined as "movement from one country, place, or locality to another [16], not necessarily on a permanent basis. We shall adopt this second definition for the purpose of this work.

2.4 Some hotspots of armed conflicts

We will now highlight some armed conflict areas in the world. The ones elaborated below are not exhaustive of all armed conflict spots but intends to establish the effects that armed conflicts have on human migration especially from the healthcare perspective.

2.5 The crisis in Central African Republic (CAR)

Since the CAR gained independence in 1960, decades of violence and instability have characterised this country [17]. The debut of the current armed conflicts dates as far back as 2013 when the Séléka Rebel coalition seized power from the then president Bozizé. In response, self-defence groups emerged with the prominent one being the Anti-Balaka group. From then till date, different armed groups and warlords now control different communities in the republic. The conflicts have been demarcated along religious lines, since the coalition of armed Muslim groups had Christians as their major target, an act which equally led to the coalition of Christian fighters to repress the advances of the Séléka coalition.

Though the conflict degenerated, religious leaders, who have strong ties to Central Africans throughout the republic can influence their faithful and mediate for peace, though the extent of their influence can fluctuate significantly [18]. Local religious leaders are on the frontlines in a different way, they live among CAR's armed groups. Collins further argues that from this position they play a careful, often overlooked, but ongoing role in managing CAR's increasingly local patchwork of conflicts, as main mediators and parties to local peace and stabilisation processes. However, the religious leaders are being accused by the government of collaborating with the armed groups in their mediation process.

The Central African Republic conflict has permeated every facet of society leading to Schools closure. Central Africans have been forced to flee their homes. A shortage of skilled health workers and medical supplies mean the health care system in Central African Republic is barely functioning. Besides, attacks against medical facilities, attacks on patients and ambulances threaten what little health care is available [19]. The humanitarian consequences of this armed conflict are lawlessness has become the order of the day throughout the country, while the population has flown to other countries as refugees in Cameroon, Sudan, DRC, Tchad, Congo, and South Sudan [20].

2.6 Crises in The Cameroon

Cameroon is plagued within the last 10 years with multicentric (tripartite) crises: the Boko Haram insurgencies in Northern Cameroon since 2014, especially around the Lake Tchad Basin [21], the Anglophone Crisis since 2016, and pressure in the eastern region in relation to the displacement and vulnerability of refugees from the Central African Republic (CAR) [22].

2.6.1 Refugee crisis in the East Region of Cameroon

The war in CAR activated an influx of refugees fleeing to zones of perceived safety. These refugees are civilians fleeing violence and abuses from the fighting men. The surge in refugee influx happened in 2014 following escalation of the violence in CAR [22]. The result was a triggering of a humanitarian crisis in the East regions of Cameroon which houses about 270,000 refugees as of 2020, a figure that rose to almost 500,000 by November 2022 [23].

With this growing refugee population, hunger continues to be a problem as more and more people are uprooted in CAR to relocate neighbouring countries, thus competing for the meagre economic resources in these countries. More than one in three refugee children under the age of 5 suffers chronic malnutrition. Meanwhile, funding to support humanitarian activities has declined significantly. In 2019, the world food program (WFP) was forced to cut its cash assistance by half. By November they had stopped altogether [24].

2.6.2 The Boko Haram Insurgency in Northern Cameroon

The Islamic sect Boko Haram, which began its remote operations in North-eastern Nigeria as far back as 2002 manifested more brutal activities by 2009 following the extrajudicial killing of its founding leader Mohamed Yusuf. Its operations became more pronounced and widespread in 2014 under the leadership of Abubakar Shekau, and spread over to Cameroon, Tchad, and Niger [25]. The group is suspected of having possible links with Al-Qaeda. As of 2015, Boko Haram's activities became more concentrated around the Lake Tchad basin. As a result, the Multinational Joint Task Force (MNJTF), that has been dormant for some time was reactivated in this same year to contain the activities of this sect [25]. Violence, abduction, and child suicide have been their major modus operandi, with significant violations of human rights. All their success is thanks to them being able to smuggle weapons and supplies across the borders, as well as recruitment of child soldiers.

The Boko Haram crisis' impact on Cameroon is compounded by Intercommunal clashes that erupted in Cameroon's Far North region in December 2021, leaving over 50 dead and driving at least 100,000 people from their homes, although the actual numbers may be much higher [26]. It is possible that people who fled the intercommunal violence fell into the dragnets of the dangerous sect. This crisis has disrupted almost every facet of the society, with healthcare facilities suffering at sometimes as the target of their attacks. Consequently, some health workers have fled the area [27], and any attempt to move health commodities to this area has been frustrated by their attacks.

2.6.3 The crisis in the North-West and South-West Regions of Cameroon

The anglophone regions of Cameroon – the North-West and South-West Regions – make up approximately 20% of the population of Cameron, but just about 9.2% of its surface area, yet these two regions play a pivotal role in Cameroon's Economy especially in agriculture and Oil industries [28].

In October 2016, teachers trade union and lawyers mobilised in a peaceful protest and presented a couple of grievances against the government. These grievances can be summarised as bad governance and marginalisation of the English-speaking Cameroonians, especially within the legal and educational systems. The challenges included, *inter alia*, the mandatory use of the French language in schools and law courts in the English-speaking regions [29], and the gradual depletion of the Anglo-Saxon culture. Failure by the Government to address the concerns attracted political activists. The activists attempted to address the concern of bad governance and the continual marginalisation of the English-Speaking population of Cameroon from the time Cameroon gained independence in January 1960. Contrary to normal expectation, the government responded harshly: the executive arm of the government resorted to issuing decrees banning even peaceful protest, and a resultant crackdown on the peaceful, armless protesters by the security forces [29] that resulted in the imprisonment of the protest leaders. This wrongful response from the government gave rise, in 2018, to armed secessionists demanding the independence of the English-Speaking Cameroons to a sovereign state.

Consequently, countless, violent armed confrontations have been recorded between the Cameroon security forces and the secessionist groups [30]. The different secessionist groups are dispersed throughout the anglophone regions, controlling different parts of the region. However, their activities are not coordinated locally, apart from the attempted coordination from the diaspora, which again brings different groups at loggerheads. The exigencies of one group are the direct opposite of the other. It therefore becomes difficult, at moment, to know who to dialogue with (even if the government was to consider this option), considering the major leaders of the movement were thrown into gaol and have, since then been held *incommunicado*. Worse still, most of the gaoled individuals were tried before military courts — in violation of international human rights law — and sentenced under the country's repressive 2014 anti-terror law [31].

The promise of a special status to the English-Speaking part of Cameroon in the "pseudo" national dialogue held in 2019 seem to have only fuelled the conflict [30]. With the persistence of the conflict, over 6000 people have been killed (though this figure could be grossly underestimated because the regions are largely inaccessible for accurate data collection [32]), while 86,000 (men, women, and children) currently live in south-eastern Nigeria [33] as refugees, being supported by the government together with the UN Refugee Agency. Others have fled to the French-Speaking region as IDPs.

The consequences of the above crises are devastating. People die at home because it is impossible to take them to any nearby health facility as roads are blocked with very heavy logs of wood; healthcare workers are caught in the web between treating wounded military (and receiving torture from separatist fighters who accuse them of collaborating with the military) and treating wounded separatist fighters (and receiving torture from the military and accusations for collaborating with the armed group). Both sides have committed regular humanitarian violations [34] during security operations. These range from rape, torture, and killings of both the young and the old not directly involved in the conflict.

Children have been deprived of the right to education for over 7 years, teachers have gone jobless for years and have had to resort to other means to earn a living, businesses have closed down, while others that attempt to continue to thrive are faced with two major challenges: exceedingly low returns, and increased expenditure due to the exigencies from the armed groups to get their services financed by the population. Transportation has quadrupled in almost all areas of the Northwest and Southwest regions, and movement is subject to multiple controls both from the Government forces and the separatist fighters.

2.7 The conflict in Somalia

Somalis are a unique community in Africa. Different from the reality in most countries, the Somalians are nearly a homogenous ethnicity [35]. The Somali people have suffered oppression and violence for prolonged periods. Interestingly and paradoxically, the violence has been from fellow Somalis, who are almost of same ethnicity. The suffering dates to the democratic, post-independence era until the military regime in 1969. According to the World Bank report, clannism and clan cleavages are a source of conflict [36]. This led to the division of Somalis, and as a result fuelled endemic clashes over resources and power, as well as mobilising militia, thus rendering broad-based reconciliation very difficult to achieve. Elmi & Barise establish that the war has multiple and complex causes that span through the political, economic, cultural, and psychological landscapes. Again, bad governance appears to play a pivotal role both in the debut and continuity of the war in Somalia, plunging the country into a very complicated situation.

Somalia, after over 2 decades of internal conflicts started re-emerging as of 2013 slowly but steadily [37]. The conflict caused over a million Somalis to migrate and became refugees in neighbouring countries with another one million internally displaced [38]. This migration did not just commence because of the war, but the aftermath of the war drastically changed the level and extent of migration in this country. The minority groups, which were initially isolated and immobile became exposed to significant levels of discrimination and marginalisation from the majority groups ethnicities; this resulted in impunity and significant suppression of these minority groups ethnicities, with the result being that the minority groups were almost completely expelled from the country.

Years of conflict, natural disasters, famine, and insecurity, all have contributed to very low scores for most humanitarian indicators. Despite high mortality caused by civil war and famine, Somalia's population is growing rapidly due to a high fertility rate [39]. This rapid population growth puts a strain on the country's poor health care and social services. About 60% of Somalia's population is younger than 25 years. These were born during the civil war, and periods of conflict have almost become a norm to them. These adverse childhood experience bring about a high prevalence of long-term health effects in adulthood. In all, Somalia's health system has been weakened by decades of conflict and recurring natural disasters, with no comprehensive Health Information Management System (HIMS) capable of electronically collecting and sharing information from community to national level [40].

2.8 The Russo-Ukrainian conflict

The Russo-Ukrainian conflict is a culmination of a tug-of-war between two camps in Europe, and deterioration of bilateral relations between Russia and Ukraine since 2014 [41]. Cheng underscores the fact that Ukraine's membership to the North Atlantic Treaty Organisation (NATO), the territorial status of Crimea and the independence of Eastern Ukraine, and security interests in Russia are the three forces that contributed to and fuel the continuity of the current war with Ukraine as the Epicentre.

After the collapse of the Soviet Union, post-Soviet states have achieved *"quasi"* independence, that caused them to be closely associated with Russia. This has been the case because Russia used comprehensive sanctions against the newly independent states which relied on Russia to export their products or import energy and other inputs [42] Thus, a Russian federation with resultant re-emergence of the Soviet Union was judged highly plausible. The United States and NATO engaged in forging closer ties with post-Soviet states to limit Russia's influence and control over these states [41]. These closer ties have evidently excluded Russia. NATO's expansion Eastwards formed a semi-circle with Russia at the centre, thus increasing NATO's membership from 16 to 30 states. Ukraine sought membership to NATO in 2014, in the wake of the Crimea rises, a request that was formalised in 2020. This Eastwards expansion of NATO has exerted military, political, economic, and cultural pressure on Russia [41].

Russia is one of the world's leading self-sufficient countries in natural resources, natural gas, crude oil, iron, apatite, gold, wheat, and a couple of others. Therefore, all the economic sanctions imposed on Russia could not bring Russia to its knees [41]. There is significant energy dependence on Russia by the EU [43], any sanctions imposed on Russia almost always result in a direct negative impact of the EU member states, with the International Monetary Fund believing Russia's economy could even grow by 0.7% in 2023.

The Russo-Ukraine war began on February 24, 2022, when the Russian President Vladimir Putin announced a 'special' military operation, claiming to protect people (the autonomous republic or Crimea) who have been subject to genocide for 8 years [44]. He attempted to take over the Ukrainian capital city of Kyiv [45], an attack that was countered by the Ukrainian forces. The fighting has continued till date with heavy losses in human life, reducing many key cities to ruins, and redressing the economic situation of Ukraine a couple of years back. A report from Office of the United Nations High Commissioner for Refugees, published by Statista, states that the estimated number of civilian casualties as of May 2023 is about 8900, a figure that could likely be less than the reality, with over 15,100 injured [46].

2.8.1 Conflict-related deaths in Ukraine from 2014 to 2021, the link with Crimea

The real figure of conflict-related deaths dates to 2014 when Russia annexed Crimea, and this sparked military conflicts between the Ukraine Government and Separatist fighters supported by the Government of Russia in Donetsk and Luhansk. Therefore, OHCHR estimates that between 14,200 and 14,400 people were killed from April 2014 to December 2021. This figure includes civilians and military personnel [46].

2.8.2 Migration in relation to the Russo-Ukrainian Conflict

From February 2022 till May 2023 the Organisation for Economic Cooperation and Development (OECD)reports that over 5.3 million Ukrainian refugees are spread over neighbouring European countries, majority of whom are housed by Poland [47]. From a population of over 43 million inhabitants as of 2021 [48], this figure reveals that close to 12% of the country's population has fled to neighbouring countries as refugees, with obvious economic impact on the countries harbouring the refugees, especially Poland.

The effect on the health system is devastating. Russia has bombed civilian residences and infrastructure such as power plants. It is not clear if health infrastructure has been targeted, but Lancet magazine claims it is becoming increasingly clear, a key characteristic of Russia's strategy has been attempts to destroy the health system, seriously undermining the Ukrainian people's right to health [49].

2.9 Armed conflict in Afghanistan

Afghanistan has been a conflict zone since 2001 when the United States and allied forces invaded the country, quickly ousting the Taliban regime. This was following their refusal to hand over terrorist leader Osama Bin Laden after the 09/11 attack on the world trade centre [50]. The conflict, which has been largely between the Government forces and Taliban forces continued till 2014 when the US-led coalition formally ended its combat mission in 2014 [51]. Then, the Afghan National Defence and Security forces (ANDSF) have been in charge of Afghan's Security.

However, the Taliban continue to perpetrate attacks on civilian populations with suicide attacks in major cities, and attacks carried out on rural districts. With these continuous attacks on the civilian populations, the United Nations Assistance Mission in Afghanistan (UNAMA) documented almost 11,000 civilian casualties in 2018 [52]. These continuous attacks resulted in complete takeover of the country in August 2021 by the Taliban. With total takeover of the country by Taliban, and their close ties with al-Qaeda, Afghanistan has literally been transformed into a terrorist haven [53]. **Figure 2** is another illustration of the conflict hotspots, indicating their concentration around North Africa and the Middle East where Afghanistan is located.

2.9.1 Afghanistan Refugee crisis

According to the UNHCR [33], an estimated 24 million Afghans are in need of humanitarian assistance. Over 6 million were forcibly displaced from their homes by the end of 2021, with 2.7 million hosted as refugees, accounting for the highest protracted refugee situation in the world. Most Afghan refugees fled to neighbouring Iran and Pakistan 80% of whom are women and children.

The effect of the Afghan war on healthcare are devastating. *The war-torn South Asian country faces an additional issue of funding as it struggles to build its healthcare system.* In this effort to rebuild the health system, there is continual spending on war. This is why, in a recent address to Afghanistan's healthcare providers, Chief Executive Abdullah Abdullah said, "With what we spend on a single day of war, we could build a state-of-the-art hospital [54]." Thus, while spending on war, Afghanistan is in need of funding for its healthcare system. To make matters worse, Health facilities in Afghanistan have come under attack from armed groups [54]. According to the World Health Organisation, there were 34 reported attacks on healthcare facilities in the first quarter of 2019, killing at least nine workers and patients and causing the closure of at least 87 medical facilities. These attacks have been recurrent over the years [55] and on civilians hors de combat.

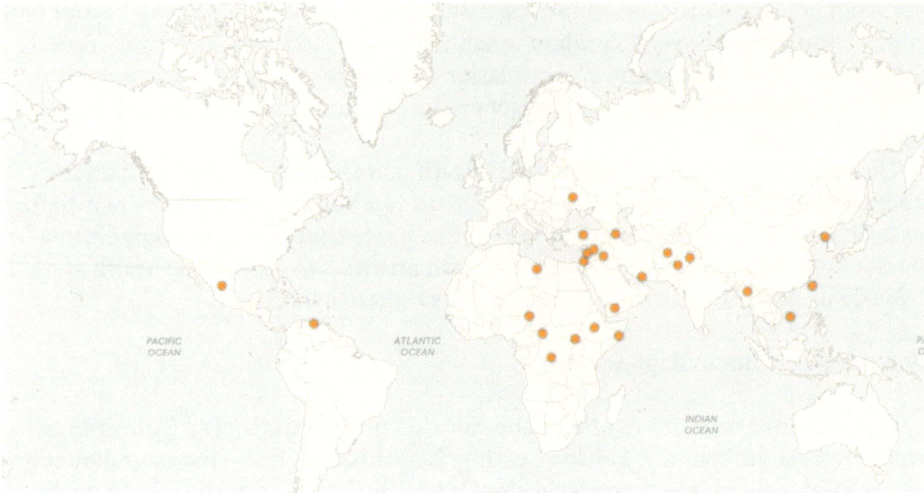

Figure 2.
Conflict spots in the world. Source: Global Conflict Tracker (https://www.cfr.org/global-conflict-tracker).

2.10 Crises in Venezuela

Venezuela is a petrostate [51], with the largest oil reserves in the world [56]. After the death of Hugo Chavez in 2013, Maduro, the Vice President took over interim position as president, and was subsequently elected to office. Because the country was in a state of economic crisis (from corruption in the reign of his predecessor), all his attempts to reverse the situation were futile, resulting in a full-blown crisis in 2015. Though not being an armed conflict per se, according to the definition mentioned earlier, the International Organisation for Migration (IOM) estimates that these crises have generated an estimated 6.1 million Venezuelans fleeing the country to neighbouring Latin America the Caribbean and Columbia [57]. The number of refugees and asylum seekers outnumber the absorption capacity of these neighbouring countries.

Though already out of the headlines, the health effect of the political and economic crisis is devastating. Available evidence shows a health system near collapse and the reversal of several decades of health gains [58]. Food and medication shortages, and the spread of infectious diseases plunged the country's health system to a chaos.

2.11 Non-international armed conflict in Yemen

The conflict in Yemen is in multiple fronts. First, there has been a longstanding conflict between the Houthis and government forces to the extent that in 2015, the Houthis took control of Yemen's capital. This forced the President Abdrabbuh Mansour Hadi to flee from the country but invited an international coalition led by Saudi Arabia, which successfully forced the Houthis out of the capital city. Since then, waves of violence have rocked the country leading to significant human losses and some cities reduced to ruins [59].

The Government is faced with yet another adversary, al-Qaeda in the Arabian Peninsula. The al-Qaeda and Houthis formed a coalition, which did not last too long due to conflicts of interest, that resulted in them fighting each other.

Besides, the Southern Transitional Council (STC) is calling for separation between the North and South of Yemen, a call which plunged the country again deeper in the already existent armed conflict [60].

About 14% of the population has been forced to flee their homes because of the crises, 75% of whom are women and children. The internally displaced live in dangerous locations characterised by food insecurity and lack of basic services, including healthcare services. According to UN Office for the Coordination of Humanitarian Affairs (OCHA), a devastated health system, disruption of water and sanitation networks, and massive numbers of displaced people have fuelled the rapid spread of diseases including cholera, diphtheria, measles, polio, and dengue [61].

2.12 The war in South Sudan

South Sudan voted to secede from Sudan in January 2011 and became a sovereign state on July 09th of the same year [62]. However, just above 2 years after its independence, a civil war emanated and frustrated most of the plans of this new and hopefully emerging country [62]. Government forces of President Salva Kir faced sudden opposition from Sudan People's Liberation Army in Opposition (SPLA-IO). This resulted in 2020 to the formation of the Revitalised Transition Government of National Unity (RTGoNU) [63]. With members of the warring parties in the new government, fighting has reduced significantly, but has not come to a halt because the peace deal and the government of national unity seemed to address symptoms, and not the root cause of the conflict [62]. As the country enters the extended 24 months of the Transitional Period, the spirit of forgiveness among the leadership of the RTGoNU is required [63].

According to Amnesty International, via its regional director for east and southern Africa [64], the cause and continuity of the armed conflict is due to ethno-political wrangling and competition among the elites over access to power and financial resources, with the mentality behind the fight that "the winner takes it all". However, in 2022, the latest cycle of violent confrontations arose, driven mainly by ferocity of national political competition, abetted by impunity from past human rights violations [65].

The USA UNHCR announced that more than 4.3 million people are in need of humanitarian assistance from South Sudan, including refugees, IDPs and asylum seekers [66]. South Sudan records the highest refugee crisis in Africa, with over 63% being under 18 most of whom are travelling alone. The women who are fleeing are survivors of violent attack and sexual assault.

The health effects of the conflict are devastating. Many weapon-wounded patients are received in the hospitals, having been air-lifted from the conflict zones that were rather hard-to-reach [67]. Sexual and gender-based violence (SGBV) has been used as a weapon of conflict, with systematic ethnically and politically motivated attacks [68]. Across the country, people have been subject to destruction, displacement, disease, and death. Violence disrupts access to healthcare, including routine vaccination, while increasing the risk of disease transmission and food insecurity, reports OCHA Services.

2.13 Overall

In all, armed conflicts have claimed millions of lives with the highest death toll recorded in armed conflict between states, followed by armed conflicts with foreign state intervention. Though the death toll from armed conflicts diminishes over the years post World War II, the figures are not negligible [69]. Quoting from Uppsala Conflict Database Program / Peace Research Institute Oslo, Roser presents the millions of lives lost so far. This is illustrated in **Figure 3** below in the average number of deaths per conflict since 1946, by type.

Contrary to the diminishing number of deaths from armed conflicts post World War II, state-based conflicts have increased drastically, claiming more lives as illustrated in **Figure 4**.

2.14 The effect of armed conflicts on human migration

Traditionally, man is a migratory being. Man moves from place to place ever since the prehistoric era in search of food and shelter. In an otherwise calm environment, the major reasons for human migration tend to shift significantly to favour the search

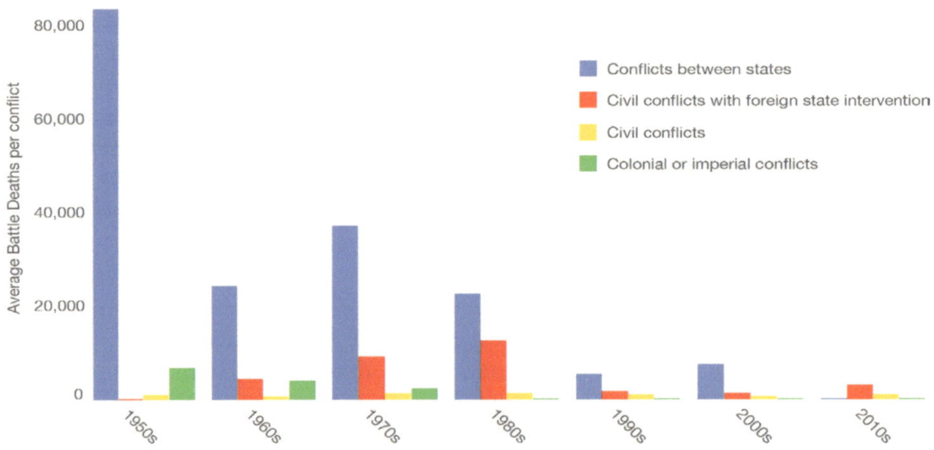

Figure 3.
Average deaths by conflict since 1946. Source: Uppsala Conflict Database Program/Peace Research Institute Oslo.

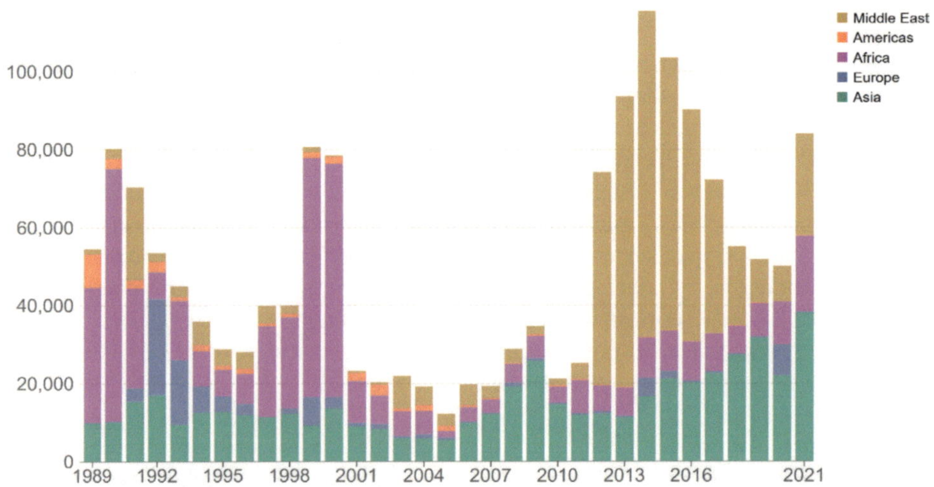

Figure 4.
Deaths in state-based conflicts by regions. Source: Uppsala Conflict Database Program/Peace Research Institute Oslo.

for better jobs, better education, better standards of living and even better health. This is usually the reason for rural-urban migration from the countryside to the cities. Rural exodus contributed to the rise in European Economies [70].

Irrespective of the cause, armed conflicts result in the vulnerable people seeking refuge in neighbouring localities or countries. Armed conflicts lead to forced migration [71]. Once migration is forced, its purpose is never just the search for food and shelter, but a place to escape being terminated. When refuge is sought within the country, the displaced are referred to as internally displaced people (IDPs). Whenever the migrating population cross national boundaries to another state, we refer to them as refugees.

Some of the reasons for forced human migration (both during war and peace) include the following:

- *The search for food*: Before globalisation reached its peak, most people depended solely on foodstuff obtained from within their countries but with globalisation, there is some level of liberalisation of cross border trade. This permits countries deficient of some food stuff to import from neighbouring countries. Conflict situations come to challenge cross border trade, internal agricultural efforts, and exposes people to adverse health and hygienic conditions. With all of these arising as a result of the armed conflicts, movement is thus significantly restricted. Food scarcity becomes acute due to increased demand and the inability of the farmers to continue with their farming activities. It thus becomes imperative for some UN agencies like the UNHCR, UNFPA, UNICEF and others to step in to assist in food provision to people displaced to neighbouring countries.

- *The search for shelter*: Armed conflicts come to destabilise whole communities and at times whole regions of a country. Mass destruction of property is not uncommon, including destruction of habitats and reducing whole localities to ruins. Those deprived of their shelter in the comfort of their homes are left with just two alternatives, either to stay in the conflict area and be exposed to death or move to a new location where there is perceived security. This has been the case with many Central African Republic citizens who fled the war to seek refuge in neighbouring Cameroon, DR Congo, and Tchad [72].

- *Agro pastoralism*: This is one of the commonest forms of migration in the arid and semi-arid regions especially of Africa North of the Sahara. In Somalia, for instance, migration becomes cyclical, deliberate, strategic, and anticipatory determined by the region's erratic rainfall patterns [38]. This causes the nomadic population to congregate in areas of permanent wells or other reliable sources of water to have access to pasture for their livestock, a pattern that reverses during the wet season.

- *Seeking medical care*: Armed conflicts can have devastating consequences on a community. Health facilities may well be functional in conflict areas within a country, but the highest challenge is to get health commodities through the last mile to the point of use. Logisticians, personnel who attempt to get health commodities through this last mile, expose themselves to stray bullets, torture, and kidnapping [73] with the resultant demand for a ransom by the warring factions in some cases. Left with these vulnerabilities, the health care system may deteriorate drastically to a level that the available institutions will not be able to meet the needs of the population. Thus, displacement to a calm area with good health care facilities assures the health of the displaced.

2.15 The notion of refugees

Refugees are people who have fled war, violence, conflict, or persecution, and have crossed international boundaries to find safety in another country. Refugees often flee with little or nothing, apart from a few clothes on the back [74]. Thus, they leave behind homes, possession, jobs and loved ones. Movement to another country imposes challenges to the refugees as well as to the host country's economy. The limited resources have automatically to be shared to harbour refugees and stop other humanitarian crises from surfacing. Therefore, armed conflicts almost always generates either refugees or IDPs.

As of mid-2022, the UNHCR estimated 103 million forcibly displaced people, 53.2 million of whom are internally displaced and 32.5 million are refugees. 4.9 million are asylum seekers, while 5.3 million are other people in need of international protection [75].

Of those displaced, 72% arise just from Syrian Arab Republic, Venezuela, Ukraine, Afghanistan, and South Sudan. 36.5 million are children while 1.5 million are children borne as refugees [76]. Launched in 1950 with an initial budget of USD 300000, the annual budget rose to over USD 1 billion in 1990, and exceeded USD 9.15 billion in 2021 [76] owing to the continuous growing number of refugees and IDPs.

2.16 Armed conflicts and disease dynamics

War and conflicts can generate and exacerbate infectious disease outbreaks over both short and long timeframes [77]. Armed conflicts generate refugees who usually concentrate in camps. Concentration in camps is thanks to the efforts of the UN agencies and local/national governments to assist the displaced who are already vulnerable in a foreign country/region. In the event of any infectious and contagious disease outbreak, it can easily become an epidemic that could evolve to a pandemic if care is not taken. This usually happens when the basic infection prevention processes like handwashing with soap and running water, and drinking of clean water are compromised.

The reality of disease dynamics and the link to armed conflicts is a direct attack on the unfinished journey to the Global Health Security Agenda (GHSA). The Global Health Security Agenda that was launched in 2014 by a group of 29 countries [78], the World Health Organisation (WHO), the Food and Agricultural Organisation (FAO), and the World Organisation for Animal Health seeks to make the world a safe place against infection diseases. With a current membership of over 70, the vision of the GHSA is to have a world safe and secure from global threats posed by infectious diseases [79]. This agenda has three key interventions in the prevention of infectious diseases [80], *prevent, detect*, and *respond* to infectious disease threats. This implies:

- Prevent avoidable disease outbreaks.

- Detect threats early enough; and

- Respond rapidly and effectively when outbreaks occur.

In conflict-affected areas, avoidable outbreaks may not easily be prevented. Normally, *vaccines, antibiotics, and antiviral drugs can play a critical role in mitigating a pandemic by reducing the infectiousness of symptomatic patients and the susceptibility of uninfected individuals* [81]. In an already fragile and fragmented supply chain for health commodities, (the reality in most armed-conflict zones around the world), it is almost impossible to respond to prevent vaccine-preventable infectious diseases and to treat the inflected to limit the spread of the infectious disease. Taking commodities to the population along the last mile may encounter numerous obstacles, and the much-needed cold chain that must be maintained with vaccines becomes difficult. The effort to provide healthcare during armed conflicts usually arises from the international community health actors stepping in to fill the gap because the state most often is unable or unwilling to provide adequate health services to the population [82].

During armed conflict, there is breakdown of the health system infrastructure, shortage of medicines and medical supplies, shortage of health workers, insufficient financial resources, as well as gaps in health data arising from the breakdown of the infrastructure [83]. It thus becomes very difficult to detect threats early enough and to determine the exact needs of the health system, and to respond with a rapid intervention.

Prevention, detection, and rapid response to outbreaks occurs within the framework of pandemic preparedness. According to WHO, pandemic preparedness should be seen as an integral part of preparedness to threats to human health caused by emergency (outbreak of any disease, or the occurrence of natural disasters of chemical incidents) [84]. “Pandemic preparedness is a continuous process of planning, exercising, revising and translating into action national and sub-national pandemic preparedness and response plans” [84]. Any level of pandemic preparedness is always compromised in conflict situation, thus compromising the Global Health Security Agenda to detect, prevent and respond to outbreaks.

In Yemen and Northern Syria, cholera outbreaks have been reported. The brutal war and armed conflicts basically damage the infrastructure of these areas, including healthcare infrastructure, besides diminishing the chances for people ever reaching healthcare and other social services. Thus, access to essential care is compromised, with less than half of the health facilities functional; and as if to worsen an already dreadful situation, the health facilities that remain open are without basic equipment [85]. Without security, adequate healthcare is impossible.

In December 2022, the International Rescue Commission (IRC) announced a 55-fold increase in cholera cases and an outbreak of measles in Kenyan refugee camp [86]. These outbreaks affected refugees largely from Somalia with three dead as of December 2022. **Figure 5** illustrates the locations and case prevalence of these cholera outbreaks.

Overcrowding, scarce clean water, and poor sanitation and hygiene practices, together with pre-existing malnutrition, comorbidities and limited access to medical care all contribute to the morbidity and mortality in the refugee population [87]. Cholera outbreaks in refugee camps was quite preponderant in the 1980s and 1990s, with almost 50% mortality in the absence of proper treatment (as opposed to the expected below 1% in normal systems where water, sanitation, and hygiene (WASH) standards are properly maintained in the health service delivery.

In a recent analysis [88], one hundred and twenty-eight (128) outbreak events involving forcibly displaced were identified over the period 1996–2016, with over 840,000 confirmed or suspected cases of measles, cholera, cutaneous leishmaniasis, dengue, and others were reported in 48 destination countries/territories. Based on the analysis of origin and destination, Desai et al. identified that Kenya experienced the highest number of distinct outbreaks, followed by Uganda, with 25% of cases imported from the location of origin of the migrated population.

Another health challenge faced by displaced people is HIV/AIDS. In emergency situations, HIV is the least concern for rescue workers in the immediate wake of a disaster

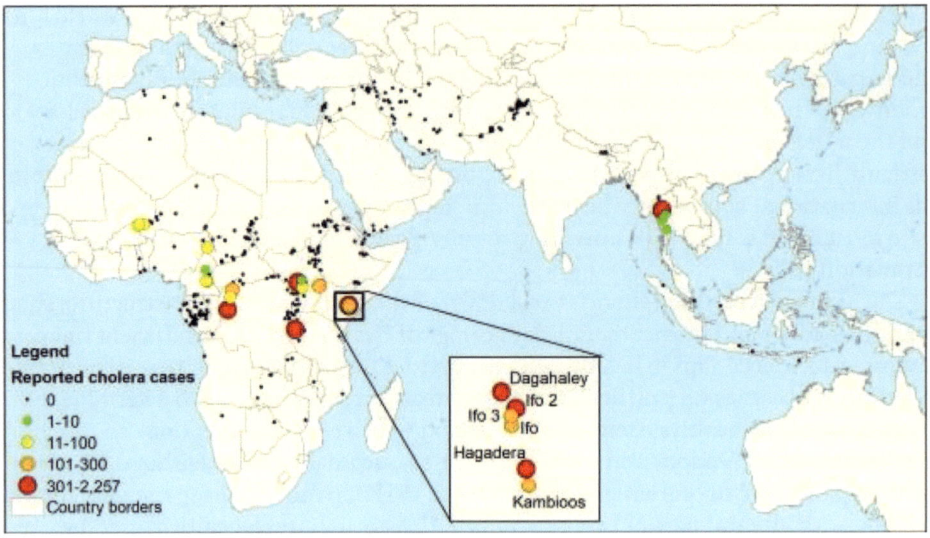

Figure 5.
Map of reporting UNHCR locations and cumulative reported cholera count, 2009–2016. Source: [87].

since more urgent needs present themselves and need to be addressed. In a UNAIDS publication that dates as far back as 1997 [89], it is highlighted that refugees are more vulnerable, especially women and children because of the risk of sexual violence, rape, and trafficking. Besides, lack of safe blood supply (in the event of transfusion), injection drug users, lack of access to condoms and to health care *inter alia* are the major causes of the high preponderance of HIV/AIDS in displaced populations (either IDPs or refugees).

Refugees do not necessarily display higher rates of HIV infection than the non-refugee population, but the trying conditions under which they live may increase their susceptibility to other diseases, HIV/AIDS inclusive [76]. Female refugees may indulge themselves in commercial sexual activity to survive, given the sometimes-harsh conditions in the host countries. Refugees usually undergo three phases in the cycle of displacement:

- Emergency Phase: Conflict or persecution causes populations to flee their homes, being thus deprived of vital resources like food, shelter, healthcare, and education.

- Post Emergency Phase: The refugees settle in a foreign country where they receive supplies of the resources that the supplying body feels they need, and which have been lost during the emergency phase.

- The final Phase: Depending on the prevailing circumstances, the refugee will choose to be repatriated to their home country, integrate, and remain in the host country, or seek asylum (resettle) in another country.

We thus see from the above analysis that armed conflicts present themselves as a threat to Global Health Security because of emerging infectious diseases and the eminent challenge to prevent, detect and respond rapidly and effectively to outbreaks. This has been evident with the SARS-CoV-2 (COVID-19) pandemic and other outbreaks in the past like Ebola, H5N1 and H1N1 pandemic. The threat to GHSA caused by armed conflict is compounded by globalisation and free movement across national and regional boarders.

2.17 Armed conflicts on the path of universal health coverage

Universal Health Coverage (UHC) means that all people have access to the full range of quality health services they need, when and where they need them, without financial hardship [90]. To achieve UHC requires people-centred Primary Health Care (PHC) well rooted in the communities they serve. It is but challenging for health systems to thrive well amid conflicts. Armed conflict is a global health challenge having consequences beyond the war-wounded, to affecting the health of the entire community [82]. Dabarre further emphasises that conflict is the ultimate social determinant of health, which causes conflict-affected communities to lag in many things including healthcare. Conflict usually affects all a country's health system from health-related infrastructure to research, policy and planning, as well as human and financial resources.

Conflict zones frustrate the last mile delivery of health commodities because of the obvious danger this poses on the logistics team. Thus, essential medicines and health technologies, an integral part of the health system cannot reach the population in a conflict zone, leading to avoidable deaths. In many countries, coverage of health services is limited by acute shortages of appropriate health workers, particularly in remote and rural areas [91]. With the few health workers exposed to continuous danger Dabarre underscores the fact that they may flee the conflict zones in search of better jobs in safer environments. It is therefore clear that the 2030 vision of UHC may not be achieved if armed conflict continues to thrive in this universe with almost all continents affected.

Armed conflicts, with the devastating effects on health systems need to be mitigated. There seems to be an established link between armed conflict and natural resources [92]. The analysis advanced by Lujala & Rustad confirm the fact that natural resources play an integral role in sparking and fuelling armed civil conflicts. According to Lujala & Rustad, oil-producing countries are 1.5 to 2 times more likely to experience armed civil conflict than nonproducers, and that when internal conflict occurs in a region that has oil reserves, it lasts twice as long as conflicts that occur in areas without oil reserves, and combatant deaths are twice as high. High-value natural resources increase the risk of conflicts in that access to revenue finances belligerent movements. Equally, grievances are created by unmet expectations or inequalities in the distribution of revenue, jobs, or other benefits. UHC required equitable distribution of wealth. When the wealth-generating resources become a reason for armed conflicts, UHC is compromised.

To mitigate the health effects of armed conflict, the first step is compliance to legislation, like the international humanitarian law (IHW) [93]. According to Lewis, IHL is clear about the protected status of medical facilities, the wounded and sick, and medical transport in armed conflicts. Failure to adhere to this legislation is either deliberate or reckless, and can amount to war crimes, provided the legislation enforces prosecution of perpetrators of such crimes. Tragic attacks have happened in medical facilities in Yemen and US strikes on Médecins Sans Frontières (MSF) facilities in Afghanistan, with evident impunity. Thus, the need to demand accountability and justice to war crimes, crimes against humanity, and violation of other international humanitarian law is warranted.

Secondly, all conflicts can be avoided. Healthcare personnel need to promote concerted global action to stop and prevent wars and promote peaceful solutions to disputes within and among nations [94]. This requires partnership and the engagement of political and economic actors to value human life over all other wants and desires to gain power and control territories, and the contribution healthcare personnel make to the society.

Third, Gebregziabher *et al* propose advocacy for access to sufficient humanitarian aid to meet population needs in conflict zones to mitigate direct and indirtect harms to heathcare delivery. This starts by recognising that every human life counts, and needs to be protected, and the protection thereof is the responsibility of heathcare personel and the governing bodies that are in place to safeguard the interests of the citizens they govern.

Dialogue seems to be the overall panacea to solve the problem of armed conflicrs and as such mitigate the negative and devastating effects on helathcare. Dialogue address various dimensions of the conflict. This is because sustainable peace depends on engaging with everyone affected by the decisions made by the people at the peace table. This initiative, if led by Global Health Leaders, can *immunise* groups from violent conflict and its downstream effects through formal and informal educational initiatives. Specifically, this approaches can include tracking early warnings of violence, creating predictive models of its outbreak, and working with local public health and medical experts to mitigate emerging conflict [95].

2.18 Armed conflicts and the sustainable development goals (global goals)

The UN Member states adopted the 17 Sustainable Development Goals (SDGs) in 2015, providing a shared blueprint of peace and prosperity on planet earth, both for now and the future [96]. The 17 SDGs, which have 169 targets, 3818 events, 1344 publications, and 7548 actions, are an urgent call for action by all countries (developed and developing) in global partnership. The 17 goals are presented below:

1. No Poverty (in all its forms everywhere)

2. No Hunger (achieve food security and improved nutrition and promote sustainable agriculture).

3. Good Health and Wellbeing (Ensure healthy lives and promote well-being to all at all ages)

4. Quality Education

5. Gender Equality

6. Clean Water and sanitation

7. Affordable and clean energy

8. Decent work and Economic Growth (promote sustained, inclusive, and sustainable economic growth, full and productive employment, and decent work for all).

9. Industry, innovation, and infrastructure

10. Reduced inequalities

11. Sustainable cities and communities (Make cities & human settlements inclusive, safe resilient & sustainable).

12. Responsible consumption and production

13. Climate action

14. Life below water

15. Life on land

16. Peace, justice, and strong institutions.

17. Partnership for the goals

Armed conflict led to forceful human migration and challenges almost all the 17 SDGs. Armed conflicts inflict poverty through the destruction of infrastructure, forced displacement of people, loss of jobs and the urgent search for shelter in a foreign land. This could reverse the economic situation of a country more than 10 years in the pre conflict situation. The COVID-19 and the war in Ukraine are a *"deadly duo"* against the attainment of SDG 1 to *end poverty* in all its forms. The number of people living in extreme poverty rose from 581 million in the pre-pandemic period to 657–676 million in 2022 [97], attributable to the *deadly duo*. We therefore see the significant contribution of armed conflicts against the realisation of this SDG.

Armed Conflict and climate change, *inter alia,* are converging to undermine *food security* worldwide. The advent of conflicts force people to migrate over regional and international boarders, leaving behind everything that has to do with their livelihood. In this new conditioned, yet uncomfortable environment, there is no guarantee for food security. It is only thanks to the effect of the UN agencies like UNHCR and UNICEF that these refugees struggle to adapt themselves to and settle in this new environment.

How can there be *good health and well-being* in the midst of conflict? Conflict frustrates all efforts of the supply chain to get health commodities through the last mile to troubled spots. Conflict destabilises the work environment such that the medics and paramedical staff cannot function optimally. In fact, Sartorius, quoting from the WHO Constitution of April 07, 1948, Defines health *"a state of complete physical, mental and social well-being and not merely the absence of disease or infirmity"* [98, 99]. Conflict challenges physical and mental health, as well as social well-being, thus compromising the realisation of this SDG goal 3. If the mental health state of the health professionals is compromised (from trauma imposed by conflict), their capacity to care for the sick and the wounded becomes as well compromised. It therefore becomes unlikely to achieve good health and well-being to all at all ages by 2030.

The first three SDGs are not the only SDGs challenges by armed conflicts and human migration. The attainment of SDG 8 is as well severely compromised by armed conflicts. This SDG aims at *promoting sustained, inclusive, and sustainable economic growth*, full and productive employment, and decent work for all. Global economic recovery is hampered, *inter alia*, by supply chain disruptions which are themselves significantly hampered by armed conflicts, either across international borders or along the last mile. Refugees very rarely have the opportunity to get engaged in the labour force and contribute to economic development, especially in the short run, until they become integrated into their new environment that they can positively contribute to economic development. According to the UN Statistics, there is rebound worker productivity from 1.6% in 2016 to 3.2%, but this is not the case in LMICs where armed conflicts are preponderant.

Armed conflicts challenge any efforts to build sustainable, safe, resilient, and inclusive human settlements -SDG 11. Ninety-nine percent (99%) of the world's urban population breathe polluted air [26]. The level of pollution increased during armed conflict situations because of significant combustion (burning), at times of whole settlements by warring parties, and decomposition of abandoned human bodies. It is not uncommon to see entire villages set ablaze during armed conflicts, especially when the Government forces perceive such an area as harbouring rebels. This has been observed in the Anglophone regions of Cameroon, in Central African Republic, in South Sudan, in Iraq, as well as other conflict areas around the globe. This renders these settlements unsafe and challenges the attainment of SDG 11. Besides, armed conflicts render the efforts of waste disposal companies impracticable. This is the reason why the UN reports that as of 2022, 55% of municipal solid waste is managed in controlled facilities, leaving 45% to accumulate and make the cities unsafe, and a potential epicentre for some epidemics like Cholera which arises largely because of eating or drinking contaminated food and water respectively. Most dwelling places for refugees could be likened to slums, adding to the over 1 billion slum dwellers.

3. Conclusions and recommendations

Armed conflicts are an evil that threaten man's existence on earth and gives little protection to man as opposed to some recently enacted laws that apparently project animal rights above human rights. The major cause of armed conflicts is either real or perceived bad governance and the intention to propagate an ideology and make it forcefully accepted by the entire population. Armed conflicts lead to forceful human migration and generates IDPs and refugees, challenging the economy of the host countries. Armed conflicts can paralyse entire Health Systems and send the economy of a country crawling on its knees.

Post conflict, aspects to consider bringing a country, its economy and the healthcare system include *inter alia*:

- Protecting health workers and health infrastructure to ensure that the entire health system does not collapse as a result of the armed conflict. The health of a people is as good as the healthcare system and the workforce. These two are major building blocks of health system strengthening and must be addressed with the necessary intentionality.

- Access to medicines and health technologies must not be interrupted in conflict situations. If there are no medicines, no health programs can thrive to produce any effects on the population. While the workforce is protected in conflict situations, due consideration must be made to allow delivery of health commodities along the last mile. Either of the warring parties can be beneficiaries of these health commodities, irrespective of the cause of the armed conflict.

- The root cause of the conflicts must be investigated and addressed to ensure lasting peace after the conflict. If the conflict is due to bad governance, as is the case in most situation around the globe, organisation of free, fair, and transparent elections with the mediation of a neutral external body may be the solution to bring about lasting peace.

- During conflict situations, the health infrastructure may be destroyed or the system collapses. When wars end, the affected areas are often left devastated. The large numbers of refugees resulting from conflict, the wounded and trauma victims needs to be rehabilitated. Reconstruction post conflict is necessary but can only succeed if it is initiated by the local population. They should have a significant say in how funding is allocated. However, before any attempt to reconstruct, it must be clear that the conflict has ended, otherwise, the efforts to reconstruct may result in mere wastage of resources which will be destroyed in the not-so-distant future.

- Reconstruction requires huge resources. Compared to the expenditure incurred during the conflict on a single day of war, we could build a state-of-the-art hospital [54]. Therefore, while huge financial resources are required to rebuild the health system infrastructure, this is usually negligible compared to the expenses incurred during the war.

- Ensuring the security of the population is paramount. Post conflict, the population becomes vulnerable, economic instability sets in, and severe poverty establishes itself. Considering that armed is a major social determinant of health, ending the conflict implies reinstating the peace of the population. To reinvigorate the population, food security will be the starting point before other needs are addressed systematically.

- Resettlement of the displaced through peaceful and planned repatriation to their home country will slowly reestablish the economy. This must be done when all the assurance is available that the displaced will return to meet a peaceful environment compared the one at the time of their departure.

If the world dreams to attain the SDGs by 2030 and Universal Health Coverage, armed conflicts must be addressed objectively, while putting aside political ambitions and potential selfish gains that most often come to the negotiation table whenever there is mediation to end an armed conflict. This way, we will align on the path to the Global Health Security Agenda.

Conflict of interest statement

No conflict of interest.

Author details

Julius Kenkoh Nkiese* and Stephanie Kininla Wirba
Mboppi Baptist Hospital Douala, Cameroon

*Address all correspondence to: nkiese.kenkoh@gmail.com

References

[1] Academy of International Humanitarian Law and Human Rights. Today's Armed Conflicts. Geneva: Academy of International Humanitarian Law and Human Rights; 2022 Available from: https://geneva-academy.ch

[2] Ero C, Atwood R. Ten Conflicts to Watch in 2023. Washington, DC, USA; 2023. Available from: https://www.crisisgroup.org

[3] Davis I, Smith D, Wezeman PD. Armed Conflict and Instability in the Middle East and North Africa. (S. I. Institute, Compiler) Stockholm. 2017. Available from: https://www.sipri.org/ yearbook/2017/03 [Accessed: June 30, 2023]

[4] Lusigi A. Africa and the Russia-Ukraine Conflict: Seizing the Opportunity in the Crisis. New York, USA; 2022. Available from: https://www.un.org/africarenewa

[5] Oyinlola M, Adeniyi O, Adedeji A. Armed Conflicts and Economic Growth in Africa. Ibadan; 2020 Available from: https://aercafrica.org

[6] Ghimire B. War in Ukraine and Its Impact on South Asia. New Delhi, India; 2023 Available from: https://www.freiheit.org

[7] Hao M, Fu J, Jiang D, Ding F, Chen S. Simulating the linkages between economy and armed conflict in India with a long short-term memory algorithm. 2020;**40**(6):1139-1150. DOI: 10.1111/risa.13470

[8] United Nations Office on Drugs and Crime. Categorisation of armed conflicts. 2018. Available from: https://www.unodc.org

[9] Uppsala Conflict Data Program. Appendix 2B. Definitions, Sources and Methods for the Conflict Data. Uppsala: Stockholm International Peace Research Institute; 2017. Available from: https://www.sipri.org

[10] ICRC. 2017. Venezuela: Protests, Armed Conflict and International Humanitarian Law. Geneva, Switzerland. Available from: https://www.icrc.org/en/] [Accessed: June 01, 2023]

[11] Macfarlane SB, AbouZahr C. The Palgrave Handbook of Global Health Data Methods for Policy and Practice. London; 2019. DOI: 10.1057/978-137-54984-6

[12] Equality and Human Rights Commission. 2019. What are human rights?. Availabe from: https://www.equalityhuman [Accessed: June 03, 2023]

[13] USA for UNHCR. Central African Republic Refugee Crises. 2017. https://www.unrefugees.org/emergencies/central-african-republic/

[14] International Committee of the Red Cross. (2018). Internally Displaced Persons and International Humanitarian Law. Geneva, Switzerland. Availabe from: https://www.icrc.org [Accessed: June 04, 2023]

[15] Encyclopaedia Britannica. Human migration. 2023. Availabe from: https://www.britannica.com/topic/human-migration [Accessed: June 04, 2023]

[16] Blakemore E. Human migration sparked by wars, disasters, and now climate. 2013. Available from: https://www.nationalgeographic.com/culture/article/migration [Accessed: June 04, 2023]

[17] Center for Preventive Action. 2023). Conflict in the Central African Republic. Washington, DC, USA. Available from: https://www.cfr.org/global-conflict-tracker/conflict/violence-central-african-republic [Accessed: June 03, 2023]

[18] Collins L. Central African Republic: A Role for Religious Leaders in Calming Conflict? Washington, DC, USA. 2020. Available from: https://www.usip.org/publications/2020/12/central-african-republic-role-religious-leaders-calming-conflict [Accessed: June 04, 2023]

[19] World Vision. Central African Republic Conflict: Fast Facts and How to Help. Monrovia. World Vision. 2023. Available from: https://www.worldvision.ca [Accessed: June 04, 2023]

[20] UNHCR. 2022. Afghanistan Refugee Crisis Explained. Washigton, DC: USA for UNHCR. Available from: https://www.unrefugees.org/news/afghanistan-refugee-crisis-explained/ [Accessed: June 01, 2023]

[21] European Commission. European Civil Protection and Humanitarian Aid Operations. 2023. Available from: https://civil-protection-humanitarian-aid.ec.europa.eu/ [Accessed: June 06, 2023]

[22] Dalrymple S. Supporting longer term development in crises at the nexus: Lessons from Cameroon. Development Initiatives. 2020. Available from: https://devinit.org/

[23] UNHCR. Cameroon Multi – Stakeholder Dialogue on Refugee. Yaoundé UNHCR; 2022. Available from: https://reliefweb.int/

[24] Lecrivain A. Cameroon: A Haven for Refugees from Conflict in the Central African Republic. Yaoundé. World Food Prograamme. 2022. Available from: https:// www.wfp.org/stories/cameroon-haven-refugees-conflict-central-african-republic [Accessed: June 05, 2023]

[25] Comolli V. The evolution and impact of Boko Haram in the Lake Chad Basin. Humanitarian Practice Network 2017. Available from: https://odihpn.org/publication/the-evolution-and-impact-of-boko-haram-in-the-lake-chad-basin/ [Accessed: June 03, 2023]

[26] UN. Cameroon: Intercommunal clashes continue to displace thousands. 2021. Available from: https://news.un.org/en/story/2021/12/1108242 [Accessed: June 06, 2023]

[27] ALIMA. Amid the displaced population crisis, the healthcare system in the far North of Cameroon has been weakened. R. Web, Compiler. 2017. Available from: https://reliefweb.int/report/cameroon/amid-displaced-population-crisis-healthcare-system-far-north-cameroon-has-been [Accessed: July 02, 2023]

[28] International Crisis Group. Cameroon's Anglophone Crisis at the Crossroads. Cameroon: International Crisis Group; 2017. Available from: https://www.crisisgroup.org/

[29] Bang HN, Balgah RA. The ramification of Cameroon's Anglophone crisis: Conceptual analysis of a looming "Complex Disaster Emergency". Journal of International Humanitarian Action. 2022;**6**:2-9. DOI: 10.1186/s41018-022-00114-1

[30] International Crisis Group. (2023). A Special Look at the Cameroon's Anglophone Special Status. International Crisis Group. Brussels, Brabant, Belgium. Availabe from: https://www.crisisgroup.org/ [Accessec May 31, 2023]

[31] Offner F. Cameroon: More than a Hundred Detainees from Anglophone Regions and Opposition Party

Languishing in Jail for Speaking Out. Yaoundé. Amnesty International. 2022. Available from: https://www.amnesty.org/ [Accessed: June 06, 2023]

[32] World Bank. The Socio-Political Crisis in the Northwest and Southwest Regions of Cameroon. 2021 10.1596/35933

[33] UNHCR. Cameroonian refugees in Nigeria – Operational. 2022. Available from: www.unhcr.org/ng

[34] Human Rights Watch. Cameroon: New abuses by both sides. 2021. Available from: https://www.hrw.org/news

[35] Elmi AA, Barise A. The Somali conflict: Root causes, obstacles, and peace-building strategies. African Security Review. 2010;**15**(1):32-54. DOI: 10.1080/10246029.2006.9627386

[36] Gajraj P, Sardesai S, Wam P. Conflict in Somalia: Drivers and Dynamics. Washington, DC; 2005. Available from: http://documents.worldbank.org/curated/en/537531468335694025/Conflict-in-Somalia-drivers-and-dynamics

[37] International Organization for Migration (IOM). Dimension of the Crisis on Migration in Somalia. Geneva, Switzerland: International Organization for Migration; 2014 Available from: http://www.iom.in

[38] IOM. Dimensions of the Crisis on Migration in Somalia. Geneva, Switzerland: IOM; 2014 Availabe from: http://www.iom.int

[39] Ibrahim M, Rizwan H, Malik MR. Mental health crisis in Somalia: A review and a way forward. International Journal of Mental Health Systems. 2022;**16**:2. DOI: 10.1186/s13033-022-00525-y

[40] WHO. Strengthening the public health system in a conflict setting: an example of a unique partnership between WHO, Sweden and Somalia working towards achieving health for all. 2022. Available from: https://www.emro.who.int/images/stories/somalia/documents/Strengthening-public-health-systems-case-study-september-2022.pdf

[41] Cheng M. The Ukraine crisis: Causes, conundrum and consequences. Auckland. 2022;**5**:95-111. DOI: 10.31014/aior.1991.05.02.350

[42] Baliga S. In: Garicano L, Rohner O, Mauro BW, editors. A Principal, Multi-Agent Model of Global Economic Consequences of the War in Ukraine Sanctions, Supply Chains and Sustainability. London, United Kingdom; 2022. Available from: https://cepr.org/system

[43] BBC News. What are the sanctions on Russia and are they hurting its economy? 2023. Available from: https://www.bbc.com/news/world-europe-60125659 [Accessed: June 04, 2023]

[44] Lister T, John T, Murphy PP. Here's what we know about how Russia's invasion of Ukraine unfolded. 2022. Available from: https://edition.cnn.com/2022/02/24/europe/ukraine-russia-attack-timeline-intl/index.html [Accessed: May 25, 2023]

[45] Ray M. Russia-Ukraine War. 2023. Available from: https://www.britannica.com/event/2022-Russian-invasion-of-Ukraine [Accessed: June 04, 2023]

[46] Statista. Number of civilian casualties during the war in Ukraine 2022-2023. 2023. Available from: https://www.statista.com/statistics/ [Accessed: June 04, 2023]

[47] OECD. The Ukrainian Refugee Crisis. 2022. Available from: https://www.oecd.org/ukraine-hub/ [Accessed: June 04, 2023]

[48] Knoema. World Atlas – Ukraine. 2023. Available from: https://knoema.com/ [Accessed: June 03, 2023]

[49] Lancet T. Russia's invasion of Ukraine: An attack on health. The Lancet. 2023;**401**:617. DOI: 10.1016/S0140-6736(23)00387-2

[50] Center for Preventive Action. Instability in Afghanistan. New York, USA: Center for Preventive Action; 2023. Available from: https://www.cfr.org/

[51] Centre for Preventive Action. Instability in Afghanistan. 2023. Available from: https://www.cfr.org/global-conflict-tracker [Accessed: May 25, 2023]

[52] UNAMA. Civilian deaths from Afghan conflict in 2018 at highest recorded level – UN report. 2019. Available from: https://unama.unmissions.org [Accessed: June 02, 2023]

[53] Center for Preventive Action. Instability in Venezuella. New York, USA: Center for Preventive Actio; 2023. Available from: https://www.cfr.org/global-conflict-tracker

[54] Latifi AM. Years of war and poverty take toll on Afghanistan's healthcare. 2019. Availabe from: https://www.aljazeera.com/news/2019/5/25/ [Accessed: May 25, 2023]

[55] UNAMA. Afghanistan, Protection of Civilians in Armed Conflict: Special Report: Attacks on Healthcare during the COVID-19 Pandemic. Geneva; 2020 Available from: https://unama.unmissions.org/sites/default/files/unama_special_report_attacks_on_healthcare_during_the_covid-19_pandemic_20_june_2020.pdf

[56] Worldometer. Oil Reserves by Country. 2013. Available from: https://www.worldometers.info/oil/ [Accessed: May 28, 2023]

[57] IOM. Venezuelan Refugee and Migrant Crisis. 2022. Available from: https://www.iom.int/venezuelan-refugee-and-migrant-crisis [Accessed: June 01, 2023]

[58] Doocy S, Page KR, Liu C, Hoaglund H, Rodríguez DC. Venezuela: Out of the headlines but still in crisis. Bulletin of the World Health Organization. 2022;**100**(8):466-466A. DOI: 10.2471/BLT.22.288269

[59] Geneva Academy. Non-international armed conflicts in Yemen. 2022. Available from: https://www.rulac.org/browse/conflicts/non-international-armed-conflicts-in-yemen [Accessed: May 30, 2023]

[60] BBC News. Yemen: why is the war there getting more violent? 2023. Available from: https://www.bbc.com/news/world-middle-east-29319423 [Accessed: May 27, 2023]

[61] OCHA. Humanitarian crisis in Yemen: Seven years on, WHO is strengthening the health system, responding to vital health needs, and saving lives. 2022. Available from: https://reliefweb.int/ [Accessed: June 03, 2023]

[62] Aufiero P, Pur NT. South Sudan at a Crossroads: Challenges and hopes 10 years after independence. 2021. Available from: https://www.hrw.org/news/2021/07/09/south-sudan-crossroads [Accessed: May 20, 2023]

[63] Gituai CT. Three Years of the RTGoNU: Unity of purpose to lead the country to enduring peace through implementation of R-ARCSS. 2023. Available from: https://jmecsouthsudan.org/ [Accessed: May 19, 2023]

[64] Chagutah T. 2023 South Sudan's conflicts are not just between communities. London, United Kingdom. Available from: https://www.amnesty.org/ [Accessed: May 10, 2023]

[65] Chagutah T. South Sudan's conflicts are not just between communities. 2023

[66] UNHCR. South Sudan Refugee Crisis. 2017. Available from: https://www.unrefugees.org/emergencies/south-sudan/ [Accessed: May 21, 2023]

[67] OCHA Services. (2023, Human Toll of Conflict and Violence Strains Healthcare System). South SudanAvailable from: https://reliefweb.int/report/south-sudan/ [Accessed: June 03, 2023]

[68] OCHA Services. South Sudan at 10: An MSF record of the consequences of violence. 2021. Available from: https://reliefweb.int/ [Accessed: June 01, 2023]

[69] Roser M, Hasell J, Herre B, Macdonald B. War and peace after 1945. 2016. Available from: https://ourworldindata.org/war-and-peace [Accessed: May 31, 2023]

[70] Baudin T, Stelter R. The rural exodus and the rise of Europe. Max Planck Institute for Demographic Research. 2022;**27**. DOI: 10.1007/s10887-022-09206-4

[71] Braithwaite A, Salehyan I, Savun B. Refugees, forced migration, and conflict: Introduction to the special issue. Journal of Peace and Research. 2018;**56**:5-11. DOI: 10.1177/0022343318814128

[72] USA for UNHCR. (2017). What Is a Refugee. USA. Available from: https://www.unrefugees.org [Accessed: June 04, 2023]

[73] Atabong AB. Nine health workers kidnapped in restive northwest Cameroon. *Reuters*. 2022. Available from: https://www.reuters.com/ [Accessed: June 02, 2023]

[74] UNHCR. What Is a Refugee. 2018. Available from: https://www.unhcr.org/ [Accessed: June 01, 2023]

[75] UNHCR. Figures at a glance. 2023. Available from: https://www.unhcr.org/us/about-unhcr/who-we-are/figures-glance# [Accessed: May 23, 2023]

[76] UNHCR. Refugees and HIV. UNHCR Global. 2023. Available from: https://www.unhcr.org/media/refugees-and-hiv-plusnews [Accessed: June 01, 2023]

[77] Sundaram M, Filion A, Akaribo BE, Stephens PR. Footprint of war: Integrating armed conflicts in disease ecology. Trends in Parasitology. 2023;**39**(4):234-241. DOI: 10.1016/j.pt.2023.01.007

[78] Osterholm MT. Global Health Security—An Unfinished Journey. Minnesota, USA; 2017. DOI: 10.3201/eid2313.171528

[79] GHSA. Global Health security agenda: A partnership against Global health threats. 2022. Available from https://globalhealthsecurityagenda.org [Accessed: July 02, 2023]

[80] USAID. Global Health Security. (USAID, Compiler) 1300 Pennsylvania Ave, NW Washington DC 20004. 2022. Available from: https://www.usaid.gov/global-health/health-areas/global-health-security [Accessed: July 01, 2023]

[81] Madhav N, Oppenheim B, Gallivan M, Mulembakani P, Rubin E, Wolfe N. Pandemics: Risks, impacts, and mitigation. In: T. I. Bank, editor. Disease Control Priorities: Improving Health and Reducing Poverty. 3rd ed. Washington, DC. Available from: https://www.ncbi.nlm.nih.gov/books/NBK525302/; 2017. DOI: 10.1596/978-1-4648-0527-1_ch17

[82] Debarre A. Hard to Reach: Providing Healthcare in Armed. 2018. Available from: www.ipinst.org

[83] Debarre A. Hard to Reach: Providing Healthcare in Armed Conflict. Stockholm: I. P. Institute; 2018 Available from:

https://www.ipinst.org/wp-content/uploads/2018/12/1812_Hard-to-Reach.pdf

[84] WHO. 2011). Pandemic Preparedness. Geneva. Available from: https://www.who.int/ [Accessed: July 02, 2023]

[85] Everett F. Under Threat: Healthcare in Conflict Zones. (T. H. Partnership, Compiler) London. 2021. Available from: https://www.healthpolicypartnership.com/under-threat-healthcare-in-conflict-zones/ [Accessed: July 02, 2023]

[86] Anyanga SB. 55 fold increase in cholera cases and an outbreak of measles in Kenya's refugee camps strain health resources, warns IRC. International Rescue Committee. 2022. Available from: https://www.rescue.org/ [Accessed: April 30, 2023]

[87] Shannon K, Hast M, Azman AS, Dominique Legros HM, Lessler J. Cholera prevention and control in refugee settings: Successes and continued challenges. PLOS Neglected Tropical Diseases. 2019;**2019**:1-11. DOI: 10.1371/journal.pntd.0007347

[88] Desai AN, Ramatowski JW, Marano N, Madoff LC, Lassmann B. Infectious disease outbreaks among forcibly displaced persons: An analysis of ProMED reports 1996-2016. (Article vumber: 49). (C. a. Health, Compiler). 2020. 10.1186/s13031-020-00295-9

[89] UNAIDS. Refugees and AIDS: UNAIDS Point of View. Geneva: UNAIDS; 1997. Available from: https:// www.unaids.org/en/resources/documents/1997/19970404_refug-pov_en.pdf [Accessed: April 29, 2023]

[90] World Health Organisation. Universal Health Coverage (UHC). Geneva, Switzerland: WHO; 2022. Available from: https://www.who.int [Accessed: June 03, 2023]

[91] Miller C, Holly L. Health workers and universal health coverage. 2012. 10.1016/S0140-6736(12)61939-4

[92] Lujala P, Rustad SA. High-value natural resources: A blessing or a curse for peace?. Sustainable Development Law & Policy y 12, Compiler). 2011. Available from: http://digitalcommons.wcl.american.edu/sdlp

[93] Lewis L. Protecting medical care in conflict: A solvable problem. (R. Web, Compiler). 2020. Available from: https://reliefweb.int/report/world/protecting-medical-care-conflict-solvable-problem [Accessed: July 02, 2023]

[94] Gebregziabher M, DeLargy P, Jumaan A, Kapila M, Rubenstein L. War prevention and mitigation are public health imperatives of our time. (c. Medicine, Compiler). 2022. 10.1016/j.eclinm.2022.101385

[95] Shapiro D, Hua C. Mitigating the global health threat of violent conflict: A preventive framework. BMJ Journals. 2020;**3**(2):409-412. DOI: 10.1136/bmjnph-2020-000114

[96] UN. The 17 sustainable development goals. 2015. Available from: https://sdgs.un.org/fr/goals [Accessed: May 27, 2023]

[97] Mahler DG, Yonzan N, Hill R, Lakner C, Wu H, Yoshida N. Pandemic, Prices, and Poverty. NW, Washington, DC: World Bank; 2022. Available from: https://blogs.worldbank.org/opendata/pandemic-prices-and-poverty [Accessed: May 15, 2023]

[98] Sartorius N. The meanings of health and its promotion. Croatian Medical Journal. 2006;**47**. Available from: https://www.ncbi.nlm.nih.gov/pmc/articles/PMC2080455/

[99] UNHCR. Central African Republic Situation. 2022. Available from: https://reporting.unhcr.org/

Chapter 5

Perspective Chapter: A Supposedly Developed Country's Response to a Healthcare Crisis – Lessons from the COVID-19 Pandemic for Future National Emergencies

Jeffrey S. Freed, Hannah S. Jacobs-El, Soo Y. Kwon and Ram Roth

Abstract

The world has just suffered through a pandemic that was responsible for the 7 million deaths. The expectation prior to this devastation would have been those countries like the United States, which are considered "developed", would have been prepared and able to ameliorate the effects of such a catastrophic event. However, this was not the case. In fact, many countries not necessarily considered underdeveloped or undeveloped weathered this crisis by mounting a much more organized response. This chapter will review the history of similar episodic epidemics, the failures that led to over a million deaths in the United States, and most importantly what is necessary to a similar event in the future to be dealt preventing the devastation that did occur in a most "developed" country like the United States. These lesions and their possible extrapolation worldwide, hoping will prevent a recurrence of the devastation we have recently experienced in the United States.

Keywords: COVID19, pandemic, disease control, politics, developed, vaccine

1. Introduction

The COVID-19 pandemic has been a stark reminder of the need for effective preparedness and response strategies in the face of global health crises. It exposed various failures and challenges in the United States' response. In this chapter, we examine the lessons learned from the pandemic, emphasizing the importance of a coordinated and unified approach to mitigate the risks and impacts of such emergencies. This analysis highlights dismissive responses by politicians, poor public understanding, flawed testing, delays in accurate testing approvals, lack of national coordination, inconsistent mask guidance, healthcare disparities, and the decentralized nature of the U.S. government. However, it also acknowledges scientific achievements, the dedication of healthcare workers, and the need to learn from these mistakes. By analyzing the successes and failures of our healthcare system, the role of politics, and the need for improved coordination between federal and state authorities, we intend to pave the way for a more resilient future.

2. Defining a developed country

One measure of a country's development is the health of its citizenry. The better the health, the longer the life expectancy and the ability to be productive. This results in economic progress and expanding wealth. The advantages of a high income "developed" country are related to an advanced healthcare system and are the foundation of the well-being of its citizens.

According to the United Nations, a *developing* country is defined as one with a relatively low standard of living and undeveloped industrial capability [1]. As measured by the Human Development Index (HDI) a developing county is considered low on the scale. The parameters of this index compare factors like poverty, literacy, education, life expectancy, and many others for individual countries around the globe. The numerical range used by the HDI index is 0.1 to 1.0. The United States has a rating of 0.921. Switzerland is at the apex with a 0.961 rating, while South Sudan is at the nadir with a rating of 0.635.

In order to evaluate whether the United States purported itself as a "developed" country in the face of the COVID-19 pandemic, we looked at the factors that are construed as being evidence of "developed". Did the confounding factors that resulted in questions about this end point, and the consequences that resulted from the level of preparedness, exist? In doing so, our major goal was not to criticize, but rather to identify where changes could be made to deal with the next catastrophic event that nature will almost assuredly make us face as the twenty-first century progresses.

The provision of healthcare during a crisis, whether the mechanism is public, private or both, is largely dependent upon public health resources identifying disease threats at population levels. This leads to the question, are high income countries like the United States sufficiently equipped and prepared to address novel disease threats like the COVID-19 pandemic? And what does a developed country need to do to be prepared for those as yet undetermined infectious disease pandemics that are almost certainly in our future.

2.1 The pandemic toll in developed countries

The World Health Organization first described the COVID-19 as a pandemic on March 11, 2020 [2]. Very few scientists or governmental officials understood the potential consequences of this deadly disease. Public health measures were instituted such as closing of some borders, but not all. Authorities issued strict stay-at-home orders, and public activity ceased. Individual nations treated the problems in different manners, but with limited resources, they were unable to deal with the overwhelming number of cases. The previously unknown virus, labeled SARS-CoV-2, an airborne virus, was transmissible prior to the presentation of symptoms in the individual. In some cases, the carrier of the virus never developed symptoms, making contact tracing more difficult. COVID infection caused severe, often fatal, disease in the elderly and vulnerable individuals (e.g., obese, diabetic, cardio-pulmonary disease patients). It was not evident how severe the illness could be until the mortality statistics began to reflect that a horrible crisis was at hand.

One of the most striking findings was that the United States had more illness and a greater number of mortalities than most developed countries. The trend was noted early in the pandemic and seemed to continue. As of this date, according to the Kaiser Family Foundation statistics, the COVID-19 virus has caused approximately 7.6 billion cases of disease and 6.85 million deaths worldwide [3]. This is equivalent to 1.4 deaths per 15 thousand cases. The population of the United States (roughly 340 million) has suffered approximately 103 million cases of disease but has had more than 1.1 million deaths. This roughly translates to one death per 100 cases, a markedly higher mortality rate.

Epidemiologic data demonstrated that the COVID-19 pandemic had a significantly higher prevalence and death rate in more developed and higher income countries, even after accounting for significant underreporting in less developed countries. Moshen Bayati used data related World Meter and per capita income from the World Bank which indicate that the COVID-19 death and prevalence rates between high income and other countries was three times higher in the former group (17,371 vs. 6180 per 1 million population). The same relationship appeared when analyzing critical cases. Dr. Bayati concluded, from simple regression analysis, that the prevalence and deaths from COVID-19 are significantly correlated to countries' per capita income. The richer a country was, the greater the loss of life. He could only surmise that high income countries had populations with more risk factors, more diagnostic tests performed, more air transport completed, and more information available. Higher reported prevalence and more deaths from COVID-19 surpassed lower-income countries [4].

2.2 A historical look at development

The ability of a country to support public health management services depends on coordination of multiple components including government health agencies at the central and local levels, donor organizations, civil society groups and directly with affected communities. These relationships are meant to provide the services necessary for successful healthcare but must also be responsible for planning for future needs and for executing programs to recognize and deal with emergencies. The Corona virus pandemic highlights the latter function as a determinant of which nations are adequately resourced, specifically prepared for this type of "attack" and which have yet to achieve that status.

Although there are a long list of parameters for defining a developed country, the observer must look not only to the present but back in history. The purpose of this exercise is to assess whether our definitions and practices have kept pace with the state of knowledge, as well as whether our actions and responses have evolved with those definitions. Surely, one of the measures of how a society has evolved is their response to an emergency, such as a pandemic. This is a reflection of their ability to learn from the past and whether those lessons and their remediation have been put into action. The COVID-19 pandemic appears to have answered the question for our global society, and the answer is that we have failed.

This type of failure is nothing new to mankind. Each time we move forward we take a step back, perhaps to re-organize, or perhaps to take a breath and reassess where we have come, and where we might want to go. Looking back for clues may be the answer. In the 2nd millennium BCE, the developed world was under the control of Egypt and Babylonia. During this period communication between groups improved significantly with the development of the alphabet. These advancements, evidence of a developed culture, allowed for transfer of information and improved commerce and the creation of a better financial status for the state. World population rose to over 100 million people, reaching a milestone that portended the potential for massive expansion, not actualized until the twentieth century [5, 6].

However, despite the developments of this period, by the end of the 2nd millennium BCE Barbarians destroyed these existing cultures and instituted social change, not necessarily improving the conditions of society.

Development waxes and wanes throughout history. Periods of rapid improvement of a given society were often followed by times of repression and ignorance. This is seen during the magnificent advances produced by the Roman Empire that were followed by the period referred to as the Dark Ages. There was an inability to carry forward the advances in all areas of human endeavor at the heights of civilization, resulting in periods of backsliding and failure to learn from the lessons of history.

2.3 Enter the Spanish flu

One only has to reflect at the events of the last 100 years to see a dramatic example of man's failure to learn from history and prepare for the devastating events that is to come. Regardless of a country's development level, effective preparedness requires proactive and cost-effective strategies. Strengthening core public health infrastructure, such as water safety measures and rapid response capabilities, is crucial. The experience of the 1918 influenza pandemic reminds us that these measures have been well-established for decades, and yet, similar mistakes were made during the COVID-19 crisis. It raises the question of why, after a century, our supposedly advanced healthcare system still faced significant challenges.

The 1918 influenza pandemic was the most devastating healthcare crisis of the twentieth century. It also demonstrated our lack of incorporation of the knowledge of past similar crises into our healthcare planning. The etiologic agent was an H1N1 virus. Although there is no universal consensus regarding the origin of the virus, its worldwide spread was catastrophic between 1918 and 1920. In the United States, it was first identified among military personnel in the spring of 1918 and spread rapidly across the country (**Figure 1**).

The 1918 pandemic, despite its name (i.e., Spanish flu), is believed to have started in the United States. Initially being reported at Fort Riley in Kansas in March 2018, it was most likely carried across the Atlantic Ocean to Europe by American soldiers on the way to fight in the Great War. Conditions like overcrowding and poor sanitation that the soldiers encountered were the perfect setting for the virus to spread like a wildfire. In fact, at Fort Riley, 522 men were diagnosed from the same severe influenza. This was soon followed by outbreaks of the flu in the army camps in Virginia, South Carolina, Georgia, Florida, Alabama, and California. The transfer of infected soldiers to Navy ships resulted in outbreaks of severe influenza and pneumonia among their crews.

2.4 The impact of politics

The initial impressions were that the flu was essentially a military personnel disease. This resulted in the impending disaster being first underestimated, then underreported and most importantly, to be spread by war in Europe. In fact, the American government intentionally suppressed press coverage of this rapidly spreading infection to avoid public panic. The flu traveled from military camp to military

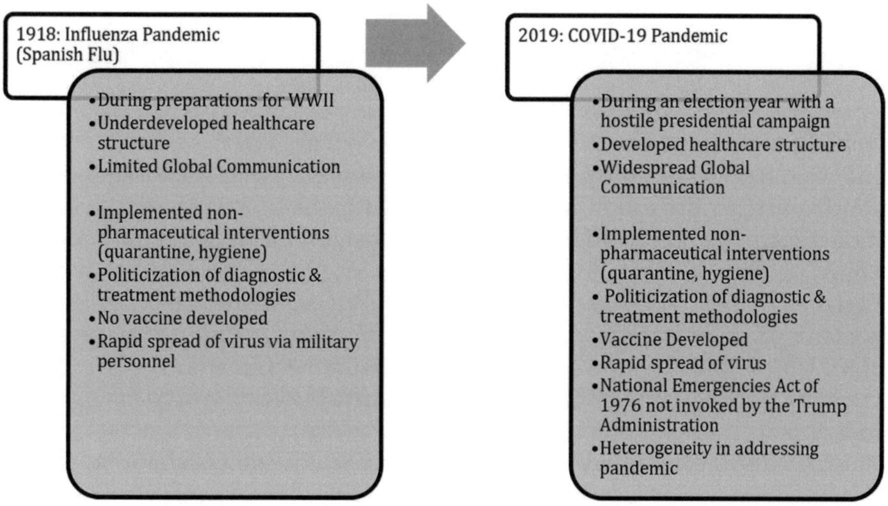

Figure 1.
Comparison of influenza and COVID-19 pandemics.

camp and then across the Atlantic. From September through November 1918, sickened 20–40% of U.S. Army and Navy personnel were sick [7]. This left American soldiers en route to the battlefields of France and Belgium to unwittingly deliver the deadly influenza virus. In this case, public health principles were based on politics. This is an error that has been repeated multiple times in history, including in the most recent pandemic of 2019.

It is estimated that more than 500 million people, or two-thirds of the world's population at that time, became infected with this virus. The number of deaths was estimated to be at least 50 million worldwide with about 675,000 occurring in the United States. Mortality was high in people younger than 5 years old, 20–40 years old, and 65 years and older. The high mortality in healthy people, including those in the 20–40-year-old age group, was a unique feature of this viral illness.

While the 1918 H1N1 virus has since been synthesized and studied [8], the properties that made it so devastating are not well understood. Furthermore, no vaccine to protect against influenza infection and no antibiotics to treat secondary bacterial infections were available at that time. Control efforts worldwide were limited to non-pharmaceutical interventions such as isolation, quarantine, good personal hygiene, use of disinfectants, and limitation of public gatherings.

Both the 1918 influenza pandemic and the 2019 COVID-19 pandemic are among the most disastrous infectious disease emergencies of modern times. There were similarities in their clinical, pathological, and epidemiological features despite being separated by more than a century. They were each met with similar public health responses. Both pandemics had lasting, psychosocial effects related to loss and hardship. In considering these two deadly pandemics, we ask: what lessons have we learned over the span of a century. Did we apply those lessons to the challenges of COVID-19 [9]? Will we be better prepared for the next pandemic?

2.5 Politics 100 years later

Of course, when comparing the world during these two pandemics, we must acknowledge at least two major differences. First, the structure of healthcare was underdeveloped and scientifically, health care systems were in their infancy in 1918. Second, these healthcare systems had limited ability to communicate on a global level in 1918. Surely 100 years later health care systems and global communication had supposedly improved dramatically preparing us for the COVID-19 pandemic.

Notably, there was one factor in both pandemics. That was the politicization of diagnostic and treatment methodologies. This was one of the major reasons that both pandemics were so difficult to confront, especially in the United States. Covid's politicization transcended the pandemic and contributed to a major rift in the political and economic stability of the United States and many other countries [10].

Even before the COVID-19 pandemic, widespread economic insecurity resulted in increasing distrust and popular discontent, ultimately damaging governance and sustainable development across the globe. It caused some countries to move toward extreme policies both on the left, (liberal) and others toward the extreme right, (conservative).

The COVID-19 pandemic eroded the veneer of social and economic security and exposed the extent of insecurity in the world. This has exacerbated societal and political instability. Even now, pandemic management should be a crucial policy priority to ensure economic, social, and healthcare security and rebuild trust. Failure to do this rapidly, will make the goals of the 2030 Agenda for Sustainable Development, the United Nations "plan of action for people, planet and prosperity", unattainable [11].

The COVID-19 crisis has dramatically signaled the extent of economic, social, and political insecurity, even in countries like the United States that previously considered themselves secure. This is likely to have profound consequences, threatening countries' ability to achieve the 2030 Agenda for Sustainable Development and its Sustainable Development Goals for developed and developing countries. If history repeats itself, as it usually does, this will impact the most vulnerable countries to the greatest extent [12]. Or at least that is the prevailing thought.

2.6 Disruption of developed countries

It is quite apparent that in one manner or another, these catastrophic world events have a significant impact on almost all aspects of society. However, the COVID-19 pandemic seems to have been particularly disruptive in developed countries. This pandemic had unique features that we must consider. First, we note a failure of traditional compartmental epidemiological models to predict the scale and dynamics of the infection in various countries. The course of an epidemic is often difficult to predict. This is especially true when it is a new emerging virus. The validity of most predictive models relies on numerous parameters, involving biological and social characteristics often unknown or highly uncertain. The COVID-19 pandemic characteristics were definitively unknown initially. Scientists who did not have a coordinated plan nor a central data center had to individually formulate an approach to gathering the necessary information and develop predictive models to understand the disease's spread [13].

3. Chaos: the best model

A different statistical approach was necessary for COVID-19. Researchers like Jones and Strigul predicted correctly that the unpredictability of this pandemic could be one of its basic properties [14]. A chaotic dynamical system model matched the method of its spread. The fundamental principle is that unpredictability comes from the fact that very similar initial conditions can often lead to very different outcomes. These researchers emphasized that if their theory was correct and the pandemic was to spread in a chaotic fashion, that policy makers would have to use this dynamic data in decision making. Unfortunately, in the United States, 50 states made individual decisions regarding the handling of the epidemic without coordination of information and resources. This resulted in a disparate response and devastating results.

Once the work on chaos dynamics and the COVID-19 was established, many epidemiological studies were completed and published rapidly. One study by Necesito et al. described the chaotic behavior of COVID-19 using a methodology referred to as State Space plots [15]. It depicted the changes in asymptotic behavior and trajectory brought about by the increase or decrease in the number of cases that resulted from the easing or tightening of restrictions and other public health measures required by governments. The Stringency index, a composite measure based on nine response indicators including school closures, workplace closures, and travel bans, was the measurements used. The authors credited the chaotic behavior of COVID-19 and the effects of population density as a potential methodology to generate more accurate COVID-19 non-linear prediction models. This, they predicted, would be used at the local and national government level to plan strategic and directed COVID-19 policies. However, during the first year of the pandemic, efforts by epidemiologists throughout the world to create models that would predict the future behavior of the deadly virus were carried out in isolation, without a central data facility or a coordination of efforts.

3.1 Quarantine still works

Prior to the development of the vaccines, quarantine models were thought to be an important methodology for disease control. Of course, this approach was employed for centuries and was once again revived when the COVID-19 pandemic struck. Mishra et al. developed three quarantine models, based on the apparent transmission characteristics of the COVID-19 virus in the human population, taking into account the compartments: susceptible population, immigrant population, home isolation population, infectious population, hospital quarantine population, and recovered population [16]. These models, and others, enabled public health officials to predict situations that were ultimately confirmed, proving that these well-established tools could be efficient and useful for public health decision making in the face of a deadly pandemic [17].

4. Election year politics

Just as the response to the influenza pandemic of 1918 by an American government preparing to enter World War I was politically influenced, the COVID-19 pandemic response was even more burdened by political influence. The latter pandemic reared its ugly head in an election year and that appears to have significantly influenced the governmental response.

Recent studies indicate that COVID-19 cases decreased the electoral support for President Trump. A "what if/then" evaluation of election data indicated that, all other things being equal, if COVID-19 cases had been 5 percent lower, President Trump would have been reelected. Data also revealed that the negative impact of COVID-19 on Mr. Trump's supporters was stronger in areas without a stay-at-home order. The impact was seen in swing states and urban counties where Trump won previously during the 2016 presidential elections. Deteriorating economic conditions did not appear to reduce electoral support for Trump. The Pandemic did. Statistical analysis showed that in most areas with increasing COVID-19 cases, candidate Biden won majority support for the election.

In searching for an explanation for the 2020 presidential election results, two possibilities emerge. First, Trump's handling of the pandemic, unlike other developed countries' leaders, was widely criticized. This reactive phenomenon is referred to as a retrospective voting approach, incumbents being punished for negative disruptions [18]. Second, the economic disruption caused by the COVID-19 pandemic most probably caused some voters to change their vote from Trump to Biden. As James Carville said in 1992, "it's the economy study". These negative economic events continue to influence our voting preferences.

There has been a continuum of negative healthcare and economic events like severe public health threats and major economic losses that have influenced local as well as national elections. These events have led to expansion of the social safety nets, including healthcare and unemployment insurance programs [19]. Of course, the underlying elements controlling the results of the 2020 election are far too complex to discuss here. It is extremely difficult to quantify which of these possibilities mentioned above was most impactful on the election. Factors like the exceptional voter turnout, which was quite high for the 2020 presidential election, voter heterogeneity in race, age, and other characteristics conditions voters' responses to the pandemic are all factors to be explored. Certainly, the COVID-19 pandemic played a significant role in the campaign for the presidency and the election results [20].

5. Many mistakes

Even though the disastrous nature of the pandemic and its enormous sequelae are relatively obvious, it is still difficult to look back and assess the major factors and their consequences that contributed to the horrendous effect on the U.S. society. Clearly, the United States had one of the highest Covid mortality rates in the world. Perhaps we can examine the factors and mistakes one by one and see how they affected the country as it struggled to deal with this new and terrifying disease that cost hundreds of thousands of lives. Tanya Lewis described many of these mistakes in her article in the journal *Scientific American* [21]. She had interviewed scientists and public health experts and teased out what they considered the biggest mistakes in the U.S.'s response. She also concludes that there are still some lingering questions that need to be addressed.

In the era of "Fake News" it is significant that scientists and public health officials failed to produce "real news" regarding the danger of the pandemic. The dismissive response by the politicians to key scientists and knowledgeable government health officials led to poor public understanding of the devastating nature of the problem and its long-term impact on American society. Using a flawed CDC-developed COVID test rather than the more robust and proven German test used by the World Health Organization, exacerbated public distrust of the U.S. government.

The FDA contributed to this failure by not swiftly approving more accurate tests and being equivocal about whether the rapid antibody test was sufficiently accurate. The United States public health services failed to nationally implement a standard for tracing, isolating, and quarantining, which are the fundamental techniques of epidemic control.

The mask guidance was particularly disorganized, the decisions being left to officials of individual states to decide rather than having a uniform national policy for an airborne spread virus. Public officials decided, without scientific support, that the spread of the virus was by large droplets, leading to the emphasis on handwashing and surface cleaning. They failed to "cover all bases" and they de-emphasized masks which are more effective in an aerosol-spread virus.

There were especially bad outcomes in remote areas and communities of color which suffered most. This can be attributed to two major factors: first, these communities have a high incidence of under-treated or non-treated comorbidities like obesity and diabetes; second, the pandemic exposed the structural racism in American healthcare, with minority communities receiving less quality care. Both these factors resulted in an increased mortality rate.

As a result of the failure of a coordinated centralized governmental response, state and local leaders made their own public health decisions and based them on inadequate data. This was due in large part to the national government's failure to have a well-conceived national strategy in place prior to the pandemic. In light the absence of a national strategy and solid scientific diagnostic and therapeutic guidelines, the states had little choice but to implement their own the pandemic plans, resulting in an uncoordinated, uncooperative, and ineffective containment of the disease. The effect was an eruption of COVID-19 cases in many locales, leading to health systems being overwhelmed. The unpredictable pattern of disease spread left no part of the country immune from this deadly disease.

Often decision makers created local and state policies that had no basis in public health. Some created policies that were often contrary to establish pandemic control measures. This enabled a self-centered approach to resource mismanagement, where in some cases, as in developing and resource poor nations, needed equipment was stored in warehouses in one state while other states were desperate for those items. A lack of national government oversight resulted in an unbalanced application of established public health measures in the United States that was not as dramatic as in other developed countries. The central administration did nothing to try to correct these errors. However, it must be remembered that our mechanism of governing is decentralized, and states individually have the right to manage crises like the COVID-19 pandemic. The President could have invoked the National Emergencies Act of 1976. Whether the political climate at the time would have allowed this, or whether it would have caused even more harm, is conjecture.

It also appears that there is a systems issue that resulted from the intrusion of politics into public health. Political affiliation emerged as a risk factor for COVID-19, evidenced by the fact that predominantly Republican counties had higher COVID-19 death rates than those with a predominantly Democrat-voting citizenry. This serves as evidence of the relationship between political party affiliation, vaccination views, and clinical cases and deaths from COVID-19 [22].

This is basically the result of the federal system of government under which we live. The states, rather than the federal government, hold the authority to make healthcare policy, independent of the federal government and other states. This creates an inconsistent and potentially dangerous situation where, in the face of a crises like the COVID-19 pandemic, states can actually be working to undo federal guidelines of the Center for Disease Control and the National Institutes of Health. This division of authority led to errors on the part of both the federal government and the states. The lack of coordination resulted in higher mortalities in some areas and higher caseloads in others. It also caused a failure of vital distribution of resources, adding to the healthcare burden in some states, and unnecessary resources abundance in other states.

During the pandemic, over 30 states passed laws contradictory to basic public health measures. This was done without scientific basis and without any coordination with other states or national healthcare authorities. This was a situation fraught with danger and was definitely counter-productive in the midst of a pandemic. It was not their conclusions that were flawed but rather their rationale.

"They knew what was best" attitude, had unpredictable outcomes. In some cases, their decisions were proven correct, as in states that opened their schools and businesses in mid-2021, and in some cases, they were completely wrong, like Alabama. In March 2020, Governor Kay Ivey issued quite "soft" orders paralleling CDC recommendations without the strict enforcement measures. On May 31st, 2021, he issued a supplemental emergency proclamation transitioning the state from an amended Safer at Home Order to a new Safer Apart Order, the third phase of COVID-19 pandemic health orders. Masks were no longer mandated statewide, but individuals were strongly encouraged to wear a mask or other facial covering when in public and in close contact with other people. That order terminated on May 31, 2021, and the state of emergency in Alabama ended on July 6, 2021. Almost 2 years later the COVID-19 cases are still substantial in Alabama, especially in the southeastern part of the state. Statistics from Johns Hopkins University show 106 deaths were reported statewide daily over the last 7 days, although some of those could have occurred earlier because of a lag in reporting. Alabama's rate of 18 deaths for every 100,000 people is far above second-place West Virginia, which had 10 deaths per 100,000 people, according to the U.S. Centers for Disease Control and Prevention [23].

6. What a developing country did well

We have discussed at length the response to the pandemic in the United States, and its failings. Let us compare our developed country's (HDI 0.921) response to an undeveloped country. To that end we will focus on the Covid-19 response undertaken by South Sudan (HDI 0.635), which did not and does not have the extensive resources that exist in the United States. South Sudan is one of the countries that continues to face a huge burden of infectious disease as well as non-infectious diseases. The country confirmed more than 20,000 cases of Covid infection and over 150 deaths by the end of 2022.

The WHO mounted a coordinated response in concert with the South Sudanese Ministry of Health to bolster preparedness and provide interventions to suppress the pandemic. To be able to provide extensive testing, almost 100 teams were trained and dispersed throughout the country. These teams were fully equipped to establish laboratories and implemented infection prevention and control operations across the countryside.

As soon as a vaccine was available (including a significant contribution from the United States), the WHO in concert with the Ministry of Health and other partners created a program to provide vaccinations for the most vulnerable communities who were plagued by floods, food insecurity, conflict and displacement. Over 1.9 million doses of the vaccine were administered by the end of 2022.

The vaccination campaign was supported by a major public campaign promoting the safety of the COVID-19 vaccines. Large numbers of South Sudanese citizens came to vaccination centers and a significant number of lives were saved.

What did South Sudan do right? First, they reached out for help to international agencies with the capability to assist them. They rapidly geared up to do testing and put public health measures in place. Public health ministry developed a program for vaccination of their population and supported this with a campaign to educate and encourage the public to be vaccinated. But most significantly, the South Sudanese government spoke with one voice through the Ministry of Health. This markedly decreased confusion and developed public confidence in the government's recommendations and participate in recommended pandemic suppression techniques and vaccinations [24].

7. Lessons from pandemics

Any comparison between the US and South Sudan is of course absurd. The authors do not believe that the complex developed United States could have achieved similar outcomes as in low-resource emerging undeveloped South Sudan. This leaves the question of what could have been done? Certainly, basic public health principles would, and should have been the very first approach to this pandemic. This was especially true when it became clear that the disease was extremely infectious leading to significant mortalities. The principles suggested here are not new and do not need further support. They have prevented a large number of cases of the disease for centuries, and a multitude of deaths. Jamison et al. described the mitigation of such an epidemic/pandemic, predating the identification of COVID-19. They wrote of "Pandemics: Risks, Impacts, and Mitigation in 2017 [25]. These principles included:

There must be:

1. *prerequisites for effective preparedness and response* to assess the problem and take steps to mitigate disease

2. Whether a country is developed or not, preparedness includes pre-emptive cost-effective strategies like *investing to strengthen core public health infrastructure*, including basic water safety and rapid response measures

3. A *coordinated response* is essential and should include situational awareness, public health messaging, transmission abatement, and care of the sick.

4. A healthcare system must have *surge capacity* proportional to the severity of the event, the pathogen, and the population at risk.

5. For many poorly prepared countries, *surge capacity often is delivered by foreign aid providers*, who may not be available in a global pandemic. This must be factored in when planning local pandemic mitigation.

These five strategies have been well established for decades. These measures were even instituted in the influenza pandemic of 1918. Mistakes were made then, as they were now.

However, one has to question why after a century, many of the same mistakes were made by our supposedly advanced healthcare system. To answer that question, we first should look at the positives our healthcare system did provide. First, we were able to produce multiple vaccines at "warp speed". The remarkable scientific achievement was unprecedented in history. The lives saved were a reflection of the ingenuity and skill of those research scientists acting unabated with essentially unlimited resources. Science prevailed.

Unfortunately, not everyone understood the benefit of the vaccines. The death rate in areas where the population was vaccinated with at least one dose and an additional booster was one quarter that of the non-vaccinated areas. This was a sad reflection of a socio-political bias imparted by ignorance and partisanship [26].

The public tried to ignore misinformation and follow health guidelines. The authors, it must be noted, have avoided any political debate in this chapter. It is for political scientists and historians to analyze and evaluate the effects that politics had on the governmental and public response to the pandemic. However, it is obvious, when speaking of public health measures, and vaccination for that matter, that information and adherence to guidelines, was inconsistently accepted and applied [27].

And lastly in the "plus" column, the healthcare workers of the United States truly stepped up when they were called upon. Through a crisis filled with uncertainties and mortal risk, these workers put their own safety aside and cared for an avalanche of patients with incredibly complex disease, many of whom were doomed from the moment of their admission to hospital. These heroes deserve a special salute for their efforts they exhibited, and the price, sometimes paid for dedication with their lives. We would be remiss if we did not note their remarkable commitment.

8. Conclusion: what now and in the future

There are many questions that remain from the pandemic that need to be answered. Will COVID-19 again mutate into a more virulent form and again cause widespread deadly disease? At the time of this writing, the virus still is causing approximately 200–300 deaths per day [28]. How often do we need to be vaccinated and will new vaccines be more effective at preventing a broader spectrum of viral illness? Why do a certain group of people develop long-term systems and how do we treat them? And, returning to our most critical question, will new animal-to-man transmitted pandemic-causing viruses appear, and will we be ready?

Clearly, some of these questions do not have immediate answers. As far as animal-to-man viruses, scientists tell us that there are hundreds of such viruses with the potential to become another COVID-19 pandemic [29].

Although our founding fathers put certain responsibilities into the hands of the states to prevent the federal government from becoming dictatorial, expanding federal powers in a defined emergency would provide a more coordinated response to such an emergency. To accomplish this Congress would have to update the Public Health Service Act. This would have to include making federal government financial support in a crisis dependent on each state adhering to established federal guidelines as dictated by the CDC and the NIH. This would allow for a seamless response of the country to such an emergency while providing necessary support to economically weaker states. This would include a refurbishing of the public health system and authority, while decreasing costly and laborious litigation regarding those established guidelines [30].

This would at least be a first step in taking politics out of pandemic response and encourage states and the federal government to work in a coordinated fashion.

Scientists around the globe are relatively sure that another pandemic or catastrophic natural disaster is in our future. If we fail to acknowledge the lessons of the COVID-19 pandemic and move to rectify the shortcomings we evidenced in our handling of it, we are doomed to repeat our errors. Albert Einstein is attributed with the quote, "Insanity is doing the same thing over and over and expecting different results." This witticism, referred to by some as "Einstein Insanity", is especially on point when speaking of the COVID-19 pandemic and any natural disaster we face in the future.

Our failures can only be forgiven if we take steps to avoid the mistakes of the recent pandemic. Lessons learned from the COVID-19 pandemic include the need for a unified, coordinated approach across the country, addressing healthcare disparities, updating legislation, and preparing for future pandemics or natural disasters. The first such step should be the acceptance that a pandemic-type event is a national problem, controllable only if we have a unified, coordinated approach across the entire country. Epidemic disease is not a problem that can be treated by government officials and politicians alone but must have the best scientists and public health experts making recommendations that have a solid scientific basis in view of the facts. Another pandemic cannot be prevented. However, only our best efforts as a nation, like those demonstrated in World War II, will allow us to avoid millions of people dying. If we do not accept this premise, it is very possible that the next disastrous event will be even worse. By rectifying shortcomings, the United States can strive toward becoming a truly developed country with a robust public health infrastructure that prioritizes the health and well-being of all its citizens.

Notes

In memory of Dr. Michael Gottlieb PhD, 1944–2021, who previously published with us on pandemic preparedness.

Author details

Jeffrey S. Freed[1*], Hannah S. Jacobs-El[2], Soo Y. Kwon[3] and Ram Roth[1]

1 Icahn School of Medicine at Mount Sinai, New York City, USA

2 University of Virginia School of Medicine, Charlottesville, VA, USA

3 Obstetrics and Gynecology, Zucker School of Medicine, New York City, USA

*Address all correspondence to: jsfmd@aol.com

References

[1] United Nations Development Programme. Country insights. Human Development Reports. Available from: https://hdr.undp.org/data-center/country-insights#/ranks [Accessed: 2023]

[2] Branswell H. Who declares the coronavirus outbreak a pandemic. Scientific American. 2020. Available from: https://www.scientificamerican.com/article/who-declares-the-coronavirus-outbreak-a-pandemic/ [Accessed: June 9, 2023]

[3] Kates J, Michaud J. Ten numbers to mark three years of COVID-19. KFF. 2023. Available from: https://www.kff.org/coronavirus-covid-19/fact-sheet/three-years-of-covid-19/ [Accessed: 2023]

[4] Bayati M. Why is COVID-19 more concentrated in countries with high economic status? Iranian Journal of Public Health. 2021;**50**(9):1929-1929

[5] Klein Goldewijk K, Beusen A, de Vos M, van Drecht G. The HYDE 3.1 spatially explicit database of human induced land use change over the past 12,000 years. Global Ecology and Biogeography. 2011;**20**(1):73-86. DOI: 10.1111/j.1466-8238.2010.00587.x(pbl.nl). Jean-Noël Biraben, "Essai sur l'évolution du nombre des hommes", Population 34-1 (1979), 13-25 (p. 22) estimates c. 80 million in 2000 BC and c. 100 million at 1200 BC

[6] Fujimura SF. Purple death: The great flu of 1918. PAHO/WHO. Pan American Health Organization; 2007. Available from: https://www.paho.org/en/who-we-are/history-paho/purple-death-great-flu-1918 [Accessed: 2023]

[7] Byerly CR. The U.S. military and the influenza pandemic of 1918-1919. Public Health Report. 2010;**125**(Suppl 3):82-91

[8] Tumpey TM, Garcia-Sastre A, Mikulasova A, et al. Existing antivirals are effective against influenza viruses with genes from the 1918 pandemic virus. Proceedings of the National Academy of Sciences of the United States of America. 2002;**99**:13849-13854

[9] Morens DM, Taubenberger JK, Fauci AS. A centenary tale of two pandemics: The 1918 influenza pandemic and COVID-19. Part II American Journal of Public Health. 2021;**111**(7):1267-1272

[10] Madhav N, Oppenheim B, Gallivan M, Mulembakani P, Rubin E, Wolfe N. Pandemics: Risks, impacts, and mitigation. In: Jamison DT, Gelband H, Horton S, et al., editors. Disease Control Priorities: Improving Health and Reducing Poverty. 3rd ed. Washington (DC): The International Bank for Reconstruction and Development/The World Bank; 2017

[11] Perry J. The politics of economic insecurity in the covid-19 era. DISD. United Nations: Department of Economic and Social Affairs Social Inclusion. 2021. Available from: https://www.un.org/development/desa/dspd/2021/01/the-politics-of-economic-insecurity-in-the-covid-19-era/ [Accessed: 2023]

[12] Transforming our world: The 2030 agenda for sustainable development. United Nations: Department of Economic and Social Affairs. 2015. Available from: https://sdgs.un.org/2030agenda [Accessed: 2023]

[13] Mangiarotti S, Peyre M, Ahang Y, Huc M, Roger F, Kerr Y. Chaos theory applied to the outbreak of COVID-19: An ancillary approach to decision making in pandemic context. Epidemiology and Infection. 2020;**148**:e95

[14] Jones A, Strigul N. Is spread of COVID-19 a chaotic epidemic? Epub. 2021;**142**:110376

[15] Necesito IV, Velasco JMS, Jung J, Bae YH, Lee JH, Kin SJ, et al. Understanding chaos in COVID-19 and its relationship to stringency index: Applications to large-scale and granular level prediction models. PLoS One. 2022;**17**(6):e0268023

[16] Mishra BK, Keshri AK, Rao YS, Mishra BK, Mahato B, Ayesha S, et al. COVID-19 created chaos across the globe: Three novel quarantine epidemic models. Chaos, Soitons & Fractals. 2020;**138**:109928

[17] Zheng H, Bonasera A. Controlling the worldwide chaotic spreading of covid-19 through vaccinations. Journal of Modern Physics. 2022;**13**(01): 1-15. doi: 10.4236/jmp.2022.131001

[18] Fiorina MP. Retrospective Voting in American National Elections. New Haven: Yale University Press; 1981

[19] Rees-Jones A, D'Attoma J, Piolatto A, Salvadori L. Covid-19 changed tastes for safety-net programs. Published online 2020:1-22. doi: 10.3386/w27865

[20] Baccini L, Brodeur A, Weymouth S. The COVID-19 pandemic and the 2020 US presidential election. Journal of Population Economics. 2021;**34**(2):739-767

[21] Lewis T. How the U.S. pandemic response went wrong-and what went right-during a year of COVID. Scientific American. 2021. Available from: https://www.scientificamerican.com/article/how-the-u-s-pandemic-response-went-wrong-and-what-went-right-during-a-year-of-covid/

[22] Wallace, J, Goldsmith Pinkham, Schwartz, JL. Excess Death Rates for Republicans and Democrats During the Covid-19 Pandemic in NBER Working Paper Series Working Paper 3051. Available from: www.nber.org/papers/w30512

[23] Impact of opening and closing decisions in Alabama - Johns Hopkins. Johns Hopkins Coronavirus Resource Center. Available from: https://coronavirus.jhu.edu/data/state-timeline [Accessed: 2023]

[24] Welcome. World Health Organization. Available from: https://www.afro.who.int/ [Accessed: May 31, 2023]

[25] Jamison DT. Disease control priorities, 3rd edition: Improving health and reducing poverty. The Lancet. 2018;**391**:10125. DOI: 10.1016/s0140-6736(15)60097-6

[26] Mathieu E, Roser M. How do death rates from covid-19 differ between people who are vaccinated and those who are not? Our World in Data. 2021. Available from: https://ourworldindata.org/covid-deaths-by-vaccination [Accessed: 2023]

[27] Nelson T, Kagan N, Critchlow C, Hillard A, Hsu A. The danger of misinformation in COVID-19 crisis. Missouri Medicine. 2020;**117**(6):510-512

[28] Centers for Disease Control and Prevention. COVID Data Tracker. Atlanta, GA: U.S. Department of Health

and Human Services, CDC. 2023. Available from: https://covid.cdc.gov/covid-data-tracker

[29] Grange ZL, Goldstein T, Johnson CK, Mazet JAK. Ranking the risk of animal-to-human spillover for newly discovered viruses. Proceedings of the National Academy of Sciences of the United States of America. 2021;**118**(15):e2002324118

[30] Gusting LO, Wetter S. Fix the backlash against public health. Science. 2023;**379**(6639):1277

Section 3

The Power to Transform: Metrics and Leveraging Technology

Chapter 6

Perspective Chapter: Application of Environmental Epidemiology for Exposure and Health Risk Assessment

Belay Desye

Abstract

Environmental epidemiology seeks to understand how various external risk factors may cause or protect against disease, illness, injuries, abnormalities, or death. Environmental epidemiology evidences suggested that there is the links between COVID-19 pandemic and environmental exposures. Environmental epidemiology provide information that can contribute to rational decision-making and resource allocation by providing quantitative estimates of risks. The environmental health issues are increasing attention and emerging globally, thus raising the environmental epidemiology concept as preventive medicine. Exposure can be assessed by using direct and indirect method approaches. Exposure assessment is important for the identification, evaluation, and control of health risks in the workplace and in the general environment. Ingenstion, inhalation, and skin contact are the main pathways for individuals to be exposed to hazardous contaminants. Exposure to biological, physical, and chemical agents in the environment can cause a wide range of adverse health consequences. Health risk assessment is the process used to estimate the nature and probability of adverse health effects in the past, current, and in the future about certain pollutants. Health risk assessment is conducted in accordance with hazard identification, dose–response assessment, exposure assessment, and risk characterization. Carcinogenic and non-carcinogenic risk assessments are used to estimate health effects due to exposure to pollutants.

Keywords: health risk, exposure, environmental epidemiology, pollutants, risk assessment

1. Introduction

Environmental epidemiology is concerned with determining how environmental exposures (physical, biological, and chemical factors) affect human health [1]. It seeks to understand how various external risk factors may cause or protect against disease, illness, injuries, abnormalities, or death. These factors may be due to natural occurring or anthropogenic. Currently, environmental health issues are increasing attention in the public, media, and government, thus raising the environmental epidemiology concept as a preventive medicine. WHO reported that 1.4 million deaths per year in Europe are due to avoidable environmental exposures [2].

The environmental evidences suggested that environmental exposures influence the severity and occurrence of COVID-19. Emerging evidences support the association of environmental exposures like air pollution, chemical exposures, climate, and the built environment and COVID-19 [3]. Environmental epidemiology can design a scientific-based mitigation strategy. It can communicate to the population about the potential advantage of control strategies by placing them in context of the hierarchy of control [4]. Environmental epidemiology requires refined and different skills to attain effectively across disciplines, implement appropriate designs and methods of analyses to identify causal relationships, and design appropriate interventions. If it is so, environmental epidemiology will continue to develop novel preventive strategies that improve the quality of life and save health care costs [5].

Environmental epidemiology is one of the main important tools used in environmental management decision-making process, development of environmental standards, and policy implementation owing to monitor and assess of environmental hazards in different settings, and quantify and estimate their health impact on the population at risk [6]. One of the founders of modern epidemiology, John Snow conducted the first environmental epidemiology study in 1854. He investigated that London residents who drink sewage-contaminated water were more likely to develop cholera than those who drink clean water [7].

The study in environmental epidemiology are most frequently observational in nature, in which the investigators can look at peoples exposures to environmental factors without intervening and then observes the patterns that emerge [8]. This is the fact that it is unfeasible to conduct an experimental studies of environmental factors in humans [9]. For example, an investigator cannot ask some of their study subjects to smoke cigarettes to see if they have poorer health outcomes then subjects who are asked not to smoke. Environmental epidemiology mostly used cohort, case–control, cross-sectional, and ecological studies [8].

Environmental epidemiologists often apply a set of criteria to decide the probability that an observed relationship between environmental exposure and health consequences is truly causal [10]. The criteria commonly used whether there is a causal relationship or not are determined using Bradford Hill criteria [11]:

- Strength of association: the larger an association between exposure and disease, the more likely it is to be causal.

- Consistency of evidence: the same results if repeat in different time, place and person.

- Specificity of association: the exposure causes only one disease.

- Temporality: exposure precedes outcome.

- Biological gradient: the presence of a dose–response relationship supports the causal association between an exposure and an effect.

- Plausibility: reasonable pathway to link outcome to exposure.

- Coherence: the cause and effect story should make sense with all knowledge available to the researcher.
- Experiment: Occasionally it is possible to appeal to experimental evidence.
- Analogy: the use of analogies or similarities between the observed association and any other associations.

These criteria are generally considered a guide to scientists, and it is not necessary that all criteria be met for a consensus to be reached [10].

2. Exposure assessment in environmental epidemiology

Exposure is the contact between a stressor (physical, chemical, and biological agents) and receptor. The stressors may come from point, line, or area sources and reach the public by way of matrices of air, water, soil, and foods. Risk is a function of exposure and hazard. For instance, even for a high hazard (extremely toxic substance), the risk of an adverse outcome is unlikely if the exposures are near zero. On the other hand, a moderately toxic substance may present a substantial risk if an individual or a population is highly exposed [12].

Environmental exposures can be proximate exposure (directly leading to health conditions) such as physical, chemical, and microbiological agents, and distal exposure (indirectly leading to health conditions) such as, socioeconomic conditions, climate change and other broadly scale environmental issues. Proximate exposure occur through inhalation, ingestion, and skin contact. Whereas, distal exposure can cause adverse health issues directly by changing proximate exposures, and indirect through changes in ecosystems and other support systems for human health [13].

Exposure can be assessed by using direct and indirect methods. A direct method measure of exposure is the best measure for assessing the effect of a specific substance on the target population (e.g., biological markers and personal monitoring) [14]. A direct approach accounted the exposures through multiple media (air, water, soil, food, etc) for through one study technique. However, a direct method approach the data collection nature is invasive and need high costs. On the other hand, indirect method measures of exposure have greater utility for source emission assessment and control, since they are capable of linking population health to specific pollution emission sources (e.g., environmental monitoring, modeling, questionnaires, and diaries). To obtain good quality and much information, it is often useful to combine two or more methods. For example, personal exposure assessments are often associated with questionnaires and diaries, and may also include biomarker measurements [15, 16] as depicted in **Figure 1**.

Exposure assessments mainly focused on prevention. It is important to know who are exposed, source of exposure, route of exposure, levels, population with the highest risk, and health effects. The important aspects or main characteristics for the determination of exposure are the nature of the agent, the intensity of the exposure, the duration of the exposure, and the frequency of the exposure. Using these basic informations, it is possible to take appropriate measures to reduce the exposure. Exposure assessment is a complex process, involving many different professions, such as occupational hygienists, toxicologist, chemists, physicians, and environmental health professionals [17].

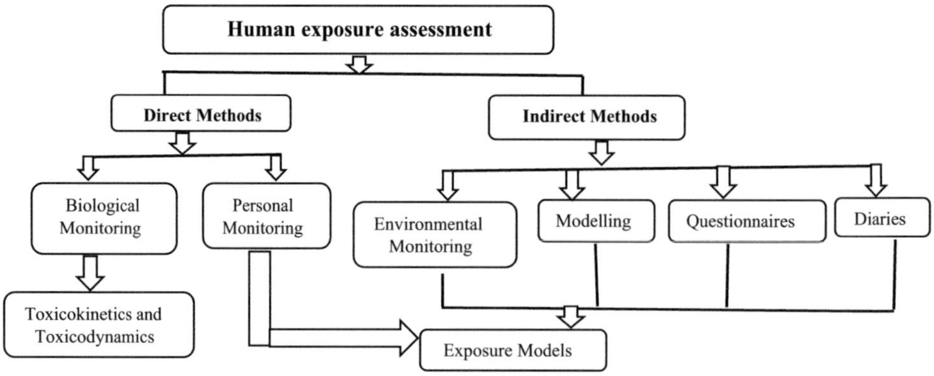

Figure 1.
Approaches to human exposure assessment methods adapted from [16].

Exposure assessment is important for the identification, evaluation, and control of health risks in the workplace and in the general environment. Ideally, it describes the sources, pathways, route, and uncertainties in the assessment. John Snow in the 1850s noted that the apparent association between the source of drinking water and the risk of dying from cholera. Although Snow was never able to see the cholera bacteria, he understood that the disease was caused by exposure to a disease causing agent in drinking water [7, 17].

In the 1950s and 1960s, the environmental exposure and health effects began. A time-series study indicated that a disease outbreaks associated with environmental pollution, such as the London fog episode due to sulfur dioxide and mercury poisoning Minamata disease in the general population of Japan and Iraq, drew attention to the relationship between environmental exposures and public health. This brought a renaissance to the realization of the significance of environmental factors for the development of diseases [17].

Exposure to biological, physical, and chemical agents in the environment can cause a wide range of adverse health consequences. For instance, heavy metal exposure through drinking water sources is a growing global concern [18]. Assessment of exposure is an important component of environmental epidemiology research. The estimation of exposure in relation to health effects is frequently difficult, and it has generally received inadequate attention. However, afield of exposure assessment is becoming an emerging issue [1, 19].

Appropriate measures of exposure can improve the ability of a study to assess adverse effects from environmental factors. Such improvements may improve the study quality and can reduce bias, but increase cost. The exposure analysis and health outcomes must be considered together to arrive at a balanced prioritization of study requirements. One of the major example achievements by environmental exposure assessment studies is possibly the decrease in lead (Pb) exposure in the general population due to the reduction of Pb in petrol and the introduction of unleaded petrol [17]. Therefore, an effective application of exposure assessment methods may improve the results of environmental epidemiology investigations.

Exposure to potential harmful agents may lead to a wide range of adverse health effects, ranging from dysfunction, discomfort, illness (morbidity) to death (mortality) [17, 20]. The relationship between source activity, exposure, and its effect on health is described in the environmental health hazard chain as depicted in **Figure 2**.

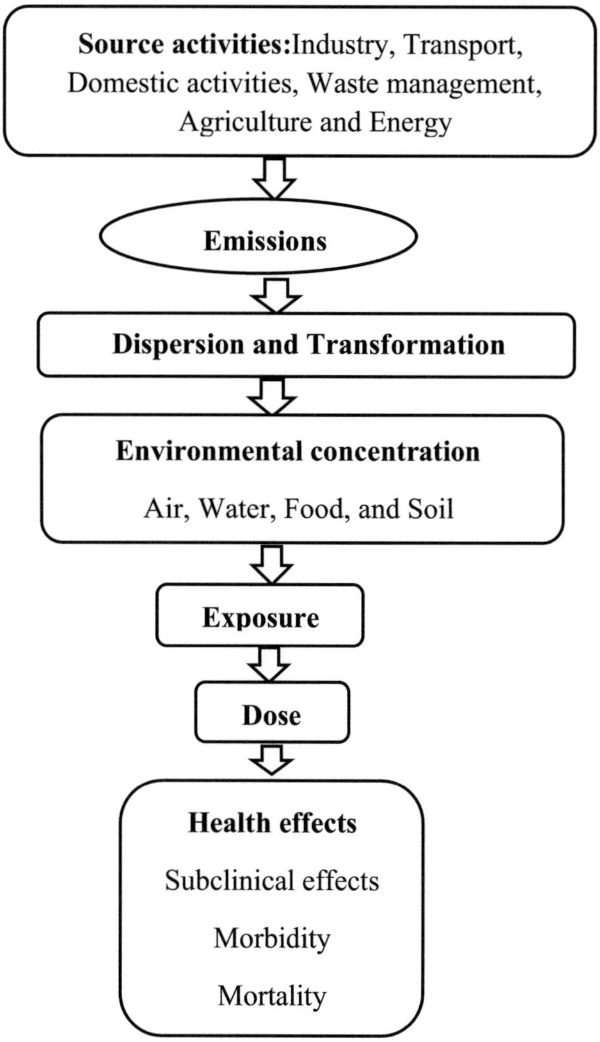

Figure 2.
The environmental health hazard chain adapted from [17, 20].

3. Health risk assessment in environmental epidemiology

Human health risk assessment is the process used to estimate the nature and probability of adverse health effects in people, groups of people, and communities, in the past, current, and in the future about certain pollutants [21]. Health risk assessment is usually carried out with a systematic approaches in response to public health concerns about the increasing incidence of health effects associated with environmental hazards due to the development of industries, urbanization, and agricultural activities [22]. Health risk assessment can provide objective scientific information and contribute to allocating resources to control exposures to environmental hazards and decision making by providing a quantitative estimation of risks [23]. However, human health risk assessment does not identify specific individuals who are exposed to a chemical, compare chemicals measured in individuals or groups of people to health outcomes, and diagnose disease.

A human health risk assessment is conducted in accordance with four steps according to United States Environmental Protection Agency (USEPA) [24]. Application of the process to different types of hazards will require different assumptions, models, and methods and these must be clearly stated at all steps.

1. **Hazard identification**: identifies adverse effects (e.g., birth defects, cancer) that might occur from exposure to a chemical or harmful agent.

2. **Dose–response assessment**: examine the quantitative relationship between exposure or dose and the probability of occurrence of adverse effects in a population (response) (described in **Figure 3**) [25], usually derived from animal toxicity tests. Some people may be more sensitive to a substance than others may. For example, children, elderlies, and peoples with existing medical conditions are more susceptible to potential hazards.

3. **Exposure assessment**: it is the process of estimating the magnitude, frequency, and duration of exposure to an agent, along with the number and characteristics of the population exposed. The main pathways for individuals exposed to hazardous contaminants are: ingestion, inhalation, and skin contact [26].

The human exposure to pollutants can calculate as follows accordingly Eqs. (1–4) which is adopted from the USEPA [24].

$$DED = \frac{\text{CxIRxEDxEFxCF}}{\text{BWxAT}} \tag{1}$$

Whereas,
DED = Daily Exposure Dose (mg/Kg-day).
C = concentration of substances, for water intake the unite C expressed in (mg/L).
IR = Intake Rate (m^3/day).
EF = Exposure Frequency (days/yr).
ED = Exposure Duration (yrs).
CF = Conversion Factor [10^{-6}].
AT = Average Time (days).
BW = Body Weight (Kg).
For oral ingestion:

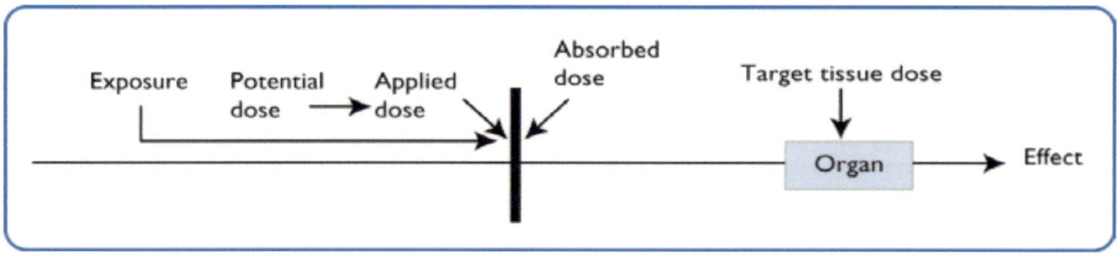

Figure 3.
Representation of dose and exposure adapted from US EPA [25].

$$I\left(\frac{\frac{mg}{Kg}}{\mathrm{d}}\right)=\frac{C\left(\frac{mg}{kg}\right)xAoFxIGR\left(\frac{mg}{d}\right)xEF\left(\frac{d}{yr}\right)xED(yr)xCF}{365(days\ in\ year)xAT(yr)xBW(kg)} \quad (2)$$

Whereas,
I = intake of substance (food, soil, water).
AoF = An oral abserction factor or bioavailability estimate (unitless).
IGR = Ingestion Rate, for water intake the unite IGR expressed in (L/d).
For inhalation of volatiles:

$$I=\frac{C\left(\frac{mg}{\mathrm{L}}\right)xIR\left(\frac{\mathrm{L}}{\mathrm{h}}\right)\mathrm{xLRxET}\left(\frac{\mathrm{h}}{\mathrm{d}}\right)xEF\left(\frac{\mathrm{d}}{yr}\right)}{365xAT(yr)xBW(kg)} \quad (3)$$

Whereas,
IR = Inhalation Rate; LR = Lung Retention factor (unitless); ET = Exposure Time.
For dermal contact with soil:

$$I=\frac{C\left(\frac{mg}{Kg}\right)xAH\left(\frac{\frac{mg}{cm^2}}{d}\right)xSA(cm^2)xAFxEF\left(\frac{d}{yr}\right)xED(yr)xCF}{365xAT(yr)xBW(Kg)} \quad (4)$$

Whereas,
AH = Soil adherance; SA = Surface area of skin exposed; AF=Skin absorption factor.

4. **Risk characterization**: it is the integration of information on hazards, exposure, and dose response to provide an estimate of the likelihood that any of the identified adverse effects will occur in exposed people. Risk characterization requires transparency, clarity, consistency, and reasonableness. Risk characterization brings together all information from earlier steps to describe the risks to different categories.

According to Zhao et al. [27] and Ma et al. [28], children are highly exposed to heavy metals than adults due to their physicochemical characteristics (higher comparative uptake, but lower toxin elimination rates). For example, children are usually more susceptible to a given hazardous substance and likely ingest significant quantities of soil due to their finger sucking behavior and exposure via breast-feeding and placental exposure, which are generally used as the main pathways of exposure for soil metals in children.

Carcinogenic and non-carcinogenic risk assessments are used to estimate health effects due to exposure to pollutants. The non-carcinogenic risk was estimated in terms of Hazard Quotients (HQs) for the elements and exposure routes using Eq. (5). The sum of all HQs is expressed as Hazard Index (HI) Eq. (6). If HQ or HI is found to be >1, there is a chance that a non-carcinogenic health effect may occur. In contrast, if HQ or HI is found to be <1, the exposed individual is unlikely to experience adverse health effects [24].

The Carcinogenic Risks (CR) are estimated by calculating the incremental probability of an individual developing cancer over a lifetime due to exposure to a potential carcinogen using Eqs. (7) and (8) [24]. Slop Factor (SF) converts the estimated daily intake of a toxin average over a lifetime of exposure, directly to the incremental risk of an individual and the risk of an individual developing cancer. For regulatory purposes, the level of acceptable cancer risk is considered $1x10^{-4}$ to $1x10^{-6}$ [29, 30].

These parameters were calculated using the following equations:

$$HQi = \frac{CDI}{RFD} \tag{5}$$

$$HI = \sum HQI \tag{6}$$

$$CRi = CDI \text{ x } SF \tag{7}$$

$$CR = \sum CRi \tag{8}$$

Whereas, CDI=Chronic Daily Intake, RFD = Reference Dose, HQi = Hazard Quotients, HI = Sum of Hazard Quotient, CR = Carcinogenic Risk, and SF = Slope Factor.

An example is how environmental epidemiology studies in health risk assessment, a study conducted in Czech Republic on potentially toxic elements pollution in agricultural soil health risk assessment revealed that of the total sample locations 6.04% non-carcinogenic and 13.05% carcinogenic to children [31]. According to Oyola et al. [32] exposure to polluted sediments through incidental ingestion and dermal contact routes was the highest risk for receptors. Another study revealed that girls were more susceptible than boys to trace metal pollutants for both carcinogenic and non-carcinogenic risk [33].

4. Conclusions

Environmental epidemiology is one of the main important tools used in the environmental management decision-making process. Environmental health issues are increasing attention and emerging globally. Exposure assessment is important for the identification, evaluation, and control of health risks in the workplace and in the general environment. Exposure to biological, physical, and chemical agents in the environment can cause a wide range of adverse health consequences. Health risk assessment is the process used to estimate the nature and probability of adverse health effects in the past, current, and in the future about certain pollutants. It is usually carried out in response to public health concerns about the increasing incidence of health effects linked to changes in environmental conditions. An effective application of exposure assessment methods may improve the results of environmental epidemiology investigations.

Author details

Belay Desye[1,2]

1 Department of Public Health, College of Medicine and Health Sciences, Adigrat University, Adigrat, Ethiopia

2 Department of Environmental Health, College of Medicine and Health Sciences, Wollo University, Dessie, Ethiopia

*Address all correspondence to: belaydesye.2001@gmail.com

References

[1] Merrill RM. Environmental Epidemiology : Principles and Methods. Sudbury, MA: Jones and Bartlett Publishers; 2008

[2] WHO. Ostrava Declaration on Environment and Health. 2018. Available from: www.euro.who.int

[3] Sly PD, Trottier BA, Bulka CM, Cormier SA, Fobil J, Fry RC, et al. The interplay between environmental exposures and COVID-19 risks in the health of children. Environmental Health. 2021;**20**(1):34

[4] Nc D, Jg A, Ptj S, Ji L. The COVID-19 pandemic: a moment for exposure science. Journal of Exposure Science & Environmental Epidemiology. 2020;**30**(4)

[5] Tonne C, Basagaña X, Chaix B, Huynen M, Hystad P, Nawrot TS, et al. New frontiers for environmental epidemiology in a changing world. Environment International. 2017;**104**: 155-162

[6] Bert B. Environmental epidemiology and risk assessment. Toxicology Letters. 202;**180**:118-122

[7] John S. Mode of Communication of Cholera (John Snow, 1855). [cited 2022 May 11]. Available from: http://www.ph.ucla.edu/epi/snow/snowbook.html

[8] Principles of Epidemiology: Home|Self-Study Course SS1978|CDC. 2021 [cited 2022 May 12]. Available from: https://www.cdc.gov/csels/dsepd/ss1978/index.html

[9] Gordis L. Epidemiology. 4th ed. Published by Saunders; January 1, 1994. Available from: https://www.amazon.com/Epidemiology-4th-Leon-Gordis/dp/1416040021

[10] Evelyn O, Talbotte GF. An Introduction to Environmental Epidemiology. 1st Published by CRC Press; 1st ed. September 30, 1995. Available from: https://www.routledge.com/An-Introduction-to-Environmental-Epidemiology/Talbott-Craun/p/book/9780873715737

[11] Hill AB. The environment and disease: Association or causation? Proceedings of the Royal Society of Medicine. 2022;**58**:295

[12] Paul Wilkinson. Environmental Epidemiology (Understanding Public Health). 1st ed. Published by Open University Press; March 1, 2006. Available from: https://www.amazon.com/Environmental-Epidemiology-Understanding-Public-Health/dp/0335218423

[13] Slikker WJ, Chang LW. Handbook of Developmental Neurotoxicology. 1st ed. Elsevier Inc; July 8, 1998. Available from: https://www.elsevier.com/books/handbook-of-developmental-neurotoxicology/slikker-jr/978-0-12-648860-9

[14] Langley A, Van Alphen M. Australia, South Australian Health Commission, Commonwealth Environment Protection Agency (Australia). In: The health risk assessment and management of contaminated sites: Proceedings of the Second National Workshop on the Health Risk Assessment and Management of Contaminated Sites. Adelaide; 1993

[15] National Research Council. Exposure Science in the 21st Century: A Vision

and a Strategy. 2012. [cited 2022 May 11]. Available from: https://nap.nationalacademies.org/catalog/13507/exposure-science-in-the-21st-century-a-vision-and-a

[16] NRC. Human Exposure Assessment for Airborne Pollutants: Advances and Opportunities |The National Academies Press. [cited 2022 May 15]

[17] Järup L, Elinder CG, Berglund M, Organization WH. Human Exposure Assessment: An Introduction. World Health Organization; 2001 [cited 2022 May 11]. Report No.: WHO/SDE/OEH/01.3. Available from: https://apps.who.int/iris/handle/10665/70570

[18] Hauptman M, Bruccoleri R, Woolf AD. An update on childhood lead poisoning. Clinical Pediatric Emergency Medicine. 2017;**18**(3):181

[19] Baker D, Kjellström T, Calderon R, Pastides H, Team WHOO and EH, Agency USEP. Environmental Epidemiology: A Textbook on Study Methods and Public Health Applications [Internet]. World Health Organization; 1999 [cited 2022 May 11]. Report No.: WHO/SDE/OEH/99.7. Available from: https://apps.who.int/iris/handle/10665/66026

[20] HEADLAMP, Health WHOO of G and IE, Programme UNE, Agency USEP. Linkage Methods for Environment and Health Analysis : General Guidelines : A Report of the Health and Environment Analysis for Decision-Making (HEADLAMP) Project. World Health Organization; 1996 [cited 2022 May 11]. Report No.: WHO/EHG/95.26. Available from: https://apps.who.int/iris/handle/10665/62988

[21] U.S. Environmental Protection Agency (US EPA). Risk Assessment Guidance for Superfund (RAGS): Part A. 2015 [cited 2022 May 11]. Available from: https://www.epa.gov/risk/risk-assessment-guidance-superfund-rags-part

[22] Zawide F. Application of environmental epidemiology in health impact assessment process. Epidemiology. 2006;**17**(6):S500

[23] ILA (International Lead Association). 2022 Available from: https://ila-lead.org/

[24] U.S. Environmental Protection Agency (US EPA). Risk Assessment Guidance for Superfund: Volume I. human Health Evaluation Manual (Part A). Washington, DC: Office of Emergency and Remedial Response; 1989

[25] U.S. Environmental Protection Agency (US EPA). Guidelines for exposure assessment. Federal Register. 1992;**57**(104):22888-22938

[26] U.S. Environmental Protection Agency (US EPA). National center for environmental assessment wd. Exposure Factors Handbook (1997, Final Report). [cited 2022 May 15]. Available from: https://cfpub.epa.gov/ncea/risk/recordisplay.cfm?deid=12464

[27] Zhao L, Xu Y, Hou H, Shangguan Y, Li F. Source identification and health risk assessment of metals in urban soils around the Tanggu chemical industrial district, Tianjin, China. Science Total Environment. 2014;**468**:654-662

[28] Ma J, Pan LB, Wang Q, Lin CY, Duan XL, Hou H. Estimation of the daily soil/dust (SD) ingestion rate of children from Gansu Province, China via hand-to-mouth contact using tracer elements. Environmental Geochemical Health. 2018;**40**(1):295-301

[29] Li Z, Ma Z, van der Kuijp TJ, Yuan Z, Huang L. A review of soil heavy metal

pollution from mines in China: pollution and health risk assessment. Science Total Environment. 2014;**15**:468

[30] Liu X, Song Q, Tang Y, Li W, Xu J, Wu J, et al. Human health risk assessment of heavy metals in soil-vegetable system: A multi-medium analysis. Science Total Environment. 2013;**463**:530-540

[31] Agyeman PC, John K, Kebonye NM, Borůvka L, Vašát R, Drábek O, et al. Human Health Risk Exposure and Ecological Risk Assessment of Potentially Toxic Element Pollution In Agricultural Soils in the District of Frydek Mistek, Czech Republic: A Sample Location Approach. 2021. [cited 2022 May 11]; Available from: https://pubag.nal.usda.gov/catalog/7598570

[32] Jiménez-Oyola S, Escobar Segovia K, García-Martínez MJ, Ortega M, Bolonio D, García-Garizabal I, et al. Human health risk assessment for exposure to potentially Toxic Elements in Polluted Rivers in the Ecuadorian Amazon. Water. 2021;**13**(5):613

[33] Rahman MA, Islam MR, Kumar S, Al-Reza SM. Drinking water quality, exposure and health risk assessment for the school-going children at school time in the southwest coastal of Bangladesh. Journal of Water, Sanitation and Hygiene for Development. 2021;**11**(4):612

Chapter 7

Contribution to the Management of Toxicological Risks in Burkina Faso: Design Process and Implementation Strategies for a Clinical Toxicology Laboratory

N. Stanislas Dimitri Meda, Normand Fleury, Ciprian M. Cirtiu, Vincent Cirimele, Cheick Armand N. Palm and Elie Kabre

Abstract

In Burkina Faso, toxicological risks have increased for more than a decade, with the irrational use of chemicals in agri-food and mining activities, as well as the consumption of psychoactive substances (PAS); and are now a public health problem. This situation has led to the establishment of a clinical toxicology laboratory, which now contributes to the diagnosis of poisoning and the prevention of risks to the health of populations through toxicological biomonitoring. The development of this initiative required a proactive approach adapted from the "interconnected chain" innovation process. The creation of a unit called the "Toxicological Analysis and Expertise Service" or "SAET" at the National Public Health Laboratory of Burkina Faso or "LNSP" is the main result of this innovative initiative in Burkina Faso's health system. If this laboratory now has a certain technical capacity or expertise, it must be strengthened through the acquisition of the additional equipment necessary to increase the supply of expertise. To do this, the strengthening of technical and financial collaborations is essential for the improvement of health security in Burkina Faso in particular and in the world in general.

Keywords: toxicology laboratory, laboratory project, innovation, SAET, LNSP

1. Introduction

For more than 50 years, the world has known about an extension of chemical products (pesticides, industrial products, drugs, dangerous products for domestic use, psychoactive substances, etc.) and their use in several fields of activity. According to the United Nations Environment Program (UNEP), international sales of chemicals would increase by around 3% per year until 2050 and there would have been an average increase of 40% in chemical production between 2012 and 2020 for Africa and the Middle East [1]. This is why the International Program on Chemical Safety (IPCS) has been in place since 1980 to assess the risks to human health and the environment that will be increasingly exposed to chemicals [2].

Indeed, man and the environment are exposed to these chemical substances, in various circumstances and to varying degrees, which can cause them acute or chronic damage. These toxic effects, which are more prevalent in the field of public health, must be subject to special monitoring [2, 3].

In addition, the chemicals to which the population may be exposed differ from one country to another, from one region to another, from one profession to another, etc. Thus in Burkina Faso, the chemical risks to which the population is exposed are mainly linked to the use of pesticides and mercury and/or cyanide, respectively, in agriculture and mining [4–10]. To these risks is added the increased consumption of psychoactive substances (PAS), specifically illicit drugs, and adulterated alcohols [6, 11–13]. As a result, the Ministry of Health of Burkina Faso is increasingly challenged by the population to deal with these ever-growing toxicological risks [14].

In order to contribute to the management of toxicological risks, our initiative had the main goal of designing and developing a project (strategic plan) to set up a Clinical Toxicology Laboratory (CTL) in Burkina Faso, in order to strengthen the system of health on the one hand in the diagnosis of intoxications and on the other hand in the assessment of the toxicological risk by biomonitoring: research, identification and/or dosage of toxins in biological and/or environmental matrices [9, 12, 15–17].

Through this chapter, we want to share our experience on a strategic approach carried out for the development of toxicological analysis in Burkina Faso, especially in the clinical field, in order to contribute to the improvement of health safety. This chapter consists of three parts. The first part deals with the context of toxicological risks and their management in Burkina Faso, the second part will unfold our strategy to develop, that is to say all the elements of a laboratory project and finally the third part will take stock of the results obtained.

2. First part: context

A toxicology laboratory in general, and a CTL in particular, constitutes an essential structure in a health system, as it is capable of providing data on the exposure to toxic substances of a population living in a given environment. This information can contribute not only to the assessment of the extent of exposure of the general population to toxic substances, but above all to the implementation of a public health intervention process aimed at analyzing and reducing toxicological risks in the population (human and environmental biomonitoring).

For several decades, the health situation related to Burkina Faso toxicology has been quite worrying. The initiative for the establishment of a CTL at Burkina Faso was mainly induced by two important public health situations:

- obvious and increasingly high toxicological risks: the existence of chemical risks to which the population is exposed in several areas of activity today constitutes a public health problem in Burkina Faso;

- a fairly limited health system in the management of toxicological risks: the absence of a Poison Control Center (PCC) and the nonperformance of clinical toxicology analyses limit Burkina Faso's health system in the assessment and management of toxicological risks, including toxicological emergencies [18].

2.1 Main toxicological risks in Burkina Faso

The toxicological risks in Burkina Faso are essentially of a chemical nature. The chemicals most often involved are pesticides, mercury, cyanide, illicit drugs, medicines, lead, arsenic and petroleum products (hydrocarbons).

These risks are most often related to:

- the use of pesticides in the food industry,
- the use of mercury and cyanide in mining (modern and/or artisanal),
- the consumption of PAS (an increasingly common practice among the general population, especially among adolescents).

2.1.1 Use of pesticides in agriculture

In Burkina Faso, agriculture occupies a prominent place in the national economy. Producers use chemical substances (fertilizers, pesticides) to increase their production and/or fight against diseases and crop pests. This situation has been promoted through a national policy known as the "Support Program for Agro-Sylvo-Pastoral Sectors." This program was developed following the decrease in agricultural productivity and therefore food deficits linked to precarious climatic conditions and attacks by crop pests.

2.1.1.1 Toxicological risks linked to the use of pesticides

If pesticides are one of the factors of agricultural development, it is good to note that their inappropriate use could be a danger brought about on several levels:

- among users, including professionals in the phytosanitary industry, farmers and their families who are exposed to the toxicity of these products during crop [19] formulation or processing activities,
- among consumers of agricultural products: the exposure is linked to the presence of toxic residues in crop products
- in the environment through the spread of pesticides in the fields. Soils, air and some surrounding water points are contaminated with these products [3–5, 9, 16, 20].

2.1.1.2 Contribution of a toxicology laboratory

With these toxicological situations/risks on these targets (users, consumers and environment), what could a toxicology laboratory bring to Burkina Faso? Indeed, the search for pesticide residues in edible products (cereals, fruits, drinking water, etc.) is already carried out in Burkina Faso, in particular at the National Public Health Laboratory (NPHL [21, 22]). This expertise could be reinforced by highlighting markers of exposure and effects through analyses of biological matrices (blood, urine) in professionals exposed to these substances and possibly in consumers.

2.1.2 Use of mercury and cyanide in mining

In addition to the increasing use of pesticides in Burkina Faso, the mining "boom" experienced by the country (in Burkina Faso in 2009, gold became the first source of foreign currency, ahead of cotton) through mining modern and artisanal is one of the major sources of exposure to highly toxic chemical substances, in particular mercury (Hg) and cyanide, both for workers, the local population and for the environment [23].

2.1.2.1 Toxicological risks

Large quantities of cyanide and mercury have often been used in a relatively short time and for a small quantity of gold. According to a report submitted by the Ministry in charge of the environment, approximately 200 tons of cyanide was used to extract 600 kg of gold only over a period of one quarter and for a single modern mining site. And during the same period, mercury was used the most (due to 1 g Hg/g of gold for a daily exploitation of approximately 25 g of gold) in artisanal mining [23].

Besides other chemical substances, such as acids (sulfuric acid, nitric acid), hydrocarbons (for blasting) and detergents are also used.

The use of these products constitutes a major toxicological risk for these workers, particularly in small-scale mining sites where health and safety measures are not often observed [5–8, 10, 23]. Also, in view of the relatively large quantities and their poor exploitation, the use of these substances is a major source of environmental pollution (contamination of water, soil, vegetation, air, etc.) and a toxic risk for the surrounding population. Indeed, these substances after exploitation in the treatment of ores or any other purpose are dumped in nature and can be conveyed by dust and rainwater (contaminant of large surfaces, water of rivers, dams, etc.). Other toxins are often generated following chemical reactions produced or released through the grinding or crushing of minerals (cadmium, lead, etc.) [6].

Although it brings a plus to the national economy, mining is a source of several diseases and risks; and therefore, constitutes a public health problem in Burkina Faso today.

2.1.2.2 Contribution of a toxicology laboratory

Faced with the health risks associated with this activity, monitoring of exposed professionals, monitoring of populations living near mining sites and monitoring of environmental pollution levels (water, soil and air) by toxicological analyses are necessary. A national toxicological biomonitoring strategy should be put in place.

2.1.3 Consumption of psychoactive substances

The consumption of PAS has now become a real public health problem in Burkina Faso, with a strong negative socioeconomic impact [11, 13]. This phenomenon is reinforced by:

- a growing precariousness within the population, especially of its young fringe (unemployment, disorientation and despair), leads to delinquency and prostitution which rub shoulders with drugs and alcohol;

- doping in the workplace to increase performance: there is a high consumption of PAS in gold panning sites (where amphetamine is the most used, alone or in combination with other substances such as cannabis and alcohols) [6].

Thus, Burkina Faso, formerly a transit country for drug trafficking, has become over the years a consumer country, causing a resurgence of insecurity in the country (acts of crime, rape, terrorism, etc.) [24].

2.1.3.1 Risks and targets

The increase in the phenomenon of drug and alcohol consumption is nowadays the cause of several cases of acute intoxication, drug addiction and other diseases such as liver and heart damage, cancers among consumers, in particular youth.

These situations challenge not only the National Committee for the Fight against Drugs (CNLD), but also all the actors who can intervene in the fight against this scourge.

2.1.3.2 Contribution of a toxicology laboratory

To contribute actively fighting against this plague, a laboratory of toxicology may provide expertise in the identification or profiling of seized products and screening for PAS through biological analyses.

2.1.4 Other chemical risk situations in Burkina Faso

Some professionals are also exposed in their work environment to potentially toxic chemical substances. We can note:

- dispensers at gas stations (called commonly gas station attendants), mechanicians and painters are exposed to hydrocarbons (gasoline fuel):

If most pump attendants do not have appropriate personal protective equipment (PPE) during work and therefore are exposed to hydrocarbon vapors (fuel); mechanicians frequently use gasoline or kerosene to clean their hands at the end of the working day.

- People working in physicochemical analysis laboratories:

These workers, especially analysts, are exposed to chemical solvents and reagents in their work environment. Indeed, most of the premises are not only not suitable (lack of ventilation, confinement of the rooms), but above all are not well equipped (absence of extractor hoods or more often nonfunctional and do not have a vacuum cleaner).

There are very few studies related to the exposure of these professionals to chemical substances and insufficient application of the regulations on the prevention of risks among these professionals [25].

Biomonitoring of workers exposed to chemical substances in their workplace: worker follow-up.

2.2 Health management of toxicological risks in Burkina Faso

2.2.1 Situation of clinical toxicology analyses in Burkina Faso

With regard to the toxicological risks described above, cases of poisoning are recorded in health facilities; however, there is no Poison control center (PCC) and the clinical toxicology analyses are not sufficient to contribute to the effective management of these cases. This constitutes one of the difficulties encountered by medical practitioners relating to the prevention and treatment of poisonings. So only symptomatic treatments are most often applied for the care of poisoning victims.

Some studies report that cases of poisoning recorded in health facilities were due to drugs, pesticides and mercury; but these studies had not been confirmed by the demonstration of the suspected toxins [4, 26–28]. However, toxicological analysis (qualitative and/or quantitative) could provide diagnostic, prognostic and even therapeutic interest in the management of emergency poisoning in hospitals.

The absence of a CTL does not make it easy to carry out biomonitoring analyses in the country. For example, biological data on a population of Burkina Faso, which we have noted in the literature, come from the laboratory of the "Institut Universitaire Romand de Santé au Travail (IST)" in Lausanne, Switzerland, relating to the dosage of urinary mercury in artisanal gold miners, carried out since 2006 [29]. Also, the dosage of lead, most often requested by mining companies, as part of the medical follow-up of workers, is subcontracted with laboratories in France. This practice is not compatible for emergency toxicology analyses (clinical and hospital), nor accessible for a large number of the population, because the delay in obtaining the results and the additional cost are not in favor of such an alternative.

There is therefore the need to set up a CTL in Burkina Faso, for a major contribution to occupational health and safety, through the assessment and monitoring of certain professionals exposed to toxic substances in their workplace through worker biomonitoring.

2.2.2 Clinical toxicology analyses carried out in Burkina Faso

These analyses are rare in Burkina Faso's health system, both at the level of public and private structures. Before 2015, only certain private clinics carried out urine screening tests for psychoactive substances (PAS) (illicit drugs) using rapid diagnostic tests (RDTs). These clinics also carried out subcontracts for certain analysis requests (blood assay for lead) with international laboratories.

Since 2011, we have seen that several requests for toxicological expertise (hospital, forensic, legal and others) are increasingly addressed to the LNSP. However, the response to these requests is most often limited to this Ministry of Health reference structure for toxicological analyses, which was created in 1999. Some examples of requests for toxicological expertise, addressed to the "Direction de la toxicologie, du contrôle de l'environnement et de l'hygiène publique (DTCE/HP)" or Direction of Toxicology, environmental control and public health summarized in **Table 1**, reveal the limits of the LNSP relating to the toxicological expert opinions requested.

For the purposes of ensuring, on the one hand, the preservation of the health of workers and consumers, the diagnosis and management of poisonings and, on the other hand, the carrying out of forensic toxicology expertise, the setting up of a clinical toxicology unit proved necessary in Burkina Faso, hence the development of a

Domain	Expertise requested	Expertise offered	Observation
Hospital	Mercury blood test	None	Not done
	Blood lead test	None	Unrealized
	Drug and medication testing	None	Service offered limit
	Therapeutic follow-up: dosage of drugs in the blood	None	Not done
	Identification of unknown substances	Pesticide research	Service offered limit
Forensic	Detection of toxic substances in autopsy specimens: alcohol, drugs, carbon monoxide or carbon dioxide	None	Not done
Judicial	Identification of a product Determination of the chemical profile of suspicious substances	Pesticide research	Service offered limit
	Determination of the toxicity of a product	None	Not done
Others	Identification of unknown substances	Pesticide research	Service offered limit
	Verification of the composition of certain building materials	Analysis based on documentary research	Service offered limit

Table 1.
Cases of toxicological analysis requests sent to the National Public Health Laboratory of Burkina Faso (LNSP) between 2011 and 2013.

project entitled "Contribution to the improvement of the health system in Burkina Faso: establishment of a clinical toxicology laboratory" [30].

2.3 Some literature review data on toxicological analysis in Burkina Faso

Through a literature review, we were able to note that most of the studies carried out in Burkina Faso on toxicology dealt with exposure factors, risks to the population or the environment linked to the use of chemicals in agri-food and mining activities, and the scourge of psychoactive substance consumption.

During the design phase of our project, we were unable to find an article dealing with clinical toxicology aspects, in terms of diagnosis or screening for intoxication, therapeutic follow-up of patients or toxicological biomonitoring of any population, through biological analyses carried out by a national laboratory. However, these studies alerted us to the existence, frequency and seriousness of these risks, with proposals for corrective and preventive measures.

Some documents dealing with toxicological risks for the population or the environment, occupational risks or risks linked to drug consumption in Burkina Faso are listed in Appendix A (**Tables A1–A3**).

However, other toxicological analyses, apart from clinical toxicology, have long been carried out in certain health facilities and university and/or research training courses. These include the LNSP, a reference health facility of the Ministry of Health, one of whose technical departments is responsible for carrying out toxicological analyses; the Institut de Recherche en Sciences de la Santé (IRSS) and Université Joseph KI ZERBO, where fundamental research in toxicology is carried out; and private health facilities that subcontract certain analysis requests to international laboratories (lead blood assay).

Significance and contribution of a clinical toxicology laboratory

A. Why a clinical toxicology laboratory in Burkina Faso

- High chemical risks in several areas of activity
- Limited health system: absence of a poison control center (PCC) and insufficient clinical toxicology analyses.

    1. Main chemical risk situations in Burkina Faso
        - Poor practice and use of pesticides in the cultivation and preservation of foodstuffs
        - Intensification of artisanal mining with the use of cyanide and mercury
        - Consumption of alcohol and drugs by young people
        - Exposure of workers to chemicals: solvents and laboratory reagents, hydrocarbons, etc.
    2. Health management of toxicological risks in Burkina Faso
        - Absence of a poison control center
        - Limited analytical capacity in clinical toxicology
        - Insufficient treatment for poisoning
        - Increase in urgent requests for toxicological analysis

B. Potential contribution of the clinical toxicology laboratory

- Improved diagnosis and management of poisoning
- Improvement in the therapeutic follow-up of patients
- Implementation of biomonitoring systems for exposed populations
- Improvement in forensic toxicology expertise: search for causes of death.

3. Second part: our project

In our project to develop a clinical toxicology laboratory, we have set goals to achieve.

The aim was to "contribute to strengthening Burkina Faso's health system by setting up a clinical toxicology laboratory". The achievement of this objective aims to make up for the shortcomings of Burkina Faso's health system in the management of toxic risks. Indeed, there is a great insufficiency in national analytical data, especially clinical data to provide evidence-based decision-making. So chronologically, three specific objectives have been set for the realization of the project:

- develop the necessary strategies for setting up a toxicology laboratory in Burkina Faso,
- strengthen the technical capacities necessary for the activities of the toxicology laboratory, and
- ensure the efficient functioning of the laboratory by carrying out clinical toxicology analyses

3.1 Design process

Our methodological approach or design process followed a proactive design process through the adaptation of acquired knowledge and the development of collaboration with several actors.

Data collection was carried out in parallel with the strategic actions developed over 4 years (2012–2015). This very often required readjustments and/or additions, reframing according to the evolution of the situation and the strategic actions carried out.

The development of the project took place in two phases:

- initially in Burkina Faso, a documentary review, exchanges with potential collaborators (industrial partners, reagent suppliers, medical practitioners, etc.) and observations on inappropriate practices or the misuse of chemicals made it possible to describe the country's health situation in toxicology,
- second in Québec (Canada), thanks to training in toxicological expertise at the Quebec Toxicology Center (CTQ) of the National Institute of Public Health of Quebec (INSPQ) (this is one of the major strategic actions of the development of our initiative), as well as interviews with partners (industrialists, suppliers, potential customers, researchers, and the like), we were able to identify and estimate the needs adapted to the context of Burkina Faso for setting up the laboratory.

By comparing our approach to those of many innovation process models described in the literature, our action strategy for setting up the clinical toxicology laboratory seems best suited to the "interconnected chain" innovation model by S. Kline and N. Rosenberg [31–33].

This is an "open" type approach to the innovation process, because technical and financial collaborations were established not only during the development of the project, but also for the implementation of the other planned actions [34–36]. With regard to collaboration, the following supports can be noted:

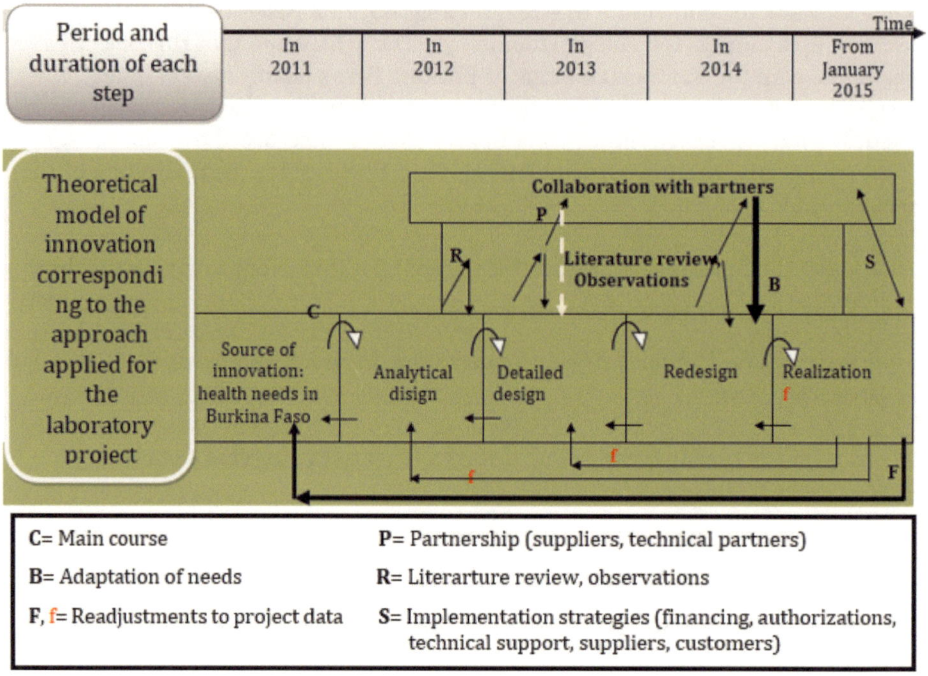

Figure 1.
Diagram adapted from the interconnected chain (S. Kline and N. Rosenberg) for the development of a clinical toxicology laboratory (CTL).

- support from the "Programme Canadien des Bourses de la Francophonie" (PCBF) or Canadian Francophonie Scholarship Program for training and project design,
- the technical support of the CTQ (INSPQ) during the design and implementation of the project,
- technical support of ChemTox in Strasbourg in France during the design, in particular on the identification and estimation of the appropriate technical needs, and
- collection of information from industrial partners specializing in the production and distribution of equipment suitable for a toxicology laboratory during design: this information is mainly related to the availability and costs of equipment.

Figures 1 and **2** summarize through this diagram our design approach and the strategic actions carried out: "Strategic approach adapted to the interconnected chain innovation model (S. Kline and N. Rosenberg, 86) for the initiative to set up a Clinical Toxicology Laboratory in Burkina Faso".

3.2 Strategies' implementation

3.2.1 Duration, orientations and planned actions

3.2.1.1 Duration

The development of the initiative is split into two phases:

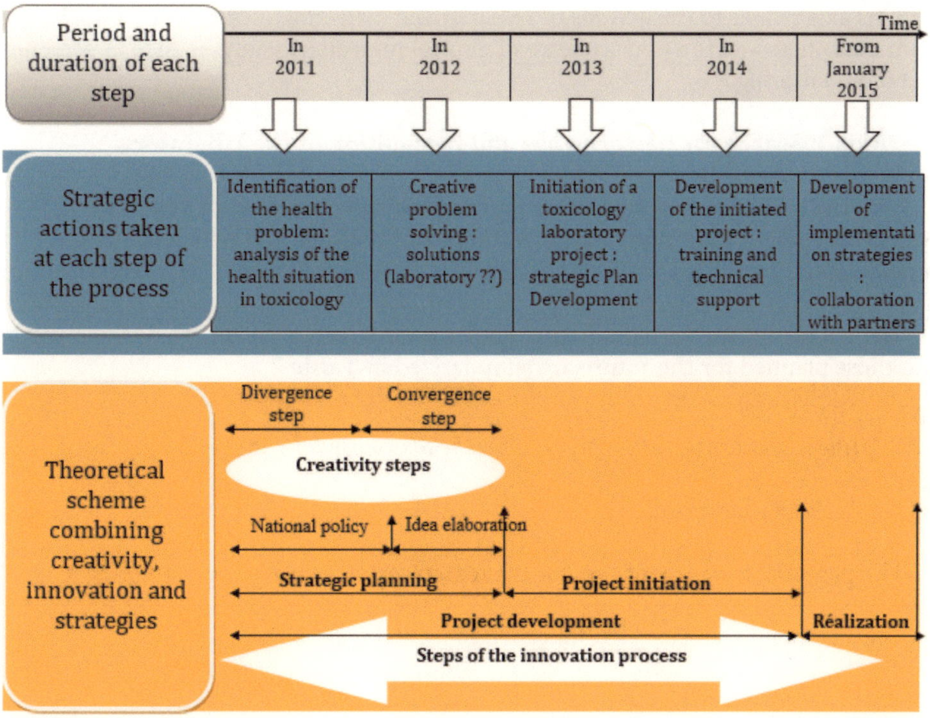

Figure 2.
Creativity and innovation combination scheme and strategic actions taken.

- Phase 1: Design phase (needs assessment) and project development (search for funding and technical partnerships);

- phase 2: Installation and operation of the laboratory.

The duration of phase 2 is planned for 5 years; however, its start depends on the end of phase 1 with the creation and obtaining of the necessary financing.

3.2.1.2 Strategic directions

For an effective implementation of the CTL, three main axes have been identified from which strategic actions have been defined:

- **Axis 1: Creation of the laboratory**

It focuses first on obtaining legal and administrative authorizations (administrative formalities, technical agreements) and second on strengthening technical capacities (financial resources (financing agreements), material (construction and fitting out of premises, acquisition of equipment, materials, reagents, etc.) and human (assignment and/or recruitment of personnel, training of assigned personnel, and so on).

- **Axis 2: Carrying out toxicology analyses**

This axis relates to the actions of research and collection of samples for analysis from customers and the performance of clinical toxicology analyses such as screening and biomonitoring.

- **Axis 3: Search for performance and recognition of the laboratory**

This last axis concerns the establishment of an effective quality assurance system with participation in interlaboratory test programs and which will be supplemented by the search for accreditation, the ultimate goal of any reference laboratory.

The main strategic actions already implemented during the design of the project and those planned for the future are summarized in **Table 2**.

3.2.2 Missions and organization planned for the toxicology laboratory

3.2.2.1 Potential assignments

The potential assignments set for the toxicology laboratory are as follows:

- ensure analyses related to clinical and hospital toxicology;

- provide analyses related to occupational and environmental toxicology: biomonitoring;

- provide forensic analyses and expertise related to forensic toxicology; and

- carry out any other activity related to toxicological expertise: research, biomonitoring and epidemiological studies.

3.2.2.2 Technical organization and potential activities of the laboratory

According to the missions mentioned above, potential customers and development prospects (future vision) on the one hand and according to the health context in Burkina Faso on the other hand, the toxicology laboratory can be organized into several technical sections [37].

Five sections have been planned in the project. These are:

- a section "reception and collection" of samples;

- a "clinical and hospital analytics" section;

- a section "analytical environment / Occupational Health and Safety (OHS)";

- a "Research and innovation" section; and

- "Quality Assurance" section.

Table 3 describes the attributions of the different technical units that have been defined, according to certain fields of application of analytical toxicology.

Execution phase	Strategic axis	Shares
Phase 1: Development of the laboratory project	AXIS 1: Creation of the toxicology laboratory	• **Project design:** o Realization of a pilot study: prioritization of toxicological analysis needs o Assessment of appropriate and adapted needs o Research and collaboration with technical and financial partners (TFPs)
		• **Setting up the laboratory/creation:** o Search for the necessary authorizations and financing o Capacity building in infrastructure and material resources o Capacity building in human resources
Phase 2: Implementation or realization of the project	AXIS 2: Carrying out toxicological analyses	• **Research and collection of analytical samples** o Information of potential customers: health structures, industries, mines, Ministry of the environment, agriculture, World Organization Health (WHO), etc. o Initiation and development of biomonitoring projects with clients
		• **Realization of qualitative and quantitative analyses** o Screening for drugs, medicines in biological or nonbiological environment o Dosage of metals in biological matrices or not (mercury, lead, arsenic, etc.) o Research and dosage of pollutants in biological media (cyanide, pesticides)
	AXIS 3: Increase in performance and search for recognition	• **Implementation of an appropriate quality assurance program:** o Adapted quality assurance system (ISO 9001 and ISO 17025) o Participation in interlaboratory controls
		• **Accreditation search for the main analytical parameters:** o Organization of audits in collaboration with reference technical partners o Submission of application for accreditation to qualified structures

REMARK: Actions can take place concurrently.

Table 2.
The main strategic actions for the implementation of a clinical toxicology laboratory (CTL).

3.2.3 Service offers and potential beneficiaries

Different service offers had been targeted (**Table 3**). They could be:

- diagnosis in intoxication, screening in the context of the consumption of psychoactive substances, as well as the therapeutic follow-up of patients will be used for the benefit of health structures, the sports environment (doping control), customs services, mining companies national and/or subregional ... ,

Unit/section of activity	Orientation/activities
Reception and collection	Collecting, receiving, registering, sorting and distributing samples
Clinic and hospital	• Toxicological emergencies: diagnosis: detection/dosage of toxic substances in a biological environment or not • Therapeutic follow-up: dosing of drugs, in a biological environment • Judicial or nonjudicial requests: analysis of autopsy samples
Environment/ OHS	• Biomonitoring of workers: analysis of metals, pesticides, cyanide and solvents in biological matrices • Population biomonitoring: health surveys, projects
Research and innovation	• Judicial requisitions: • detection/dosage of toxins in biological or nonbiological matrices and • evaluation of the toxicity of a sample. • Epidemiological studies: health surveys (with other units) • Development of analytical methods • Training of staff and trainees
Quality assurance	• Implementation and development of a quality policy

Table 3.
Organization and potential fields of activity of the toxicology laboratory.

- toxicological biomonitoring and health surveys planned as part of public health studies and/or health programs for the benefit of the authorities, national and international organizations for the promotion of health and the protection of the environment (World Organization Health (WHO), United Nations Environment Program (UNEP), International Labor Organization (ILO), etc.)

- forensic medical expertise for the benefit of forensic doctors and judicial police officers (JPOs).

NB: Diagnosis, screening and follow-up therapeutic will be the category of the most frequent service offer with regard to the absence of PCC and requests for analyses from health practitioners in the context of the management of poisoning. Health structures and societies mining should be the greatest beneficiaries of the activities of the toxicology laboratory.

The analytical parameters targeted for these different offers have been identified according to the toxicological risks identified. The potential target parameters that may be set depending on the type of service are summarized in **Table 4**.

3.2.4 Needs identified for the establishment and operation of the laboratory

The needs identified within the framework of the clinical toxicology laboratory project relate essentially to technical needs, in particular human and material resources.

3.2.4.1 Needs in qualified human resources

Several categories of technical personnel are needed to effectively carry out the activities of a toxicology laboratory, the analysts being the most important. The technical profiles to be mobilized are technologists, chemists and toxicologists. Technologists (50% of the total laboratory workforce) and chemists or biochemist (25% of

Service offer	Settings of interest targeted	Devices
Screening and follow-up therapeutic	Illegal drugs	Organic and nonorganic
	Medications	Organic and nonorganic
	Alcohols	Organic and nonorganic
Biomonitoring	Arsenic	Organic and nonorganic
	Mercury	Organic and nonorganic
	Lead	Organic and nonorganic
	Pesticides	Organic
Health research and surveys	Any parameter possible in the laboratory	Organic and nonorganic
Forensic expertise	Any parameter possible in the laboratory	Organic and nonorganic

Table 4.
Service offerings and priority analysis parameters.

the total laboratory workforce) should be the most represented profiles. The toxicologists and the support staff (maintenance technician, equipment upkeep and cleaning staff) in reduced numbers (20% of the total laboratory staff) will have to supplement the number of technical staffs. The mobilization of this technical staff should be progressive, due to at least 50% of each profile the first 2 years and the rest the following years according to the planned duration of the project (i.e., 5 years).

3.2.4.2 Material resources requirements

Infrastructure and material needs (equipment, consumables, laboratory reagents) must be adapted to the planned toxicological analysis activities.

For infrastructure, it will be necessary that the constructions and fittings of the premises meet certain quality and safety standards. However, this should depend on the chosen implantation site.

The main needs of a laboratory are analytical instruments. These devices should be able to cover all the analytical parameters of interest. Chromatographs and atomic absorption devices are the most targeted (**Table 5**).

3.2.5 Budget estimate

The overall budget for all needs (human and material resources) and for operation for 5 years is estimated at United States Dollars (US$1,907,590 (**Tables B1–B5**)).

This budget covers five investment headings, each with a defined proportion in relation to the overall budget. The acquisition of analytical devices occupies the largest share of the overall budget with 57% (**Figure 3**).

The average annual investment is estimated at US$317,911.79 or about 17% of the total estimated budget. The fourth year of the laboratory establishment process should see the largest proportion of investment with approximately 93% of the overall budget (**Figure 4**).

Depending on the source of funding, the technical and financial partners (TFPs) could support the project up to about 30–40% of the overall budget.

Analytical technique	Device identified	Possible analytes	Estimated quantity	Expected vesting period
Immunochemistry	RSS II (+RDT drugs)	Drugs, medicines	1	Year 1
	Immunochemical automaton	Drugs, medicines	1	Year 1
Atomic absorption	CV-AAS: FIMS 100	Mercury	1	Year 2
	GF-AAS AAnalyst 600	Metals	1	Year 2
Chromatography	GC-MS	Drugs, medicines, pesticides, cyanide ...	1	Year 3
	HPLC-MS	Drugs, medicines, pesticides, cyanide ...	1	Year 4

CV-AAS, cold vapor atomic absorption spectrometry; FIMS, flow injection mercury system; GF-AAS, graphite furnace atomic absorption spectrometry; GC, gas chromatography; HPLC, high-performance liquid chromatography; MS, mass spectrometry; RSS, rapid slide scanner.

Table 5.
The main analytical devices identified and their acquisition scheme.

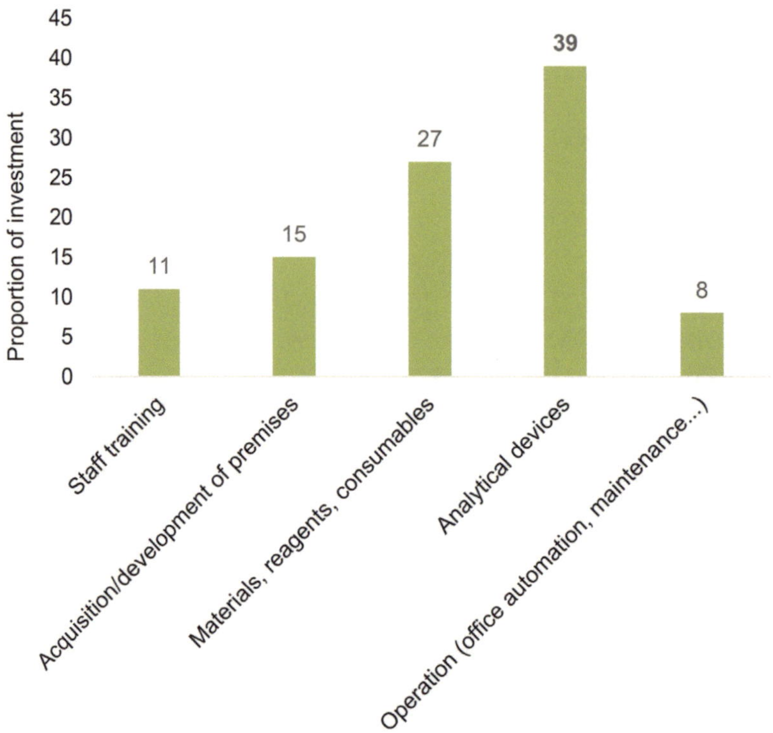

Figure 3.
Breakdown of the budget according to investment headings.

3.2.6 Determination of the location of the laboratory

There were several possibilities for setting up a clinical toxicology laboratory in Burkina Faso. Several hospitals and others can house this type of laboratory. However,

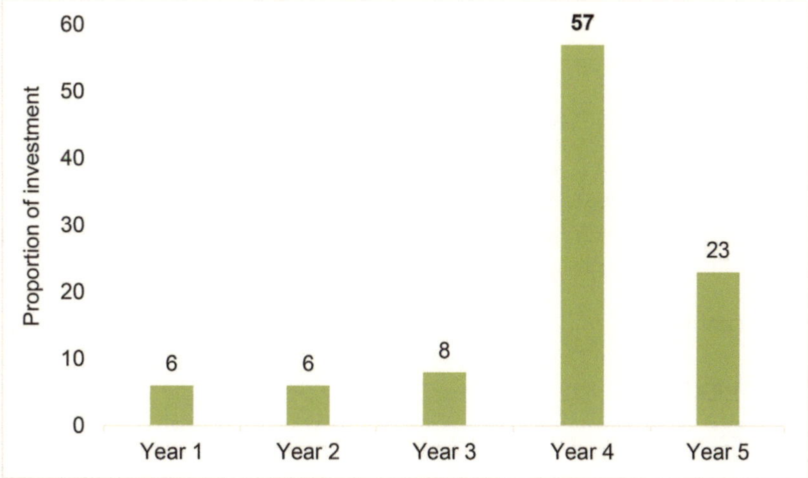

Figure 4.
Breakdown of the budget by year.

according to the existing analytical potential, the LNSP was the most favorable site of choice in terms of minimizing costs and reducing implementation times. During the development of the initiative, the LNSP already had the following assets:

- a relatively advanced technical platform (materials and devices available): Chromatographs (GC-MS, HPLC), biochemical analysis automaton,
- infrastructure and premises,
- a space available for possible construction of new premises,
- the missions of the clinical toxicology laboratory meet certain attributions or missions of the DTCE/HP of the LNSP,
- the clinical toxicology laboratory project is part of the LNSP's 2014–2018 strategic plan,
- the LNSP is the supervisory structure of the initiator of the project, having benefited from training at the CTQ for the establishment of the laboratory, and
- the project was already introduced to the authorities of the Ministry of Health for the creation.

3.2.7 Implementation constraints or risks for the project

The risks associated with the development of this project were the refusal or noncommitment of the health authority, the insufficiency or absence of the necessary funding. The lack of cooperation from potential customers (other health structures, mines, etc.) was also noted as an element that could slow down the progress of the implementation of the project.

To deal with these risks; mitigation measures had been planned, such as:

- the involvement of health authorities in the implementation, and of resource persons,
- the development of a financing and advocacy plan with financial partners according to their potential and orientations.
- developing a communication, information and awareness-raising plan for medical clinicians, mining companies and others, to incorporate toxicological analyses into their practices.

Project summary

A. Project objectives

- develop strategies for setting up a toxicology laboratory in Burkina Faso,
- strengthen the technical capacities necessary for the activities of the toxicology laboratory, and
- ensure the efficient functioning of the laboratory by carrying out clinical toxicology analyses

B. Methodological approach to main chemical risk situations in Burkina Faso

- Proactive approach, inspired by the "interconnected chain" innovation model of Kline and Rosenberg, 1986
- Design was carried out in two phases (in Burkina Faso and in Québec) based on documentary review, observations, training and interviews, from 2011 to 2015.

C. Implementation plan

- Two stages:
    - phase 1: design and development of the project and
    - phase 2: installation and operation of the laboratory.
- Three axes of strategic orientation
    - axis 1: creation of the laboratory,
    - axis 2: performing toxicology analyses and
    - axis 3: search for accreditation for the laboratory.

D. Organization and missions and projects for the laboratory

- Reception and sample collection section
- Clinical and hospital analytical section for analyses relating to clinical and hospital toxicology

- Environment/OHS analytical section for analyses relating to occupational and environmental toxicology: biomonitoring
- Research and innovation section for any other activity related to toxicological expertise: research, toxicovigilance and forensic expertise
- Quality assurance section for setting up quality systems.

E. Service offers and potential beneficiaries of the clinical toxicology laboratory

- Screening and therapeutic monitoring for health structures mainly
- Biomonitoring for health authorities and organizations, mines and industries
- Health studies and surveys for research institutes, authorities and health organizations
- Forensic medical expertise for judicial authorities and others.

F. Resources required

- Technical human resources required: technologist, chemist and toxicologist
- Necessary analytical equipment: chromatographs ++

G. Estimated budget

- Overall budget for 5 years: US$1 907 589,65
    - average annual investment US$317 911,79
    - thirty-nine percent of the overall budget to be invested in year 4
    - fifty-seven percent for analytical devices
- Potential sources of financing: TFPs identified (WHO, UNEP, ILO, etc.)
    - forty percent of the overall budget
    - proactive approach, inspired by the "interconnected chain" innovation model of Kline and Rosenberg, 1986
- Design carried out in two phases (in Burkina Faso and in Québec) based on documentary review, observations, training and interviews, from 2011 to 2015.

H. Choice of the laboratory site

- National Public Health Laboratory of Burkina Faso for its many potentialities:
    - o high-level technical platform: chromatographs and others available,
    - o infrastructure and premises available, and
    - o space available for possible construction of new premises

I. Implementation risks and mitigation measures

- Main risks:
    - o noncommitment of the health authority and
    - o insufficient or no necessary funding
- Main mitigation measures:
    - o involvement of health authorities in the implementation,
    - o development of a financing plan, and
    - o advocacy with financial partners for funding

4. Part three: project implementation status

The initiative to set up a CTL arose from our professional ambition to contribute to strengthening toxicological expertise in Burkina Faso. While the subject was being considered, this need was expressed by the Ministry of Health in an administrative note addressed to the LNSP, with the subject "assessment of the operational capacity of the National Public Health Laboratory in the field of environmental and clinical toxicology" [38]. While the LNSP was a benchmark for its technical capacity in environmental toxicology, in terms of water and soil monitoring and health aspects, this was not the case for clinical toxicology, for which we had just proposed setting up this expertise. This memorandum reinforced our initiative, which led to it being included as one of the key points in the National Public Health Laboratory's (LNSP) 2014–2018 strategic plan [39]. In addition to this, in response to this note from the Ministry of Health, the first draft of the initiative entitled "Projet de renforcement des capacités du Laboratoire national de sante publique en analyses toxicologiques: mise en place d'une Unité de toxicologie (UNITOX-LNSP)" or Project to strengthen the capacities of the National Public Health Laboratory in toxicological analysis: setting up a toxicology unit was submitted to it [40]. These were the first administrative actions that led to the creation of the STM, which later became SAET.

This part will deal with the inventory and the results obtained in the implementation of the clinical toxicology laboratory project. First of all, we will present the results of the implementation over the period of 5 years, that is to say from 2015 to 2019, then we will come to the difficulties encountered and finally the situation at the current state (2023) and prospects.

4.1 Implementation review

Toxicological Analysis and Expertise Service has become a national reference in toxicology, and above all in Burkina Faso's health system. Today, SAET is involved in a number of toxicological assessments. After 5 years of operation, we carried out an evaluation of SAET's performance, especially in the context of increasing demand. This evaluation, carried out in 2020, was intended to take stock of the current situation, assess the level of efficiency and define prospects for improvement.

Some of the data from this evaluation, which show the considerable contribution made by SAET at national level, are summarized in the following points.

4.1.1 Number of toxicological expertise requests received

The LNSP, through SAET, received and processed more than 238 requests for toxicological expertise between 2015 and 2019, of which 62% (n = 147) were of a judicial nature. These data were considered as a statistical basis of toxicological expertise needs in Burkina Faso, even if some data could not be recorded or dismissed for technical insufficiencies. We also noted that the number of requests each year gradually increased from 2015 (n = 39) to 2019 (n = 58). This situation could essentially be justified either by a wide dissemination of information on the availability of this toxicological expertise offer at LNSP or by a reinforcement and improvement in the quality of this service offer at LNSP.

4.1.2 Applicants for toxicological expertise

In 81.93% (n = 195) of cases, the main clients for toxicological assessments were public institutions. Among these, JPOs were strongly represented (over 70%). This situation may reflect the use of analytical solutions to JPO requests in the processing of legal cases. In addition, the number of recourses by private structures has gradually increased over the years, to exceed the frequency of recourse by public institutions in 2019 (62% private structures vs. 38% public structures). This considerable proportion of referrals from private facilities could be explained by the improvement in LNSP's technical offering through SAET's activities.

In addition, the Ministry of Health has progressively called on the SAET's expertise in the investigation of poisoning cases, particularly those of a collective nature that have occurred in recent years in the country.

4.1.3 Data on samples analyzed

Over 1650 samples were processed between 2015 and 2019, an average of 332 per year. These samples mainly included food, chemical, biological and pharmaceutical products, as well as substances of unknown nature.

Food products were the most represented (70%) of the samples analyzed. This was justified by the fact that food products were the most incriminated in cases of suspected poisoning or chemical submission, and in cases of involuntary intoxication.

SAET's various analytical reports on these samples led to the reinforcement of the monitoring system for food products, particularly those produced locally at national level [21, 41].

Biological samples, mainly urine and blood, are most often taken in response to requests for diagnosis in clinical toxicology, forensic toxicology (autopsy sampling) and occupational health and safety (mining company workers). In the latter field, SAET contributes to the screening and monitoring of PAS consumption by mining site professionals on an ongoing basis.

Pesticides, drugs and chemical screening were the main analyses carried out. Pesticides were identified as the main etiology of emergency intoxications with fatalities. In addition, for the same assessment period, a review of 194 samples submitted for drug testing revealed a positivity rate of 33.69% (n = 65), of which 80% concerned biological samples. Amphetamines and cannabinoids were the most frequently detected PAS.

4.1.4 SAET efficiency level

Through this study, we were able to note that 40% of the requests processed had provided a satisfactory analytical solution to the request submitted; i.e., precise guidance had been given to the requestor. These are situations in which, a causal relationship between exposure and the toxic effects observed in the intoxications had been established. In other cases, where the response was incomplete, the insufficiency was most often linked not only to the absence of certain materials (equipment, standards and reagents), but also to the low sensitivity and the low sensitivity and specificity of certain techniques and methods. Over the years, however, SAET has strengthened its technical capabilities through the introduction of new analytical methods, increasing the frequency of complete responses to over 52% in 2019. The assessment made in 2022 indicates that the level of efficiency is over 60% [24, 42–44].

To further boost efficiency, SAET should work on developing suitable methods with even lower detection limits, to detect as many toxic substances as possible in a sample. This could be achieved by implementing and exploiting certain chromatographic techniques (gas chromatography coupled-mass spectrometry (GC/MS)), liquid chromatography coupled-high-resolution mass spectrometry (LC/MS-MS) and inductively coupled plasma mass spectrometry (ICP-MS)).

4.2 Difficulties encountered and prospects

The constraints and limits in the implementation of the laboratory project are of several orders.

4.2.1 On the administrative level

As the LNSP is a public administration institution, financial procedures are one of the major constraints in the process of acquiring the necessary material resources. Also, a relatively small budget has been allocated for the acquisition of the necessary equipment.

In addition, the instability and small size of the SAET's technical staff make it impossible to plan the development of the laboratory's activities.

4.2.2 On the technical side

Several aspects can be identified, which handicap the activities of the toxicology laboratory:

- Insufficient maintenance of equipment (chromatographs) most often causing recurring breakdowns,

- absence or insufficiency of some materials and reagents, and

- insufficient capacity building of technical staff.

4.3 Outlook

Currently, several types of clinical toxicology analyses can be carried out at SAET, but they must be improved and reinforced (**Tables C1** and **C2**). To do this, we plan to:

- continue the development of analytical toxicology through the implementation of new methods and parameters analytically,

- continue and strengthen technical collaboration with the CTQ, United Nations Office on Drugs and Crimes (UNODC), and

- advocate with TFPs for technical capacity building support.

The establishment of a PCC and the development of a national toxicological biomonitoring strategy will greatly contribute to strengthening the activities of the CTL [45].

5. Conclusion

The increasing and uncontrolled use of chemicals (pesticides, mercury, cyanide, illicit drugs, adulterated alcohols, etc.) in Burkina Faso, in various sectors of activity, has always been a major health concern, with many risks of exposure to dangerous substances. Unfortunately, the health system of Burkina Faso presented a rare availability, if not difficult accessibility, to clinical toxicological analyses for monitoring the exposure of the population or for a better management in case of intoxications.

But, since 2015, with the creation of the SAET, which has a clinical toxicology laboratory, the health system has been strengthened by performing certain clinical toxicology analyses locally. The performance of these analyses has enabled the Ministry of Health to deal with certain toxicological health situations.

Today, the CTL contributes to the diagnosis, screening and therapeutic monitoring of patients in health facilities. It is therefore a valuable solution for doctors in the management of intoxications. It is also involved in the monitoring of populations exposed in their working or living environments [46]. Today, the SAET is involved in all health incidents with toxicological suspicions and provides its expertise in investigations.

Beyond the health field, the SAET makes an enormous contribution to the forensic, regulatory and judicial fields by analyzing suspect samples in cases (attempted poisoning, autopsies, product counterfeiting, fraud, etc.) [47–51].

The SAET initiative now has an impact on health security at several levels:

- At the socioeconomic level, the SAET's expert assessments make it possible to better identify risk areas and take appropriate preventive measures (awareness and training) for the benefit of the population. As a result, the number of cases of acute poisoning is reduced, as well as the number of victims. Healthy people are much more productive and the Ministry of Health (State) saves money by reducing the number of emergency interventions, which are extremely costly.

- From an environmental point of view, the knowledge of the circumstances in which poisoning occurs and of the products involved has made it possible to take measures to protect and preserve the environment and the quality of life.

- In terms of health safety and public health, the SAET data provide an overview of toxicological risk management in Burkina Faso, reliable real-time data on poisonings and a greater capacity for anticipation on the part of health services in the face of toxicological emergencies. We also note the strengthening of controls on consumer products, the prohibition or withdrawal of adulterated products, etc.

- On the scientific front, the sharing or dissemination of SAET data through scientific productions (congresses, articles and others) contributes to the improvement of health safety in Burkina Faso and worldwide.

However, this unit encounters difficulties most often of a technical nature, such as the lack of adequate equipment. This is why an advocacy program for obtaining the necessary support has been drawn up with the aim of submitting it to the various potential partners. The capacity building of this laboratory will further strengthen Burkina Faso's health system in particular, and thus contribute to improving health security in the world in general [2, 15].

Acknowledgements

I express my gratitude to the authorities of Burkina Faso, in particular to those of the Ministry of Health and the National Public Health Laboratory for the authorization to set up clinical toxicology analyses and for all the efforts made for the development of toxicological expertise in Burkina Faso.

I take the opportunity through this document to express my gratitude to the Canadian Government, particularly to the Department of Foreign Affairs, Trade and

Development (DFATD), which fully funded my training in toxicological expertise at the CTQ, through the Canadian Francophonie Scholarship Program (CFSP) or PCBF. It was during this training that much of the project was designed.

Also, my greetings go to the managers of the PCBF at this time, specifically to Jeanne Ghallager, senior manager of the PCBF in Canada and to Mrs. NEBIE at the Canadian Embassy in Burkina Faso, who could be considered as coauthors of the design of the laboratory project.

I salute the authorities of the "Institut national de santé publique du Québec" and thank the entire team of the Center de Toxicologie Québec for the acceptance in their institution, the welcome and the sympathy.

I particularly thank all the staff of the toxicology laboratory for their professional cooperation and all the scientific lessons they gave me during this training.

I salute the first manager and all the staff of the LNSP for their support in the development of toxicological expertise at SAET.

I particularly thank all the technical collaborators at SAET who have contributed and are still working to strengthen the technical offer related to clinical toxicology analyses: Dr. SOURABIE P. Bernadette, Dr. DOULGOU Daouda, Dr. KOMI Albert, Dr. GAMBO Odile and all those whose names I could not mention.

Conflict of interest

"The authors declare no conflict of interest."

Notes/thanks/other declarations

The following abbreviations, LNSP, SAET, DTCE/HP and STM, are kept as such in the document because they are established designations within the establishment and also adopted by technical and financial collaborators (reagent suppliers and other service providers). So, any translation would result in a distortion of their denomination.

It is essential to note that the "LNSP" has more recently become "ANSSEAT" (i.e., National Agency for Environmental, Food, Occupational and Health Product Safety). We have kept "LNSP" because it is under this name that the project was developed.

Annex

A. Documentary related to the toxicological situations in Burkina Faso

See **Tables A1–A3**.

Documentary references	Toxicological situations/risks and targets
Adama TOE (rapport): Approche méthodologique et conceptuelle d'évaluation de l'impact environnemental et social pour la construction de cinq magasins de stockage des pesticides dans la région du Sahel – Burkina Faso, 2013 (Revue Africaine de Santé et de Productions Animales, © 2013 E. I.S.M.V. de Dakar)	• Cases of poisoning among producers after application of the product in the cotton field • Risks of exposure to pesticides for: • producers (lack of compliance with safety and hygiene measures: nonuse of protective equipment, noncompliance with hygiene rules), • the rural population, • professionals in the phytosanitary industry, • the consumer of crop products, and • the environment.
Adama TOE. (rapport): Étude pilote des intoxications dues aux pesticides agricoles au Burkina Faso, 2010	
Adama TOE et coll: (rapport): Etude d'impact environnemental et social pour la construction d'un magasin de stockage de pesticides à Gorom-Gorom (province de l'Oudalan), 2010	
Alain P.K. Gomgnimbou (article): Usage des intrants chimiques dans un agrosystème tropical: diagnostic du risque de pollution environnementale dans la région cotonnière de l'est. du Burkina Faso, 2009 (Base volume 13 (2009) numéro 4)	
Baba OUATTARA (article): Effet des pesticides sur l'activité microbienne d'un sol ferrugineux tropical du Burkina Faso, 2010 (Cameroon Journal of Experimental Biology 2010 Vol. 06 N° 01, 11–20.)	
Moustapha OUÉDRAOGO: (article) Étude des facteurs de risques d'intoxications chez les utilisateurs de pesticides dans la région cotonnière de Fada N'Gourma au Burkina Faso; 2009	
Moustapha OUÉDRAOGO: Pesticides in Burkina Faso: Overview of the Situation in a Sahelian African Country, 2011(Pesticides in the Modern World-Pesticides Use and Management, Dr. Margarita Stoytcheva (Ed.), ISBN: 978-953-307-459-7, InTech	
NGANOAH Victoire Sylvie (mémoire): Étude des risques environnementaux et sanitaires liés à l'utilization des pesticides chimiques de synthèse dans la culture du coton à l'Ouest du Burkina Faso, 2009	
Richard OUEDRAOGO et al. 2014: Risk of workers exposure to pesticides during mixing/loading and supervision of the application in sugarcane cultivation in Burkina Faso, 2014 (*International Journal of Environmental Science and Toxicology* (ISSN: 2315-9927) Vol. 2(7) pp. 143-151, July, 2014)	

Table A1.
Documentary references related to the use of pesticides in agriculture.

Documentary reference	Risks and targets
Aboubakar H. OUEDRAOGO (article): L'impact de l'exploitation artisanale de l'or (orpaillage) sur la santé et l'environnement, 2006	• Workers and residents of modern and artisanal mining sites are exposed to multiple health risks: o exposure to mercury, cyanide, o exposure to lead, cadmium, chromium, ... , and o exposure to hydrocarbons • Environmental pollution
Dr Gountiéni Damien LANKOANDE 1 et Dr. David Maradan (rapport). Coût de l'inaction de la gestion des produits chimiques dans le secteur minier et agricole. Rapport final Ministère de l'Environnement et du Développement Durable (MEDD) Initiative Pauvreté Environnement (IPE). Juin 2013; page 48	
Edith SAWADOGO: L'impact de l'exploitation artisanale de l'or: cas du site de Fofora dans la province du Poni.2011	
Issaka DIALGA: Du boom minier au Burkina Faso: opportunité pour un développement durable ou risque de péril pour les générations futures? 2013	
MBALLO Boubacar (mémoire) impacts possibles des activités minières sur les ressources en eau en Afrique de l'ouest: cas des mines aurifères du Burkina Faso, 2012	
MINISTÈRE DE L'ENVIRONNEMENT ET DU CADRE DE VIE (rapport): contribution du Burkina Faso a l'étude sur le plomb et le cadmium, 2005	
MINISTERE DE L'ENVIRONNEMENT ET DU CADRE DE VIE: rapport de synthèse de l'atelier national de sensibilisation, d'information et d'éducation du public sur le mercure (hg) au Burkina Faso, Ouagadougou du 09 au 11 Novembre 2009	

Table A2.
Literature references relating to toxicological risks in mining.

Documentary references	Risks and targets
Aboubakar H. OUEDRAOGO (article): L'impact de l'exploitation artisanale de l'or (orpaillage) sur la santé et l'environnement, 2006	• Risk of acute poisoning, drug addiction and other diseases (hepatic, heart damage, cancer, etc.) for consumers within the population (rural population, in particular youth, gold washers)
Dr Gountiéni Damien LANKOANDE1 et Dr. David Maradan (rapport). Coût de l'inaction de la gestion des produits chimiques dans le secteur minier et agricole. Rapport final Ministère de l'Environnement et du Développement Durable (MEDD) Initiative Pauvreté Environnement (IPE). Juin 2013; page 48	
Edith SAWADOGO: L'impact de l'exploitation artisanale de l'or: cas du site de Fofora dans la province du Poni.2011	
Issaka DIALGA: Du boom minier au Burkina Faso: opportunité pour un développement durable ou risque de péril pour les générations futures? 2013	
MBALLO Boubacar (mémoire) impacts possibles des activités minières sur les ressources en eau en Afrique de l'ouest: cas des mines aurifères du Burkina Faso, 2012	
MINISTÈRE DE L'ENVIRONNEMENT ET DU CADRE DE VIE (rapport): contribution du Burkina Faso a l'étude sur le plomb et le cadmium, 2005	

Documentary references	Risks and targets
MINISTERE DE L'ENVIRONNEMENT ET DU CADRE DE VIE: rapport de synthèse de l'atelier national de sensibilisation, d'information et d'éducation du public sur le mercure (hg) au Burkina Faso, Ouagadougou du 09 au 11 Novembre 2009	

Table A3.
Documentary references relating to the consumption of psychoactive substances

B. Project budgeting

See **Table B1**.
NB:

- PTF: Canada, France, European Union (EU), WHO and UNEP
- Equity: Personal investments of the project initiator

Overall budget of the project: 1152776780 West African CFA francs (XOF francs)
See **Table B2**.
A. Project financing plan: Project budget by axis and by year
See **Table B3**.
B. Budget plan according to the two phases of the project
a. Budget for the first phase of the project
The budget for this phase covers the following points:

- Training course in toxicological analysis at the CTQ

Budget Section	Estimated amount (×1000)	Completion period	Potential sources of funding
Study trip/training course	24,698.6	Stage 1	PCBF (already funded)
Acquisition and fitting out of premises	65,256	Stage 1 + Stage 2	TFP
Laboratory equipment, materials and consumables	77,471.7	Stage 1	TFP
Equipment (FIMS, FAAS, GC/MS and LC/MS)	655,078.5	Stage 2	TFP
Reagents and reference standards	15,666.98	Stage 2	TFP
Pilot study: priority parameters	6195	Stage 1	TFP
Training (advanced courses)	51,200	Stage 1 + Stage 2	PCBFs and others
Functioning	252,610	Stage 2	TFP
Research and collaboration with TFPs	4600	Stage 1 + Stage 2	Equity
Total	**1,152,776.78**		

Table B1.
Budget summary: Summary of the overall budget for the implementation of the clinical technology laboratory (CTL).

Objective	Stock	Cost (XOF Francs x1000)
Create a toxicology unit	Design	—
	Internship in a toxicology laboratory	24,698,6
	Research and collaboration with TFPs	4600
	Pilot study: Determination and prioritization of toxicological analysis needs	6195
	Submission and validation of the project and with the authorities	—
	Organization/reorganization or modification of the organization chart.	—
Strengthen the capacities of the LNSP in toxicological analysis	Acquisition and development of premises	65,256
	Acquisition of equipment and materials, reagents	748,217,18
	Staff recruitment/remuneration/training.	129,900
	Training (advanced course)	51,200
Carry out toxicological analyses	Information from potential customers	62,910
	Identification and dosage of drugs and medicines in biological media	
	Dosage of metals in biological media	
	Identification and dosage of drugs in nonbiological media	
	Identification and dosage of environmental pollutants in biological media	
	Monitoring and evaluation	57,600
	Implementation of a quality assurance system: participation in inter-laboratory testing	2200
Total budget		**1,152,776,78**

Table B2.
Estimated overall budget: Provisional budget for the main actions.

AXIS	Year (in XOF francs, ×1000)					
	2011–2015	**Year 1**	**Year 2**	**Year 3**	**Year 4**	**Total per axis**
Axis 1	31,893.6	700	700	700	700	34,693.6
Axis 2	86,7852	132,035.98	239,975	389,777	18,800	867,373.18
Axis 3	16,400	44,477.5	67,277.5	55,277.5	67,277.5	250,710
Total per year	**135,078.8**	**177,213.48**	**307,952.5**	**445,754.5**	**86,777.5**	**1,152,776.78**

Table B3.
Project budget by axis and by year.

- Establishment of the laboratory (development of premises, part of the acquisition of equipment and materials, recruitment of staff).

See **Table B4**.

Budget section	Amount/Unit cost (x1000)	Quantity	Estimated amount	Potential sources of funding
Study trip/training course	24,698.6	1	24,698.6	PCBF (already funded)
Pilot study	6195	1	6195	PCBFs, other PTFs
Course development	12,800	1	12,800	
Acquisition and fitting out of premises	35,256	1	35,256	TFP
Acquisition of equipment	99085.2	1	99085.2	TFP
Functioning	18,300	1	18,300	
Research and collaboration with TFPs	1800	1	1800	Equity
Total			198,134 .8	

Table B4.
Budget for the first phase of the project.

b. Budget for the second phase of the project
The budget for phase 2 concerns the following points:

- Functioning
- Training (advanced course)
- Part of the acquisition of equipment
- Project monitoring and evaluation
- Implementation and monitoring of the quality system

See **Table B5**.

Budget Section	Amount/Unit cost (×1000)	Quantity	Estimated amount	Potential sources of funding
Advanced courses	12,800	3	38,400	PCBFs, other PTFs
Acquisition and fitting out of premises	30,000	1	30,000	TFP
Acquisition of equipment	633,465	1	633,465	TFP
Reagents and reference standards	15,666.98 _ _	1	15,666.98 _ _	TFP
Functioning	234,310	1	234,310	PTF and Laboratory
Collaboration with TFPs	700	4	2800	Equity
Total			954,641, 98	
TOTAL BUDGET (phase 1 + 2)			1,152,776.78 _ _	

Table B5.
Budget for the second phase of the project.

C. Assessment according to the strategic orientations

See **Tables C1** and **C2**.

Strategic axis	Shares	Status of implementation

AXIS 1: Creation of the toxicology laboratory	Project design	• Project designed
		  ◦ Existence of the final project document with all the details
		  ◦ Existence of technical collaboration with the CTQ

	Setting up the laboratory/ creation	• Official creation of the Medical Toxicology Service at the LNSP
		  ◦ Existence of a creation order (Ref.: Order No. 2015/344/MS/CAB creating a medical toxicology department at the LNSP)
		  ◦ Staff and premises assigned to the service

AXIS 2: Carrying out toxicological analyses	Research and collection of analytical samples	• Samples received from several structures
		  ◦ Hospital structures
		  ◦ Judicial police officers
		  ◦ Others

	Realization of qualitative and quantitative analyses	• Analyses carried out • Search for PAS in blood, urine and others • Screening for pesticides in blood, urine and others • Dosage of metals in blood and urine not yet effective
AXIS 3: Increase in performance and search for recognition	Implementation of an appropriate quality assurance program	• Quality system in place • Standard adopted: ISO 9001:2105 and ISO 17025:2017 • Participation in UNODC interlaboratory tests
	Accreditation search for the main analytical parameters: drugs, metals, pesticides.	• Unrealized

Table C1.
Assessment of the implementation of strategic actions.

Analytical technique	Device identified	Analytes identified	Analytical situation
Immunochemistry	RSS II (+RDT drugs)	Drugs, medicines	Feasible
	Immunochemical automaton	Drugs, medicines	Feasible
Atomic absorption	CV-AAS: **FIMS 100**	Mercury	**Not yet feasible**
	GF-AAS AAnalyst 600	Metals	Not yet feasible
Chromatography	GC-MS	Drugs, medicines, and pesticides	Feasible
	GC-FID	Alcohol	Feasible
	HPLC-DAD	Drugs, medicines, and pesticides	Feasible

Table C2.
Technical offers relating to clinical toxicology currently available at the Toxicological Analysis and Expertise Service (SAET).

Author details

N. Stanislas Dimitri Meda[1*], Normand Fleury[2], Ciprian M. Cirtiu[2], Vincent Cirimele[3], Cheick Armand N. Palm[4] and Elie Kabre[4]

1 National Public Health Laboratory, Ouagadougou, Burkina Faso

2 Quebec Toxicology Center, National Institute of Public Health of Quebec, Québec, Canada

3 ChemTox Laboratory, Strasbourg, France

4 National Public Health Laboratory, Ouagadougou, Burkina Faso

*Address all correspondence to: dimmedas@yahoo.fr

References

[1] PNUE. Global chemical outlook: Towards sound management of chemicals. 2012

[2] OMS, OIT, PNUE. Lignes directrices de lutte contre les intoxications, Programme International de Sécurité Chimique. 1988

[3] Fournier et Bonderef. Les produits antiparasitaires à usage agricole. Conditions d'utilisation et toxicologie. Paris: Tec. et doc. Lavoisier; 1983

[4] Toé A et al. Contribution à la toxicologie agro-industrielle au Burkina Faso: étude des intoxications d'agriculteurs par les pesticides en zone contonnière du Mouhoun: résultats, analyse et proposition de prise en charge du problème,, *Revue de médecine du travail.* Vol. 29, n° % 1unique. 2002

[5] Lankoande GD, Maradan D. Coût de l'inaction de la gestion des produits chimiques dans le secteur minier et agricole, Rapport final Ministère de l'Environnement et du Développement Durable (MEDD), Ouagadougou. 2013

[6] Sawadogo E. L'impact de l'exploitation artisanale de l'or: cas du site de Fofora dans la province du Poni. 2011

[7] Human Rights Watch. Un mélange toxique: Travail des enfants, mercure et orpaillage au Mali. 2011

[8] IPE/Burkina Faso. L'utilisation irresponsable de produits chimiques au Burkina Faso. 2014

[9] Jepson PC et al. Measuring pesticide ecological and health risks in West African agriculture to establish an enabling environment for sustainable intensification. Philosophical Transactions on Royal Society. 2014;**B 369**:18

[10] Artisanal Gold Council. La santé dans l'orpaillage et l'exploitation minière artisanale: Un manuel pour instructeurs. [En ligne]. 2015. Available: https://www.unido.org/sites/default/files/files/2017-11/AGC_Health_training_textbook_French.pdf. [Accès le 05 mai 2023]

[11] ABSP (Association burkinabè de santé publique). Enquête sur le tabac chez les adolescents en milieu scolaire de Ouagadougou et de Bobo Dioulasso. 2003

[12] Commission économique et social des Nations Unies. Rapport du secrétariat: situation mondiale en ce qui concerne le trafic de drogues, Cinquante-septième session, Vienne, 13–21 mars 2014

[13] ONUDC. Rapport mondial sur les drogues 2012. 2012

[14] Le Quotidien. Journée mondiale de lutte contre la drogue. 2015

[15] FEM (Fonds pour l'environnement mondial). Bâtir des partenariats pour la gestion sans dangers des produits chimiques; 40

[16] Ministère de l'agriculture de l'hydraulique et des ressources halieutiques du Burkina Faso. Plan de gestion des pesticides au Burkina Faso. 2004

[17] Ministère de l'environnement et du cadre de vie du Burkina Faso. Profil national du Burkina Faso pour la gestion des produits chimiques. 2008

[18] Lheureux P, Maes V, Askenasi R. Du Bon Usage Du Laboratoire De

Toxicologie 1re partie: Aspects techniques. Réanimation Urgence. 1996; **5**(12):87-95

[19] Ouédraogo M et al. Étude des facteurs de risques d'intoxications chez les utilisateurs de pesticides dans la région cotonnière de Fada N'Gourma au Burkina Faso. Environnement, Risques & Santé. 2009;**8**(14):343-347

[20] Gomgnimbou APK et al. Usage des intrants chimiques dans un agrosystème tropical: diagnostic du risque de pollution environnementale dans la région cotonnière de l'est du Burkina Faso. Biotechnologie, Agronomie, Société et Environnement. 2009;**13**(14): 499-507

[21] Dimitri Meda NS et al Niveau de contamination des eaux conditionnées produites au Burkina Faso par les pesticides, chez Congrès d'épidémiologie et de santé publique, Lomé (Togo). 2022

[22] Meda NR et al. Pesticide residues in commonly consumed food from five localities of Burkina Faso: occurrence and health risk assessment. Environmental Monitoring Assessment. 2022;**195**(11):160

[23] Ministère de l'environnement et du cadre de vie du Burkina Faso. Projet Initiative Pauvreté Environnement (IPE): analyse économique du secteur des mines liens pauvreté et environnement; Rapport final du 31 mai 2011

[24] Dimitri Meda NS et al. Recherche de substances psychoactives: bilan de cinq ans d'expertises toxicologiques au Laboratoire national de santé publique du Burkina Faso, chez Congrès international d'épidémiologie et de santé publique, Lomé (Togo). 2023

[25] Bationo B, Doulgou D, Dimitri Meda NS. Évaluation du risque chimique dans le service des contaminants, des pesticides et des engrais d'un laboratoire dans la ville de Ouagadougou., chez 1er congrès de la Société Burkinabè de médecine du Travail (SOBUMET), Ouagadougou. 2021

[26] Koueta F. Les intoxications aigues accidentelles de l'enfant: aspects épidémiologiques, étiologiques et évolutifs au CHU pédiatrique Charles-de-Gaulle de Ouagadougou (Burkina Faso). Cahiers Santé. 2009;**19**(12)

[27] Ouédraogo M et al. Acute intoxications in two university hospitals in Burkina Faso. 2012;**486**(14):483-486

[28] Dimitri Meda NS et al. Épidémiologie des urgences toxicologiques d'origine alimentaire au Burkina Faso. Revue d'épidémiologie et de santé publique (RESPE). 2022; **70**(1):S3

[29] Ouedraogo AB. L'impact de l'exploitation artisanale de l'or (orpaillage) sur la santé et l'environnement. 2006

[30] Meda NS, Fleury N, et al. Initiative innovante pour l'amélioration du système de santé au Burkina Faso: stratégies de mise en place d'un laboratoire de toxicologie clinique. Toxicologie analytique et clinique (ToxAC). 2015;**27**(12S)

[31] OCDE. La mesure des activités scientifiques et technologiques principes directeurs proposés pour le recueil et l'interprétation des données sur l'innovation technologique. Oslo: Manuel d'Oslo; 2005

[32] Kline SJ, Rosenberg N. An Overview of Innovation. 2009

[33] Forest J, Micaëlli JP, Perrin J. Innovation et conception: pourquoi une

approche en terme de processus?, chez Congrès International Franco-Québecoise de Génie Industriel, ALBI (France). 1997;**10**

[34] Hjertvikrem N. Collaboration in Research and Innovation Networks. 2020

[35] Conseil de la science et de la technologie. Innovation ouverte-Enjeux et défis pour le Québec, Rapport de conjoncture 2009, Québec. 2010

[36] OCDE. Synthèses: Innovation ouverte dans des réseaux mondiaux. Paris: Éditions de l'OCDE; 2008. p. 8

[37] CTQ. Organisation et gestion, section 4 du Manuel des procédures du système qualité, ISO/CEI 17025, 9e Edition. 2014

[38] Ministère de la Santé du Burkina Faso. Note n¤2013-1604 MS/SG/DGS du 24 juillet 2013 du Secrétaire Générale du Ministère de la Santé, Ougadougou: Archives LNSP, juillet. 2013

[39] LNSP. Plan stratégique LNSP 2014-2018. Ouagadougou, Burkina Faso: Archives LNSP; 2014

[40] LNSP. Projet de renforcement des capacités du Laboratoire national de sante publique en analyses toxicologiques: mise en place d'une unité de toxicologie (UNITOX-LNSP). Ouagadougou, Burkina Faso: Archives LNSP; 2014

[41] Meda N-SD et al. Sécurité sanitaire de l'aliment: évaluation du risque toxicologique d'origine alimentaire dans les cantines scolaires au Burkina Faso. Toxicologie analytique et clinique (ToxAC). 2021;**33**(13S):S60

[42] Palm CAN, Nacoulma AP, Dimitri NS et al. Validation d'une méthode de dosage de la morphine dans les urines, chez XXIe Journéees des Sciences de la Santé de Bobo Dioulasso (JSSB), Bobo Dioulasso (Burkina Faso). 2022

[43] Meda NSD, Cheick NR, et al. Investigations toxicologiques dans un cas d'intoxication alimentaire collective d'une famille au Burkina Faso. Toxicologie analytique et Clinique (ToxAC). 2022;**34**(13)

[44] Dimitri NS, Palm CAN, Bambara O et al. Contribution à la gestion des risques sanitaires au Burkina Faso: bilan de cinq (2015-2019) ans d'expertises toxicologiques au Laboratoire national de santé publique, chez XXIe Journées des Sciences de la Santé de Bobo Dioulasso (JSSB), Bobo Dioulasso (Burkina Faso). 2022

[45] Capolaghi B et al. Stratégies analytiques en toxiclogie d'urgence. Annales de Toxicologie Analytique. 2000;**XII**(4):274-281

[46] INSPQ. Lignes directrices pour la réalisation des évaluations du risque toxicologique d'origine environnementale au Québec. 2012

[47] Dimitri NS, Palm CAN, Meda NR et al. Intoxication alimentaire mortelle dans une famille au Burkina Faso: apport des analyses toxicologiques dans la recherche des causes de décès, chez Deuxième Congrès Burkinabè de Santé Publique (CBSP), Ouagadougou. 2021

[48] Dimitri NS, Palm CAN, Youl O. et al. Contribution du Laboratoire national de santé publique dans la prise en charge des intoxications alimentaires au Burkina Faso de 2015 à 2019, chez XXe Journées des Sciences de Santé de Bobo Dioulasso (JSSB), Bobo Dioulasso (Burkina Faso). 2020

[49] Palm CAN, Dimitri NS et al. Apport des analyses toxicologiques dans les investigations post-mortems, chez XXIe Journées des Sciences de la Santé de Bobo Dioulasso (JSSB), Bobo Dioulasso (Burkina Faso). 2022

[50] Dimitri NS et al. Stratégies et méthodes analytiques utilisées pour la recherche des substances psychoactives au Laboratoire national de santé publique du Burkina Faso, chez XXIe Journées des Sciences de la Santé de Bobo Dioulasso (JSSB), Bobo Dioulasso (Burkina Faso). 2022

[51] Gambo O et al. Validation d'une méthode de dosage de la chloroquine dans le sang par chromatographie liquide haute performance, chez XXIe Journées des Sciences de la Santé de Bobo Dioulasso (JSSB), Bobo Dioulasso (Burkina Faso). 2022

Chapter 8

Point-of-Care Testing in Rural and Remote Australia: An Emerging Technology to Address Global Health Challenges, Crises and Security

Mark Shephard, Susan Matthews, Louise Causer, Belinda Hengel and Rebecca Guy

Abstract

Point-of-care (POC) testing enables rapid pathology results to be utilised in primary care settings for timely clinical decision-making and treatment during a patient consultation and can contribute to public health surveillance and responses. Large-scale POC testing networks (supporting 100 or more rural and remote health services) now operate for chronic, acute and infectious diseases across the length and breadth of Australia. Sound operator training, quality management and digital connectivity systems, in addition to strong clinical and cultural governance, underpin these networks, mitigate risks to patient safety, and facilitate scalability. Real-world examples from our Australian-based POC testing networks highlight how contemporary global health problems, such as diabetes, acute medical crises and the COVID-19 pandemic response can be addressed by the judicious application of POC testing in primary care settings. The recent role POC testing played in supporting First Nations communities of Australia during the pandemic serves as a template for and provides learned experiences that can be translated or adapted to other countries should or when future global security issues arise. The potential to use POC testing as an adjunctive diagnostic tool to support and enhance global health security needs to be balanced against the limitations of using this innovative technology.

Keywords: point-of-care testing, governance, risk mitigation, translational research, emergency response, pandemic

1. Introduction

Point-of-care (POC) testing is a transformational medical technology that is the fastest growing sector of the pathology industry globally; the global market size was estimated to be US$33 billion in 2022 and growing to US$100 billion by 2032, with a compound annual growth rate of 12.2% [1]. POC testing enables pathology tests to be performed on a patient during a medical consultation in a setting outside the clinical laboratory with results available in a short time frame that facilitates timely clinical decision-making and treatment, leading to improved patient outcomes. POC testing can also contribute meaningfully to public health surveillance and actions in the face of ongoing or emerging epidemics or pandemics, by facilitating diagnosis in high- or special-risk population sub-groups or local communities that are not readily serviced by traditional pathology services.

The settings in which POC testing can be undertaken is ever increasing and includes primary care facilities such as general practices and First Nations medical services as well as pharmacies, workplaces, sports medicine, military services, extreme environments (including polar research stations), and contexts such as disaster management and (as will be described later in this chapter) epidemic or pandemic responses [2].

The advantages of conducting POC testing in primary care settings are profound. The patient-centredness of the POC testing process provides a convenient, accessible and accepted service for consumers, while the speed of result delivery reduces patient anxiety and facilitates more timely diagnosis and appropriate clinical management. The trained POC testing operator who performs the test for their local community has an increased sense of responsibility and empowerment. The consulting medical practitioner can make an evidence-based, informed clinical decision based on the results provided and institute management more rapidly. Operational efficiencies for health service workflow including averted medical evacuations can be achieved, while the portability of POC testing devices also enables them to be used in community outreach, mobile vans or localised outbreak settings. Across a network of primary care services, a significant local workforce capacity with readiness, resilience and competence to perform POC testing can be created [3].

Point-of-care (POC) testing has specific relevance for rural or remote primary care environments, where geographic isolation and long distances from the nearest pathology service can lead to traditional laboratory processes being compromised; sample integrity becomes a major issue due to harsh transport conditions while long turnaround times for results to be returned to remote services result in loss to follow-up of patient care [4, 5].

While performed in variable patient and community centric settings and offering enhanced portability compared to traditional laboratory pathology services, at its core, POC testing remains a medical science discipline; requiring specialised training and competency assessment of non-laboratory health professionals and adherence to standard operating procedures and technical requirements to reduce pre-analytical, analytical and post-analytical errors associated with the test result/s. Such processes are paramount to ensure that results generated by POC testing technologies are analytically valid and pose minimal risk to patient safety. The continuous surveillance of operator competency, device function and analytical quality through the field use of routine laboratory practices such as quality control (QC) and external quality assurance testing (EQA, also known to as proficiency testing)—where services test samples with assigned values of an analyte—underpins the use of POC testing in primary care environments.

2. POC testing in Australia

Australia has been a pioneer and leader in both the application of POC testing in primary care—particularly services supporting Aboriginal and Torres Strait Islander (now more commonly referred to as First Nations) communities—for the past 25 years. Large-scale POC testing networks (involving close to 100 or more rural and remote First Nations health services) now operate for chronic, acute and infectious diseases across the length and breadth of Australia (**Table 1**); these are managed for the Australian Government by specialist POC testing network providers including the Flinders University International Centre for Point-of-Care Testing and the Kirby Institute, University of New South Wales, in collaboration with peak First Nations bodies and leadership groups, rather than by traditional pathology laboratories [2, 4–6].

The QAAMS (Quality Assurance for Aboriginal and Torres Strait Islander Medical Services) Program enables POC testing for the diagnosis and management of diabetes as well as the detection of early renal disease in over 200 First Nations communities throughout Australia. The Program, managed by the Flinders International Centre for Point-of-Care Testing, has been funded continuously since 1999 by the Australian Government and remains the largest POC testing network in Australia. The analytical quality of POC testing in this program has been shown to be equivalent to that of Australasian laboratories and has met profession-derived analytical benchmarks for the past 20 years for both haemoglobin A1c (HbA1c) and urine albumin:creatinine ratio (UACR) [7, 8]. Statistically significant improvements in glycaemic control have been observed in First Nations patients with diabetes both within and between communities [9, 10]. The QAAMS Program has led to health policy change, whereby POC testing is now embedded into pathways for the diagnosis and management of First Nations people with diabetes. This includes the reimbursement of POC test cartridges through the Australian government medical rebate scheme, which is available to actively enrolled QAAMS participants.

The Northern Territory (NT) POC Testing Program operates in every remote health facility in the Northern Territory of Australia. The Territory's land mass,

Disease focus	Program name	Duration of program	POC tests performed	Number of services	Managed by
Chronic	QAAMS	24 years (since 1999)	HbA1c^ and Urine ACR#	238	Flinders ICPOCT*
Acute	NT POC testing	15 years (since 2008)	Electrolytes, Blood Gases, Troponin I, Creatinine, Glucose, Haemoglobin, INR	94	Flinders ICPOCT*
Infectious	National emergency syphilis response (ESR)	5 years (since 2018)	Syphilis	112	NACCHO** and Flinders ICPOCT
	Aboriginal and Torres Strait Islander COVID-19 POCT program	3 years (since 2020)	SARS-CoV-2+	101	Kirby Institute*** and Flinders ICPOCT

^Haemoglobin A1c.
#Albumin:creatinine ratio.
+Severe Acute Respiratory Syndrome Coronavirus-2.
**Flinders University International Centre for Point-of-Care Testing.*
***National Aboriginal Community Controlled Health Organisation.*
****Kirby Institute, University of New South Wales.*

Table 1.
Examples of large-scale POC testing networks in Australia.

5.5 times larger than the United Kingdom, is extremely remote and sparsely populated and is amongst the most challenging environments in Australia to conduct POC testing. The NT POC Testing Program, funded by the Northern Territory Government since 2008 and managed by the Flinders International Centre for Point-of-Care Testing, has revolutionised pathology service delivery in the Territory, particularly for acute medical emergencies such as acute myocardial infarction, acute respiratory disorders, acute renal disease and acute blood loss [11, 12]. The ability to perform opportunistic tests for cardiac troponin, blood gases, electrolytes and creatinine, and haemoglobin, respectively, have enabled efficient triage of acutely ill patients [13]. The device's international normalised ratio (INR) test also enables the management of patients on warfarin therapy. Through the on-site capacity to rule in or rule out the need for the medical evacuations of a patient, the NT POCT Program is estimated to save the Northern Territory Government more than AUS$21 million per annum [14]. In a further health policy change, POC testing has also been integrated into clinical pathways for acute care in Northern Territory local clinical guidelines [15].

The National Emergency Syphilis Response (ESR) and the Aboriginal and Torres Strait Islander COVID-19 POC Testing Programs were initiated and funded by the Australian Government (then) Department of Health during the past 5 years and delivered in partnership with National Aboriginal Community Controlled Health Organisation (NACCHO).

The ESR program responded to an outbreak of infectious syphilis and its subsequent rapid spread through First Nations communities across northern, central, western and southern Australia. POC testing using lateral flow technology (manual test strips for the detection of *Treponema pallidum* antibodies) was implemented to increase the uptake of syphilis screening in these communities. With information on past syphilis history from the jurisdictional registers, a patient with a reactive POC testing result was able to be offered immediate intramuscular treatment with antibiotics (benzathine benzylpenicillin) in an attempt to break onward or vertical transmission of the disease. The reactive POC test was followed up with confirmatory laboratory testing to differentiate between active and past syphilis infection. An independent report on the program commissioned by the Australian Government found that the program (through the National Aboriginal Community Controlled Health Organisation [NACCHO] and its partners, including the Flinders University International Centre for Point-of-Care Testing (who managed the training and quality systems for field POC testing) had developed a highly successful blueprint for the design of future First Nations health and wellbeing initiatives [16].

The Aboriginal and Torres Strait Islander COVID-19 POC Testing Program was implemented by the Australian Government through the Aboriginal and Torres Strait Islander COVID-19 Advisory Group as part of the emergency response to the COVID pandemic which swept the world (including Australia) in early 2020 [6]. Leveraged from knowledge and expertise gained through an existing smaller molecular-based POC testing program for sexually transmitted infections (refer Section 3.2 for details), the COVID-19 POC Testing Program was managed and delivered on behalf of the Government by the Kirby Institute at the University of New South Wales (the Kirby) and the Flinders University International Centre for Point-of-Care Testing (ICPOCT). The COVID-19 pandemic took molecular-based POC testing into unchartered waters. The POC testing response needed to be swift, flexible and adaptable to the changing requirements (and subsequent testing frameworks and public health responses) as the pandemic evolved in Australia, while remaining complementary to high throughput, urban laboratory test facilities. All the while, this program took place in an environment where global cartridge supply was limited. As a global security issue, the world had not faced such a level of 'uncertainty' or 'unknown' for more than 100 years since the Spanish influenza epidemic that killed 50 million people and infected a third of the world's population (500 million) in 1918 [17]. On this basis, global medical device regulatory bodies fast-tracked molecular-based SARS-CoV-2 diagnostic tests (and later SARS-CoV-2 antigen and antibody tests) from development to market through the application of emergency-use only (EUO) authorisation and cartridge supply allocations. This enabled rapid access and distribution of SARS-CoV-2 POC tests facilitating early adoption of POC testing in empowering First Nations health services to enable swift results which then triggered prompt community-based, public health responses. As such, this POC testing model serves as a testing framework template that can be readily adopted in high-risk populations to complement other broader testing strategies should future global security issues arise.

The core elements of the QAAMS, NT POC Testing and Aboriginal and Torres Strait Islander COVID-19 POC Testing Programs are similar and represent the progression of the field of POC testing across the last two and a half decades; they include:

- A defined clinical or public health need
- Political will and funding support from Government
- Strong clinical and cultural governance
- Targeted site selection to improve equity of access to diagnostic testing for high and special risk populations with linkage to care
- Engagement with key stakeholder groups (including partners and community)
- Documentation of policies, guidelines, risk assessment and mitigation strategies and quality management processes
- Sound training and competency assessment for POC testing operators
- Analytical quality surveillance systems*
- Scientific and technical support services
- Supply logistics (for testing cartridges/strips and other consumables), and
- Connectivity and reporting systems (the electronic transfer of POC test results into patient management systems and/or notification systems).

**However, it should be noted that due to the EUO authorisation of SARS-COV-2 POC tests and the need for rapid scale-up, extensive in-situ, post-market assay verification studies were performed to a lesser extent prior to field implementation in the COVID-19 POC Testing program, than for the QAAMS and NT POC Testing programs.*

Table 2 compares and contrasts these key elements across the QAAMS (chronic disease), NT POC Testing Program (acute care) and the Aboriginal and Torres Strait Islander COVID-19 POC Testing (infectious disease) networks.

With the core quality elements implemented and the networks operating routinely, clinical, cultural, operational and cost benefits can be realised through accessing POC testing technology. Further, the research impacts of POC testing permeate many research types and levels, as shown in **Table 3**.

Core element	QAAMS program	NT POC testing program	Aboriginal and Torres Strait Islander COVID-19 POC testing program
Clinical/Public health need	Rates of diabetes three-fold higher in First Nations people; Diabetes-related mortality in First Nations people four-times higher than non-Indigenous population [18]	Acute medical episodes leading cause of mortality/morbidity in the Northern Territory; High costs of medical retrievals [11, 14].	Emergency response to global COVID-19 pandemic; First Nations people more susceptible to severe illness/ complications from COVID-19 [6]
Funding source	Australian Government	NT Government	Australian Government
Governance	Program Management Committee including Clinical Support Officer and First Nations Leadership Forum	Program Management Committee including Clinical Support Officer and representative from peak First Nations body	Overseen by National Aboriginal and Torres Strait Islander COVID-19 Advisory Group; Program Clinical Advisory Group
Site selection	Targeted at high-risk population subgroups in services with diabetes as a health priority	Initially prioritised to larger health services serving larger population sizes, but now operating in every remote health service in NT	Site inclusion criteria developed to target high- and special risk remote populations, with sites approved by jurisdictional and national governance committees
Stakeholders (examples)	Industry (Siemens) Peak State/Territory First Nations bodies	Industry (Abbott) Peak Territory First Nations body (AMSANT)	Industry (Cepheid) Peak National First Nations body (NACCHO), Jurisdictional pathology services and public health departments
Policies, guidelines and risk/quality management	Aligns with latest NPAAC Requirements for POC Testing in Australia (2021) [19]	Aligns with latest NPAAC Requirements for POC Testing in Australia (2021) [19]	Aligns with latest NPAAC Requirements for POC Testing in Australia (2021) [19] and policies from PHLN [20] and CDN Australia [21]
Training	Flexible training options, including face-to-face, annual training workshops and web-based training available 24 hrs per day/7 days per week; Written and practical competency assessment	Flexible training options, including face-to-face training and web-based available 24 hrs per day/7 days per week; Written and practical competency assessment	Face-to-face training not available due to travel restrictions to First Nations health services during pandemic; Prerequisite modules on infection control and personal protective equipment; Written and practical competency assessment, Practical using Facetime on mobile phone
Device/ technology	Siemens DCA system/ immunoassay	Abbott i-STAT 300/ mainly electrochemical	Cepheid GeneXpert /molecular-based (PCR)

Core element	QAAMS program	NT POC testing program	Aboriginal and Torres Strait Islander COVID-19 POC testing program
Analytical quality	QC and EQA (both monthly)	QC (monthly) and EQA at selected hub sites (monthly)	QC (both 'positive' and 'negative' controls) and EQA (2 samples quarterly)
Scientific support	Working week 9 am–5 pm	Working week 9 am–5 pm	Working week 9 am–5 pm and telephone hotline 24 hrs per day/7 days per week for review of positive (or presumptive positive) patient results
Supply logistics	Provided by Siemens	Provided by Abbott	Provided by Logistics Support team from Kirby Institute
Connectivity	Uni-directional capture of de-identified results required, but not universally implemented due to different PMSs used across Program	Uni-directional capture of de-identified results (from device to central database at Flinders University); manual entry of results by operator into Territory-wide PMS	Uni-directional capture of de-identified results (to central database at Kirby) and identified data to multiple end-users (including PMS, pathology repositories, and jurisdictional departments of health); Public-facing and internal-facing dashboard reports; Mandatory reporting of (identified) notifiable infections

NPAAC = National Pathology Accreditation Advisory Council; NACCHO = National Aboriginal Community Controlled Health Organisation; AMSANT = Aboriginal Medical Services Alliance Northern Territory; QC = quality control; EQA = external quality assurance; PHLN = Public Health Laboratory Network; CDN = Communicable Disease Network; PMS = patient management system.

Table 2.
The key elements of three working POC testing networks in Australia.

Research	Elements
Medical science research	Device evaluation—pre- and post-field evaluation and implementation, ease-of-use, comparison to previous technologies.
	Analytical equivalence to the laboratory and ability to meet analytical benchmarks—most fundamental and most important in terms of patient risk/safety.
Implementation science research	Training and quality surveillance systems—innovation/creativity. Discrete end-user acceptability studies—patient, clinician, health service, community levels. Linkage to care.
Translational research	Transferability of networks across chronic, acute and infectious diseases
	Transferability of networks between services, between jurisdictions (national) and internationally.
	Scalability of networks from pilot to national to international models.
Public health research	Impacts at community level—equity of access/stakeholder acceptability.
	Impacts at health service level—building workforce capacity/resilience.
	Impacts at health system level—economic benefits. Impacts at health system level—disease burden, population health and wellbeing; early warning for disease surveillance and emerging. Pandemics. Impacts on health system policy and identification of sustainable funding.

Table 3.
Examples of multi-faceted research impacts of POC testing.

3. The Aboriginal and Torres Strait Islander COVID-19 POC testing program—A template for addressing future global security events

3.1 Setting the scene

Coronavirus disease (COVID-19) is a highly infectious disease caused by the severe acute respiratory syndrome coronavirus 2 (SARS-COV-2). While the origin of the virus remains problematic, the first cases of the virus appeared in Wuhan, China in December 2019 and spread rapidly across the globe. In Australia, the first case was reported on 25 January 2020 [22]. The World Health Organisation (WHO) declared the outbreak a 'public health emergency of international concern' 5 days later and a global pandemic on 11 March 2020 [23]. Across the subsequent 30 months, there have been a series of peaks and troughs in the number of COVID-19 infections in Australia, corresponding most often to the appearance of new coronavirus variants of concern. By August 2023, the WHO Coronavirus (COVID-19) dashboard reported that there had been over 769 million confirmed cases of COVID-19 globally, including 6.95 million deaths due to the virus [24]. Within Australia, the WHO dashboard reported over 11.5 million cases and 22,618 deaths [24]. While the virus is still circulating in the Australian population, its impact on the general population following widespread vaccination roll-out continues to subside for the present.

Despite widespread international travel restrictions, when the virus first hit Australian shores, the Australian Government were particularly concerned about the potential risk of severe impact of the virus on the country's First Nations people [6, 25]. First Nations people, particularly those living in remote communities, experience high rates of comorbidities including diabetes, cardiovascular disease and obesity, rendering them at higher risk of contracting serious illness and/or complications from the virus, similar to those documented in these communities during the H1N1 influenza outbreak in 2010 [26]. Many First Nations people in remote communities live in large households, making physical distancing problematic and culturally challenging and increasing the risk of infectious disease transmission. As explained previously, people living in remote communities are geographically isolated from regional pathology laboratories and therefore have limited access to testing when needed. Further, early in the pandemic, there was a limited understanding of the mechanisms of disease progression, a high burden on emergency and intensive care equipment and resources, minimal experimental treatment regimens and no vaccines available for the disease; as a result, expected mortality rates would be higher than if these options were available. The National Aboriginal and Torres Strait Islander COVID-19 Advisory Group was convened early in 2020, and recognised the importance of ensuring rapid, robust, and tailored COVID-19 responses for remote communities that were led by First Nations peoples.

3.2 A pivotal role for POC testing

To overcome justifiable concerns about the impact of COVID-19 on First Nations people, the Australian Government sought to support POC testing as a significant tool in the community-led emergency response in regional and remote settings. Firstly, through QAAMS, the NT POC Testing Program, the ESR Syphilis program and an existing molecular STI POC testing program called TTANGO (Test, Treat and Go) [27, 28], POC testing was a well-accepted technology in First Nations communities that had proven culturally safe, clinically and operationally effective and cost effective. Secondly, through TTANGO, molecular-based POC testing using the Cepheid GeneXpert system (the same system on which SARS-CoV-2 testing could be performed) had been systematically introduced into remote First Nations communities over the past decade for sexually transmitted infections (STI) for chlamydia, gonorrhoea and trichomoniasis at primary health services. The TTANGO POC testing network was being managed for the Australian Government through the Kirby-Flinders ICPOCT partnership and had been scaled-up from a randomised controlled trial (involving 12 sites) through a translational research phase and, at the start of the pandemic, to a routine implementation phase across 31 communities [27, 28]. There was also already a significant STI POC testing operator workforce in place who were competent in the operation of the GeneXpert system and had sound knowledge of quality management practices. Suitable and adaptable support infrastructure was also in place (supply chain logistics and connectivity). The Government therefore leveraged this established POC testing network to implement and rapidly expand a new program for SARS-CoV-2 testing using these same and additional GeneXpert devices. Importantly, the peak regulatory body overseeing medical devices and diagnostic tests in Australia—the Therapeutic Goods Administration (TGA)—had approved the use of a new SARS-CoV-2 assay for EUO on the GeneXpert system in March 2020 [29]. Two months later (May 2020), the WHO issued a statement that the GeneXpert SARS-CoV-2 assay (and other molecular-based technologies) could be performed 'on the bench, without the need for a biosafety cabinet, when the local risk assessment so dictates and proper precautions [re infection control] are in place' [30]. Further operator safety options were available within the COVID-19 POC Testing program through the direct provision of personal protective equipment (PPE) for enrolled health services and later the validation of a specific molecular transport media (rather than the recommended viral transport medium), capable of inactivating high titre (greater than 1×10^7 copies/mL) SARS-CoV-2 virus within 2 minutes of contact between the sample swab and media [31].

The GeneXpert system comprised a four-module GeneXpert device (allowing four tests to be performed at the same time), a laptop with proprietary software to enable the testing process, and a barcode scanner. In some larger community health services, or during local outbreaks, two GeneXpert devices were synchronously linked to form a higher throughput eight module device. A single-use, self-contained, disposable test cartridge performed a real-time, reverse transcriptase polymerase chain reaction (RT- PCR) test *in situ*, initially identifying nucleic acid material (RNA) from the SARS-CoV-2 virus (specifically the nucleocapsid (N-gene) and the viral envelope (E-gene) targets) and amplifying this material through thermal cycling to generate a fluorescent signal in a positive sample [6, 32]. Initially, test results (positive [detecting both N and E-gene targets], presumptive positive [detecting E-gene only], or negative) were available in just 45 minutes. Initially, a nasopharyngeal swab sample was collected (this was later expanded to include oropharyngeal and deep nasal swabs), placed into a 3 mL molecular transport medium tube, before mixing, and then loading into the testing cartridge using a transfer pipette. Further development of the Cepheid GeneXpert SARS-CoV-2 assay included validation for specific variants of concern as the pandemic progressed.

3.3 Which services to prioritise?

In addition to those services already with a GeneXpert device being used for STI POC testing, remote health services which were located a significant distance from a laboratory, and which had SARS-CoV-2 testing capacity, were prioritised for a device. Specifically, they needed to be more than 2 hours' drive from the closest laboratory, have at least three staff members to ensure capacity to perform testing, and either service a community of at least 500 First Nations people (a so-called 'hub' site) or provide centralised testing to 'spoke' communities with a total population of more than 500 people [6, 25].

3.4 Ramping up the program in rapid time!

The Kirby Institute and Flinders ICPOCT were formally contracted by the Government in April 2020 to deliver the program [6, 25]. As mentioned, the Government purchased additional GeneXpert devices to supplement those already in operation through the TTANGO STI Program and announced the COVID-19 POC Testing Program would begin operation in May 2020.

An intense period of work between April and May 2020, including extensive engagement with stakeholders, resulted in the development of policies and procedures regarding governance, the development of comprehensive training resources, quality management procedures, risk assessment and mitigation strategies, and specifications for a connectivity system not only to report results into multiple patient management systems (PMS) but also into jurisdictional public health notification systems. It was imperative that all these documents met standards that were expected by key stakeholder groups including the National Pathology Accreditation Advisory Council (NPAAC), who oversaw national requirements for the conduct of POC testing in Australia as well as produced a complimentary guidance document for POC testing during the pandemic; the Public Health Laboratory Network (PHLN), an expert panel of microbiologists representing Australasian laboratories; and the Communicable Diseases Network (CDN), who had disseminated national guidelines on COVID-19. The quality and value-add of molecular COVID-19 POC testing (and other COVID-19 testing practices such as waste-water surveillance testing) was under intense scrutiny by these bodies, who were responsible for developing and revising a national COVID-19 testing framework throughout the pandemic.

The program was overseen by the National Aboriginal and Torres Strait Islander COVID-19 Advisory Group; this group compromised senior representatives from NACCHO, CEOs and public health medical officers from Aboriginal Community Controlled Health Services (ACCHS), State/Territory ACCHS peak bodies and health representatives from federal and State/Territory Governments. In addition, a Program Clinical Advisory Group monitored the program on a more regular basis. The operational teams from the Kirby Institute and Flinders ICPOCT, responsible for day-to-day activities of the program, reported to both groups as required.

The development of flexible training resources and a competency assessment process for trained operators was particularly challenging given the short scale-up timeframe available in combination with the restricted travel into remote communities early (prior to widespread COVID-19 vaccination regimes). Prior to GeneXpert POC training, all trainees had to first complete prerequisite training modules in infection control, hand hygiene and the donning and doffing of personal protective equipment (PPE), which were separate to the GeneXpert training program developed by Flinders ICPOCT. Underpinned by detailed risk assessments and standard operating procedures including key risk mitigation steps, GeneXpert operator training resources included a PowerPoint presentation, a series of visual posters which provided step-by-step guides on how to perform patient, QC and EQA testing and how to interpret and action GeneXpert SARS-CoV-2 results (with assistance from a scientific hotline). As travel to First Nations communities was prohibited during the pandemic, training was delivered via an online platform by a team of Flinders ICPOCT scientists. Competency assessment involved both written and practical components; with face-to-face training not being a viable option during the pandemic, ICPOCT scientists observed POC testing trainee operators conduct a QC test in real-time via a mobile phone app (FaceTime). Flinders ICPOCT commenced online training on 14 May 2020.

The GeneXpert training and competency process, as well as the external prerequisite training, was time consuming, relatively intensive and often difficult to schedule; however, the trade-off was the high quality of test results, as evidenced by a very low rate of unsuccessful tests (0.7%) and excellent performance with QC and EQA testing; for the latter testing mode, the mean concordance with expected EQA results was greater than 98% for both 'positive' and 'negative' samples [33].

False negative test results (from either the laboratory or POC testing) were of particular concern during the pandemic in Australia, as such a patient with COVID-19 could be unsuspectingly transmitting the infection throughout the community while assuming they were 'negative'. In contrast, a false positive result could initiate an unnecessary public health response including, in some settings where isolation was not available or feasible, the evacuation of an individual from community and relocation to a designated COVID-19 quarantine facility.

The training framework for POC testing in primary care settings must align with regulatory frameworks in a given country, with the complexity of the POC test process and the personal or public health risk classification assigned to the test determining the intensity/level of training needed [34]. For a simple lateral flow test of low complexity and low personal and/or no public health risk, for example a pregnancy test, which has minimal steps and is easily read, operator training and competency assessment can be relatively basic and can potentially be delegated to 'advanced' trainers or local 'POC testing champions'. However, for a test of high complexity with high public health risk (such as SARS-CoV-2, HIV or hepatitis B/C), training and competency assessment needs to be targeted and rigorous.

A quality management system to support SARS-CoV-2 patient testing was rapidly implemented and involved services conducting both QC and EQA testing. For EQA testing, two blinded samples were tested every 3 months; these samples were prepared by the Royal College of Pathologists of Australasia (RCPA) Quality Assurance Programs Pty Ltd., one of two accredited EQA providers in Australia [33]. Both QC and EQA results were regularly reviewed by the scientific team and corrective action initiated if required. Strict maintenance, cleaning and risk mitigation procedures were also implemented at the service, which later extended to 'single-bagging' of the disposable sample transfer pipette (placing the used pipette into a specimen bag and sealing prior to disposal) or 'double bagging' of each used cartridge (placing the used cartridge into two specimen bags and sealing prior to disposal). These enhanced disposal procedures have been drafted in consultation with the manufacturer for inclusion in an improved IFU (instructions for use) sheet to further reduce biological and/or amplicon contamination risk.

Technical and scientific support for field operators was established from 9 am to 5 pm Monday to Friday by ICPOCT scientists, and a 24-hour telephone hotline service was operated initially by an ICPOCT scientist and later by Kirby staff to support services when a 'positive' case was identified and facilitate the local public health response.

Logistic support provided by Program staff included support for the initial software and hardware set-up of GeneXpert devices and the supply of testing cartridges, full PPE (gowns, gloves, face shields, masks) and consumables. Due to a global shortage of cartridges, cartridge supplies were procured at the national level and allocated accordingly to laboratories and to the Aboriginal and Torres Strait Islander COVID-19 POC Testing Program, with a sharing of cartridge resources between all stakeholders to accommodate high throughput testing sites and local outbreaks. Supplies were then managed and distributed to services dependent upon anticipated need by the Program logistic team. The program was also flexible in responding to the need to deploy GeneXpert resources to services experiencing transient outbreak levels of COVID-19 infections.

A connectivity reporting system, based on that established for the STI program [35], was modified and expanded to ensure de-identified patient SARS-CoV-2 results were captured in real-time by the program's central database, integrated into the service's patient management system and also directed to jurisdictional health departments for integration into their notifiable infections databases for mandatory public health surveillance purposes.

3.5 Rolling out the program

POC testing for SARS-CoV-2 in First Nations communities began in May 2020 and a program website with information for participants and training resources was launched in June. From June to October 2020, 80 health services were systematically integrated into the program, with over 5000 tests performed. By November 2020, all 86 sites initially selected to join the program were active, just under 7400 tests had been performed and the first positive cases in the community were identified. Positive test results were immediately followed up and actioned by the program with an ensuing rapid public health response implemented by the responsible clinician and public health team as required which included isolation of the community member and rapid testing of close family contacts to prevent the spread of infection in the community.

By August 2022, 105 services were engaged in the program, more than 900 operators had been trained and the cumulative number of SARS-CoV-2 patient tests performed exceeded 72,600 (**Figure 1**).

With the introduction of lateral flow rapid antigen point-of-care testing (RATs), prioritisation of molecular POC testing was tailored accordingly to support management of more severely ill patients and maintain staffing in remote clinics.

3.6 Impact and benefits of the Aboriginal and Torres Strait Islander COVID-19 POCT program

The Australian Government committed a total of $27 Million dollars to the COVID-19 POC Testing program. This investment provided a more than solid return. An independent review of the program, commissioned by the Government, prepared a report on the program in December 2022 (which was released publicly in July 2023) [25]. The report concluded:

> *"In summary the Program has been highly successful. It has achieved its intended aim of improved health outcomes for First Nations people through better access to COVID-19 testing. It is estimated that the Program has averted* **between 23,000 and 122,000 infections** *that would be likely to have arisen in the 40 days after the first infection was identified in a remote First Nations community. It is estimated that the Program has avoided* **between AUS$337 million and $1.8 billion in health costs**. *The key factors that underpinned this success were well informed and culturally competent governance, the GeneXpert system and the technical support given by the Kirby Institute and Flinders University, and the model of care provided by the ACCHS sector".*

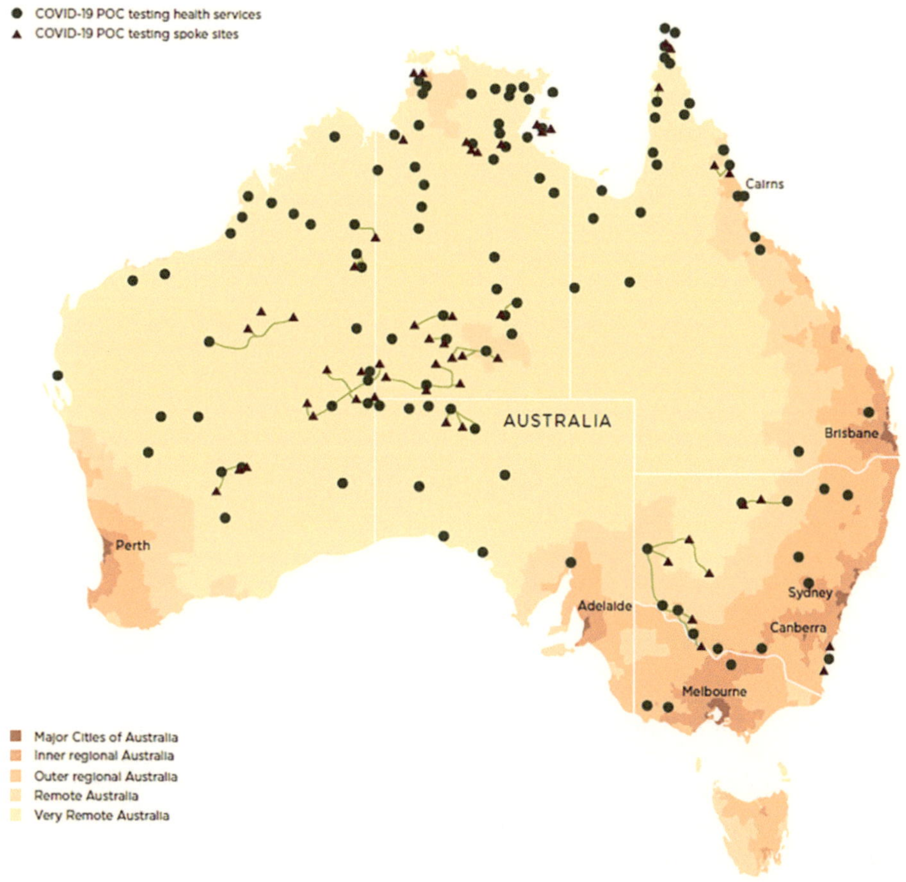

Figure 1.
Map showing general location of hub and spoke sites participating in the Aboriginal and Torres Strait Islander COVID-19 program.

A summary of the Program's key outcomes, adapted from this report [25], is provided in **Table 4**.

4. Lessons learned and their transferability to other countries

While considered generally low throughput and higher cost (compared to laboratory testing), POC testing can be a practical adjunctive diagnostic tool to support a timely response to a global health security issue, whether it be an infectious disease pandemic (as the world has just experienced) or a major natural or human-initiated disaster. POC testing forms part of an overall diagnostic solution and has niche application in such events, particularly in circumstances where laboratory testing is not readily available (e.g. remote communities), a rapid time to result is required, high- and special-risk subpopulations exist and where the rate of community transmission of the disease places burden on or exceeds the local pathology laboratory capacity. This applies particularly to low- and middle-income countries (LMIC and MIC) where access to traditional laboratory testing is often limited by geographic remoteness and loss to follow-up can be high.

Outcome	Short-term	Long-term
For patients	• Morbidity and mortality associated with COVID-19 was reduced.	• High quality care was received in the most appropriate setting.
For community	• The spread of COVID-19 transmission was broken in these communities. • Sustainability of health services in remote communities during the pandemic was improved.	• Confidence in the communities' capacity to handle COVID-19 was improved. • Confidence in the health service was improved and people were more willing to engage with treatment and care.
For the health system	• Unnecessary medial isolations or evacuations were avoided. • POC testing devices were rapidly deployed to other locations of epidemiological concern.	• Costs and impacts on other health services (e.g. hospital admissions, primary care interactions) were reduced. • Provision of support to remote health services created networks and built knowledge of support ('resilience') for future pandemics. • Capacity and autonomy in the testing of other infectious diseases was enhanced.

Table 4.
Key short- and long-term outcomes from the program.

The dynamic nature of global disease transmission or disaster events and the need to learn 'on the run' often in the face of a paucity of evidence, as occurred with the recent COVID-19 pandemic, means that POC testing needs to be nimble and adaptive in its application. 'Just in time' training, the ability for POC testing to be rapidly scaled up in a cost-effective and timely manner, and capacity to leverage both existing technology that may already be available in the field and a workforce ready POC testing operator base are examples of strategies that can enhance health security preparedness and responsiveness.

Planning and preparedness for using POC testing as a supplementary tool in global health security scenarios is the key to the ultimate effectiveness of this technology. In the post-COVID era now upon the world, most countries are reflecting on how to prepare for future infectious diseases and significant adverse events. Planning for how and when to use POC testing optimally should be a crucial component of preparedness and should be built into regional, national and international policy documents on global security incident management. POC testing should be integrated to meet local, specific community as well as broader public health needs, while also complying to general pathology regulation requirements. How well that planning is undertaken—particularly the identification of enablers and barriers to uptake—will have a significant bearing on the clinical usefulness and efficiency of POC testing in the field. Embedding POC testing in remote primary care practice (as has occurred in our Australian models) has not only raised awareness of the broad clinical, cultural and operational utility of POC testing but also built an experienced and resilient workforce of POC testing operators who were able to adapt readily to the new and immediate challenge presented by COVD-19.

Key lessons learned from the Australian experience of utilising POC testing, which can be transferable to other settings around the world, are summarised as a checklist in **Table 5** [36].

Checklist	Comment
Government	• Political and funding support from government is critical.
Governance	• Strong governance structure involving multidisciplinary stakeholders, including government, clinical, public health, industry, health services and consumer advocates is essential.
Engagement with community	• Investment in community engagement and awareness of the benefits of introducing POC testing for its intended purpose is paramount.
Linkage to policy	• Embedding POC testing practice into national health policy for addressing global security issues must be prioritised.
Linkage of POC devices and test clusters to clinical pathways	• Streamlining the use of POC testing device and test clusters into established clinical management pathways for triage and treatment is important.
'Fit for purpose' POC devices and test clusters	• POC devices and test clusters that are analytically 'fit for purpose' should be selected and evaluated; that is, they are appropriate for the clinical setting in the context of the population to be tested and the clinical conditions to be considered. • The original ASSURED and now redefined REASSURED criteria [37, 38] are simple tools developed for primary care and community settings in LMIC. In particular, these criteria recognise that 'no diagnostic tool is perfect' and that it is important to assess the 'trade-off' between accuracy, accessibility and affordability when selecting a 'fit-for-purpose' POC testing opportunity.
Complexity/risk of POC test systems	• In past years, there was an assumption that POC testing in primary care settings should be restricted to devices of low complexity (e.g. rapid diagnostic test strips); however, the Australian example has shown that devices of high complexity linked with tests with high public health risk (e.g. SARS-CoV-2) can be performed safely in community settings in the event of a major disease outbreak.
Linkage between specialist POC network providers and laboratory pathology providers	• Supportive and complementary relationships between these two groups should be built, particularly if 'front-line' POC testing requires follow-up laboratory testing and/or confirmation, other supplementary tests (e.g. multiplex respiratory test panels) or specific referral testing (e.g. genotyping).
Management of reagent stocks and consumables	A successful and responsive POC testing network must prioritise: • Established relationships/processes with industry suppliers for supply of devices, reagents and quality testing products at competitive pricing. • Contingencies for stockpiling and prioritisation when supplies are limited during periods of surge capacity. • Strategies for maintenance of supply chain during transport. • Consideration of refrigeration/power requirements at health service level. • Supply of ancillary equipment e.g. personal protective equipment.
Training and competency	Training and competency must involve: • Pre-event preparedness training to build an informed and event-ready workforce, including regional POC testing champions. • 'Just in time' training for rapid mobilisation of testing workforce when an event occurs. • Innovative mechanisms for observed competency assessment, when travel to remote health services is restricted or not possible. • Contingency training options for when face-to-face training is not available (e.g. during community lockdowns).

Checklist	Comment
Risk mitigation and quality management	• A risk management matrix should be used to assess risks to operator and patient safety versus perceived benefits of introducing POC testing. • POC testing should be undertaken within a documented and systematic quality management framework, which conforms to in-country regulatory requirements. • Automated early warning systems for anomalous results and trends should be implemented and monitored. • Escalation of incidents/adverse events for review at the clinical governance level (e.g. through a safety review committee) and reporting to regulatory bodies (as required) is critical. • POC testing quality management procedures should be embedded into preparedness activities in advance of a global event occurring.
Connectivity solutions	Elements of a practical connectivity solution should include: • Environmentally robust connectivity capability (to work e.g. in extremes of temperature which may occur in a global event). • Barcoding to facilitate positive patient identification. • Strategies to deal with patients who are unable to be identified. • Flexible connectivity systems, including jurisdictional notification where required.

Table 5.
Checklist to maximise the potential of POC testing in a global security event.

5. Acknowledging the limitations of and barriers to the adoption of POC testing

While the evidence that POC testing can be a complementary diagnostic tool in global events is clear, several limitations and barriers remain as an obstacle to the widespread uptake of this technology.

Certainly, if all the enablers listed in the previous table are not in place to support POC testing uptake—notably lack of political will; poor governance; disengagement of stakeholders; and lack of policy, regulation or quality management procedures—then it is certain that POC testing will fail. Other factors that limit effectiveness also need to be considered and are summarised in **Table 6**.

Limitations	Comment
Maintaining a sustainable workforce	• Staff turnover, especially in remote locations, represents the most significant challenge for sustainable POC testing. • Flexible training options (both for delivery of training and for training resources) that are tailored to the needs of the health professionals being trained can be part of the solution to reduce the impact of staff turnover. • Opportunities for retraining beyond initial competency expiratory dates must be part of POC testing policy to minimise risk to patient safety.
Awareness of limitations of the POC test method used	• Common limitations of and interferences for individual test methods should be noted from manufacturer's IFU (instructions for use) and recorded in quality management documents. • Temperature and humidity limits for device operation should also be noted/documented as field conditions may preclude routine device operation if these parameters are exceeded.

Limitations	Comment
Potential for overuse/misuse of POC test	• POC test should only be used for its intended clinical purpose, as defined in policy documents. Outside this scope should be considered 'off label' use, which requires additional validation as an in-house, in-vitro diagnostic test.
Unavailability of suitable quality materials to monitor analytical performance	• For some POC tests, particularly in the event of a new disease outbreak e.g., commercially available, robust QC and EQA materials may not be manufactured or available. • Engagement of field operators regarding the importance of QC and EQA testing is critical; without an understanding of why quality testing is needed and subsequent investment from operators, the POC test system may fail and risk to patient safety is increased. • Non-conformance with agreed procedures for QC and EQA testing can increase risk to patient safety.
Cost of introducing a POC test system	• Without government support in terms of block funding or rebates for testing, costs of introducing POC testing may be prohibitive. If so, scalability of POC testing networks to regional or national levels in the event of an outbreak may be impracticable.

Table 6.
Limiting factors for the uptake of POC testing in a global security event.

6. Concluding remarks

Utilising a variety of analytical methodologies and device types, point-of-care testing has proven a valuable tool in improving equity of access to pathology services in high-risk, remote communities within Australia and has been an invaluable and complementary diagnostic aid in assisting the COVID-19 pandemic surveillance and public health response in this country.

Specifically, molecular-based POC testing offers rapid detection of individual active infection and thus has broad application in the context of future global security, especially considering the predicted upsurge in emerging infectious diseases, the development of multiplexed assays to detect related disease types simultaneously and the possible device simplification and miniaturisation of POC tests through the application of microfluidic technologies (e.g. that may combine molecular-based methods in a lateral flow type format). Ideally, post-market assay evaluation and verification studies are required for the provision of integral, robust evidence prior to scaling-up quality POC testing. Such studies should be comprehensively performed and reported prior to the widespread implementation of any new diagnostic test or technology. However, in the advent of rapid diagnostic toolkits for disaster management, new infectious disease outbreaks or future pandemics, extensive field evaluation performed outside of the laboratory setting is often not possible. Under these circumstances, it is even more pertinent that POC testing is underpinned by robust training and quality management systems specifically adapted for different environmental settings using non-laboratory staff, combined with appropriate clinical governance and linkage to care.

In conclusion, POC testing has the potential to deliver equity of access to pathology testing in remote communities and broader public health impact in high- and special-risk populations during events of global significance. Fundamental to the successful implementation of POC testing is recognition that POC testing is founded in medical science and requires the following complimentary elements: strong leadership and investment from Governments; a solid governance structure to support POC testing field programs; sound preparation for implementation of POC testing including comprehensive training and competency, quality management and connectivity systems, the flexible and nimble repurposing of multiplex devices if available, adaptable redistribution and reprioritisation for testing cartridges when supplies are low. In this context, the real-world application of POC testing serves as a complementary, yet important, diagnostic tool should or when future global health security issues arise.

Acknowledgements

This book chapter is written on behalf of the large, multidisciplinary POC testing teams at the Kirby Institute and the Flinders University International Centre for Point-of-Care Testing. The authors acknowledge and thank the Australian Government Department of Health and Aged Care for their support in funding the QAAMS, ESR, TTANGO and Aboriginal and Torres Strait Islander COVID-19 POC Testing networks. The Northern Territory Government is also acknowledged for funding the NT acute care POC testing program. The authors acknowledge the contribution to these networks of many stakeholders including the National Aboriginal Community Controlled Health Organisation (NACCHO); Indigenous Leaders Forum and Groups, participating Aboriginal community controlled and government health services; national, jurisdictional and local Aboriginal Community Controlled Health Organisations; national, State and Territory health departments, and other government services; our industry and academic partners; pathology providers and most importantly, the dedicated health professional staff working as POC testing operators in our networks.

Conflict of interest

The authors have no conflict of interest to declare.

Author details

Mark Shephard[1*], Susan Matthews[1], Louise Causer[2], Belinda Hengel[2] and Rebecca Guy[2]

1 Flinders University International Centre for Point-of-Care Testing, Adelaide, Australia

2 Kirby institute, University of New South Wales, Sydney, Australia

*Address all correspondence to: mark.shephard@flinders.edu.au

References

[1] Precedence Research, Ottawa, Canada. Healthcare: Point-of-Care Testing Market. Report Code 2270 [Internet]. 2023. Available from: https://www.precedenceresearch.com/pointof-care-testing-market [Accessed: 26 August 2023]

[2] Shephard M, Shephard A, Matthews S, Andrewartha K. The benefits and challenges of point-of-care testing in rural and remote primary care settings in Australia. Archives of Pathology and Laboratory Medicine. 2020;**144**(11):1372-1380. DOI: 10.5858/arpa.2020-0105-RA

[3] Shephard M. An introduction to point-of-care testing and its global scope and application. In: Shephard M, editor. A Practical Guide to Global Point-of-Care Testing. Melbourne, Australia: CSIRO Publishing; 2016. pp. 1-14

[4] Shephard M, Matthews S, Markus C, de Courcy-Ireland E, Duckworth L, Haklar I, et al. Pathology testing at the point of patient care: Transformational change for rural communities. In: Rusangwa C, editor. Rural Health - Investment, Research and Implications. London, UK: IntechOpen; 2023. pp. 1-29. DOI: 10.5772/intechopen.109769

[5] Spaeth B, Matthews S, Shephard M. Patient-centred point-of-care testing: A life-changing technology for remote health care. In: Onal A, editor. Primary Health Care. London, UK: IntechOpen; 2021. pp. 1-15. DOI: 10.5772/intechopen.100375

[6] Hengel B, Causer L, Matthews S, Smith K, Andrewartha K, Badman S, et al. A decentralised point-of-care testing model to address inequities in the COVID-19 response. The Lancet InfectiousDiseases.2020;**21**(7):e183-e190. DOI: 10.1016/S1473-3099(20)30859-8

[7] Shephard M, Shephard A, McAteer B, Regnier T, Barancek K. Results from 15 years of quality surveillance for a national Indigenous point-of-care testing program for diabetes. Clinical Biochemistry. 2017;**50**:1159-1163. DOI: 10.1016/j.clinbiochem.2017.07.007

[8] Regnier T, Shephard M, Shephard A, Graham P, DeLeon R, Shepherd S. Results form 16 years of quality surveillance of urine albumin to creatinine ratio testing for a national Indigenous point-of-care testing program. Archives of Pathology and Laboratory Medicine. 2020;**144**:1199-1203. DOI: 10.5858/arpa.2020-0106-OA

[9] Shephard M. Clinical and cultural effectiveness of the 'QAAMS' point-of-care testing model for diabetes management in Australian Aboriginal medical services. Clinical Biochemist Reviews. 2006;**27**:161-170

[10] Spaeth BA, Shephard MDS, Schatz S. Point-of-care testing for haemoglobin A1c in remote Australian Indigenous communities improves timeliness of diabetes care. Rural and Remote Health. 2014;**14**:2849. Available from: http://www.rrh.org.au/articles/printviewnew.asp?ArticleID=2849

[11] Matthews S, Spaeth B, Duckworth L, Richards J, Prisk E, Auld M, et al. Sustained quality and service delivery in an expanding point-of-care testing network in remote Australian primary care. Archives of Pathology and Laboratory Medicine. 2020;**144**(11):1381-1391. DOI: 10.5858/arpa.2020-0105-RA

[12] Shephard M, Spaeth B, Mazzachi B, Auld M, Schatz S, Loudon J, et al. Design,

implementation and initial assessment of the Northern Territory point-of-care testing program. Australian Journal of Rural Health. 2012;**20**:16-21. DOI: 10.1111/j.1440-1584.2011.01243.x

[13] Spaeth BA, Shephard MDS, Omond R. Clinical application of point-of-care testing in the remote primary health care setting. Quality in Primary Care. 2017;**25**:164-175

[14] Spaeth BA, Kaambwa B, Shephard MDS, Omond R. Economic evaluation of point-of-care testing in the remote primary health care setting of Australia's Northern Territory. ClinicoEconomics and Outcomes Research. 2018;**10**:269-277. DOI: 10.2147/CEOR.S160291

[15] Remote Primary Health Care Manuals. Manuals [Internet]. 2022. Available from: https://remotephcmanuals.com.au/ [Accessed: 26 August 2023]

[16] Equity Economics. Blueprint for the Future: Evaluation of NACCHO's Role under the Enhanced Syphilis Response. A Report Prepared for the National Aboriginal Community Controlled Health Organisation (NACCHO). 2021. pp. 2-5

[17] Centers for Disease Control and Prevention. Pandemic (H1N1 Virus). 1918. Available from: https://www.cdc.gov/flu/pandemic-resources/1918-pandemic-h1n1.html [Accessed: 26 August 2023]

[18] Ride K, Burrow S. Review of diabetes among Aboriginal and Torres Strait Islander people. Journal of the Australian Indigenous HealthInfoNet. 2022;**3**(2):3. DOI: 10.14221/aihjournal.v3n2.1

[19] National Pathology Accreditation Advisory Council (NPAAC). NPAAC Requirements for Point of Care Testing. 2nd ed. Australian Government Department of Health [Internet]; 2021. Available from: https://www1.health.gov.au/internet/main/publishing.nsf/Content/35DE5FC4786CBB33CA257EEB007C7BF2/$File/DT0002469%20-%20NPAAC%20-%20Requirements%20for%20point%20of%20care%20testing%20Second%20edition%202021%20-%2020211215.pdf [Accessed: 26 August 2023]

[20] Public Health Laboratory Network. PHLN Guidance on Laboratory Testing for SARS-CoV-2 (The Virus that Causes COVID-19). Available from: https://www.health.gov.au/sites/default/files/documents/2022/01/phln-guidance-on-laboratory-testing-for-sars-cov-2-the-virus-that-causes-covid-19.pdf [Accessed: 26 August 2023]

[21] Communicable Disease Network Australia. Coronavirus (COVID-19). CDNA National Guidelines for Public Health Units. Available from: https://www.health.gov.au/resources/publications/coronavirus-covid-19-cdna-national-guidelines-for-public-health-units?language=en [Accessed: 26 August 2023]

[22] Ministers. Australian Government Department of Health and Aged Care. First Confirmed Case of Novel Coronavirus in Australia. Media Release January 25, 2020. Available form: https://www.health.gov.au/ministers/the-hon-greg-hunt-mp/media/first-confirmed-case-of-novel-coronavirus-in-australia [Accessed: 26 August 2023]

[23] Australian Government Department of Health and Aged Care. About Coronavirus (COVID-19). Available from: https://www.health.gov.au/topics/covid-19/about#:~:text=The%20World%20Health%20Organization%20(WHO)%20declared%20the%20

novel%20coronavirus%20(pandemic%20 declaration%20is%20still%20active [Accessed: 26 August 2023]

[24] World Health Organization Coronavirus (COVID-19) Dashboard. Available from: https://covid19.who.int/ [Accessed: 26 August 2023]

[25] Nous Group. Department of Health and Aged Care. Evaluation of COVID-19 Point-of-Care Testing in Remote and First Nations Communities. 2022. Available from: https://www.health.gov.au/sites/default/files/2023-05/evaluation-of-covid-19-point-of-care-testing-in-remote-and-first-nations-communities_0.pdf [Accessed: 26 August 2023]

[26] Flint SM, David JS, Su J-Y, Oliver-Landy EP, Rogers BA, Goldstein A, et al. Disproportionate impact of pandemic (H1N1) 2009 influenza on Indigenous people in the top end of Australia's Northern Territory. Medical Journal of Australia. 2010;**192**:617-622. DOI: 10.5694/j.1326-5377.2010.tb03654.x

[27] Causer LM, Guy RJ, Tabrizi SN, Whiley DM, Speers DJ, Ward J, et al. Molecular test for chlamydia and gonorrhoea used at point of care in remote primary healthcare settings: A diagnostic test evaluation. Sexually Transmitted Infections. 2018;**94**:340-345. DOI: 10.1136/sextrans-2017-053443

[28] Guy RJ, Ward J, Causer LM, Natoli L, Badman SG, Tangey A, et al. Molecular point-of-care testing for chlamydia and gonorrhoea among Indigenous people attending primary health services: A cross-over cluster randomised controlled trial. Lancet Infectious Diseases. 2018;**18**:1117-1126. DOI: 10.1016/S1473-3099(18)30429-8

[29] Australian Government Department of Health: Therapeutic Goods Administration. COVID-19 Test Kits Included on the ARTG for Legal Supply in Australia. Available from: https://www.tga.gov.au/resources/covid-19-test-kits/xpertr-xpress-sars-cov-2 [Accessed: 26 August 2020]

[30] World Health Organization. Laboratory Biosafety Guidance Related to Coronavirus Disease (COVID-19). Interim Guidance. May 13, 2020. Available from: https://www.who.int/publications/i/item/laboratory-biosafety-guidance-related-to-coronavirus-disease-(covid-19) [Accessed: 26 August 2023]

[31] van Bockel D, Munier CML, Turville S, Badman SG, Walker G, Stella AO, et al. Evaluation of commercially available viral transport medium (VTM) for SARS-CoV-2 inactivation and use in point-of-care (POC) testing. Viruses. 2020;**12**(11):1208. DOI: 10.3390/v12111208

[32] Al-Kindi N, Al-Shukri I, Al-Rashdi A, Al-Siyabi N, Al Mahruqi S, Al-Kindi H, et al. Validation of GeneXpert testing for SARS-CoV-2 RNA in eight hospital laboratories in Oman. The Pan African Medical Journal. 2021;**40**. Article 2. DOI: 10.11604/pamj.2021.40.2.27224

[33] Andrewartha K, Shephard M, Milic, M, Miller K, Malinsky E, Byers D, et al. Quality assurance testing for SARS-CoV-2 RNA detection in the Aboriginal and Torres Strait Islander COVID-19 point-of-care testing program. In: Presented as a Poster at the 1st Australasian Conference on POC Testing for Infectious Diseases (POC 23 Conference); 14-15 March 2023; Sydney, Australia. Available from: https://researchnow.flinders.edu.au/en/publications/quality-assurance-testing-for-sars-cov-2-rna-detection-in-the-abo

[34] Therapeutic Goods Administration. Classification of IVD Medical Devices. Available from: https://www.tga.gov.au/sites/default/files/classification-ivd-medical-devices.pdf [Accessed: 26 August 2023]

[35] Saha A, Andrewartha K, Badman S, Tangey A, Smith K, Sandler S, et al. A flexible and innovative connectivity solution to support national decentralised infectious diseases point-of-care testing programs in primary health services in Australia. Journal of Medical Internet Research. 2023;**25**:e46701. DOI. 10.2196/46701

[36] Shephard M, Arbon P, Kost G. Point-of-care testing for disaster management. In: Shephard M, editor. A Practical Guide to Global Point-of-Care Testing. Melbourne, Australia: CSIRO Publishing; 2016. pp. 378-392

[37] Mabey D, Peeling RW, Ustanowski A, Perkins MD. Diagnostics for the developing world. Nature Reviews Microbiology 2002;**2**:231-240. DOI: https://doi.org/10.1038/nrmicro841

[38] Land KJ, Boeras DI, Chen X-S, Ramsay AR, Peeling RW. REASSURED diagnostics to inform disease control strategies, strengthen health systems and improve patient outcomes. Nature Microbiology. 2019;**4**:46-54. DOI: 10.1038/s41564-018-0295-3

Section 4

Leadership, Workforce Development and Finance

Chapter 9

Global Health Security: An Evaluation of Public Health Expenditure, Health Status and Economic Development in Nigeria

Ngozi Chioma Ewurum and Samuel Oseloka Okafor

Abstract

This chapter examines the intersection of public health expenditure, health status, and economic development in Nigeria and their implications for global health security. Drawing on a comprehensive dataset spanning the period, 1981-2021, the study utilizes a simultaneous equation model, employing three-stage least squares for data estimation. We developed an innovative composite economic development index (EDI) that integrates the Seers' Three-Pillars Model of Development encompassing poverty, inequality, and unemployment using principal component analysis (PCA). Additionally, the study crafted a health status index, utilizing indicators such as infant, under-five, maternal mortality rates, and crude death rate. Utilizing PCA allows for a comprehensive evaluation of economic development that encompasses both socio-economic and health dimensions. Other control variables used were adopted from the six WHO health system building blocks. Findings reveal bidirectional causal relationships between public health expenditure and health status, with a unidirectional causal relationship observed from health status to economic development. There is no direct causal link between public health expenditure and economic development, indicating an indirect impact through health status. This inferred that the impact of public health expenditure on economic development works through the health status channel. Policy recommendations include increasing budget allocations to health sector, subsidizing health services, and addressing poverty, inequality, and unemployment issues by improving health infrastructure, income levels, enhancing equitable healthcare accessibility and affordability, bolstering human resources for health in the healthcare sector and reliable power generation. These interventions are essential for fostering sustainable and inclusive economic development in Nigeria, enhancing the country's resilience to health crises, reducing vulnerability to mortality rates and diseases, thereby contributing to global health security efforts.

Keywords: public health expenditure, health status, composite economic development index, global health security, three-pillar model of development, simultaneous equation, three-stage least square (3SLS)

IntechOpen

1. Introduction

Economic development has become pervasive that the pursuit of economic progress and its impact have permeated multiple dimensions of society. The persistent global concern and attention towards sustainable economic development have spurred various efforts by countries especially developing nations, to prioritize health policies, programs and agendas alongside their economic growth strategies. Globally, healthcare especially child health is identified as a core factor for long-run economic development [1]. Thus, Investing in health initiatives such as the sustainable development Goals (SDGs) adopted by UN member states in 2015, aiming to address various global challenges, including poverty, hunger, and inequality within and among countries is vital for ensuring healthy lives and promoting overall well-being for all citizens at all ages, as they are essential components for a sustainable economic development. In the context of global health security, economic development is closely tied to a nation's ability to invest in and maintain a strong healthcare system. However, economic development often leads to improved infrastructure, including healthcare facilities, which can enhance a country's ability to respond to emergencies and outbreaks. Conversely, weak health systems in any country, including Nigeria, can pose a threat to global health security. Diseases can easily cross borders, and insufficient healthcare infrastructure may hinder a country's ability to respond effectively to outbreaks.

Strong, resilient, and inclusive health systems are crucial foundations for addressing the most pressing health challenges worldwide [2]. It includes achieving the Sustainable Development Goal (SDG) target of Universal Health Coverage (UHC) as well as ensuring national, regional, and global health security (https://sustainabledevelopment.un.org/SDG3) [3]. They are essential for improving health outcomes, promoting social and economic development, and building healthier, more resilient societies [2, 4].

Global health security has become a critical concern in the twenty-first century, with infectious diseases, pandemics, and other health challenges and emergencies posing significant threats to populations worldwide. In this context, understanding the dynamics of public health expenditure, health status indicators, and economic development in individual countries is essential for effective preparedness and response to health crises. Nigeria, as the most populous country in Africa, faces unique challenges in ensuring health security for its citizens and contributing to global health stability. Health constitutes a fundamental human right, and ensuring effective global public health security hinges upon a collective responsibility [5]. The collective responsibility for global health involves cooperation among nations to address various challenges like infectious diseases, maternal and child mortality rates, pandemics, and healthcare access. It requires sharing resources, knowledge, and technology to build resilient healthcare systems and respond effectively to health emergencies. By prioritizing investment in healthcare, Nigeria can contribute to addressing global health challenges while also advancing its own inclusive economic development agenda [6, 7].

Health is a fundamental determinant of an individual's overall quality of life, with broader implications for global well-being and safety. The interconnectedness of national health dynamics carries profound ramifications for global health and safety. The imperative lies in fostering international collaboration, fortifying robust health systems, and ensuring effective governance. This imperative trifecta forms the linchpin for adeptly managing the intricate interplay of global health implications; thereby advancing a collective framework for sustained well-being on a global scale. However, the correlation between health and economic development is consistent with the worldwide endeavors aimed at attaining the sustainable development Goals (SDGs), with a specific focus on Goal 3 (Good Health and Well-being for all at all ages) and Goal 8 (Decent Work and Economic Growth). Achieving these goals by 2030 involves reducing global maternal mortality ratio to less than 70 per 1000 live births, preventing newborns and child deaths to at least as low as 12 per 1000 live births and 25 per 1000 live births respectively, and in turn fostering sustainable development (United Nations-sustainable Development Goals; https://sustainabledevelopment .un.org/SDGs3). However, increase investment in health systems is needed to support countries in their recovery and build resilience against future health threats. Therefore, advancement in healthcare not only enhances individual well-being but plays a pivotal role in fostering the sustainable success of broader development initiatives.

In the dynamic landscape of global health security, nations stand at the crossroad of public health resilience, the well-being of their populations, and economic development. Public health resilience refers to a nation's capacity and ability to effectively manage, prepare for, respond to, and recover from health crises. However, the overall welfare of the citizens underscores the comprehensive nature of well-being, including physical and mental health, access to education, and a satisfactory quality of life. Nations must consider the holistic welfare of their populations as an integral component of their broader health security and development agendas. Global health security involves collaboration among nations to ensure the health and well-being of people worldwide. However, a well-functioning and resilient health system is fundamental to achieving a regional, national and global health security. Sustained progress on global health security cannot be made without functioning and resilient health system capable of protecting all people, including the poorest and most marginalized from health threats [8].

An essential element of economic development of a country is its people state of health. Economic development can be understood as a multifaceted process that involves sustained economic growth, expanding human freedoms, and creating an environment that supports people's well-being [9]. As articulated by Sachs [10], economic development delineates the trajectory through which nations transcend poverty and attain higher levels of economic and social well-being which encompasses improvement in quality of life, income per capita, employment opportunities, access to healthcare, education, social services and a general enhancement of societal conditions. Thus, economic development is referred to as a process of sustained increased in the real per capita income of a country, accompanied by structural transformation and diversification of the economy, improvement in living standards and reduction in poverty and inequality [11–13].

Health in the Post-2015 Agenda [14], a report of the Global Thematic Consultation on Health, recognizes health as a critical contributor to, and outcome of, sustainable development and human well-being. Health status refers to the overall health and well-being of individuals within a population. Thus, Makuta and O'Hare [15] sees improved health status as not only a goal but a prerequisite for the development process, since good health and wellbeing is a life asset globally and an important form of human capital. Therefore, to make the biggest impact on development, then, the government must empower and invest in citizens by increasing health expenditure and devoting substantial funds to its health sector to support its healthcare need [16].

Public health expenditure involves funding for various health-related activities such as healthcare services, preventive measures, healthcare infrastructures, personnel, medicines, and research. Adequate funding for healthcare is crucial for the development of a robust health system, capable of handling a higher volume of patients during emergencies and providing effective preventive measures. It involves having a robust healthcare system, emergency response mechanism, and the ability to manage and control the spread of diseases. Unfortunately, in developing countries like Nigeria, the percentage allocation for health is habitually minuscule, resulting in poor health outcomes [17]. Okafor [18] confirms that Nigeria health situation is of growing concern especially in the area of children, women/mothers and most vulnerable in the society while Amiri and Gerdtham [19] argue that significant investments are needed to improve women and children's health, arguing that they are fundamental to development. However, despite the investments and some improvements made so far on health sector, Nigeria's health indices remain weak and this is a significant challenge stating that Nigeria's average life expectancy was 54.3% in 2018 and the infant mortality rate stood at 74.2 per 1000 live births in 2019 [20–22]. Weak health systems in any country, including Nigeria, can pose a threat to global health security. Disease can easily cross borders, and insufficient healthcare infrastructure may hinder a country's ability to respond effectively to outbreaks.

In Nigeria, challenges such as corruption, mismanagement, and insufficient allocation of funds have historically affected the healthcare sector. Insufficient funding can lead to a lack of essential resources and services, impacting the overall health of the population and global health security at alrge. Consequently, the health infrastructure in Nigeria faces various challenges, including inadequate facilities, a shortage of healthcare professionals, and uneven distribution of resources. Strengthening and expanding healthcare infrastructure are essential for improving overall health security. Indeed, the World Bank noted that the Nigeria's government expenditure on health is the lowest in the world. The budgetary allocation to health in 2018 by the Federal Government was only 4.5%, compared to 7.1% for education and 7.8% for power, works and housing. In 2019, the budgetary allocation to health was 4.7%; in 2020 and 2021, it was 4.14% and 4.18% respectively. This marginal increase to 4.18% in 2021 budget was as a result of the sudden outbreak of COVID-19 pandemic. Therefore, it is not surprising that health outcomes in the country are among the poorest in the world [23, 24].

Despite these challenges, health remains a critical tool for promoting a sustainable economic development in a rapidly changing world by advocating for an investment in health sector through allocation of a sizeable fund to health sector which will reduce mortality rates and in turn lead to poverty, inequality and unemployment reduction in other to attain economic development. Conversely, Dudley Seers theory of development has made significant contributions to the discourse on development by highlighting the importance of considering social dimensions alongside economic growth.

The objective of this chapter is to examine the relationship among public health expenditure, health status, and economic development in Nigeria and its broader implication for global health security. It seeks to advance conceptual instruments based on Dudley Seers' developmental approach. It advocates for a multidimensional perspective that includes poverty, inequality, unemployment, and other socioeconomic factors. This necessitates the creation of measurement indices capturing these dimensions for a more holistic understanding of development outcomes. Building upon Seers' concepts on development known as Seers' Three-Pillar Model of development which is a combination of poverty, inequality, and unemployment as key dimension, this chapter introduces and developed a new composite index, the composite economic development index (EDI), tailored to assess the specific development level in Nigeria. This economic development index aims to provide a more comprehensive and context-specific evaluation of economic development in the country. The composite economic development index (EDI) is considered a novel concept of measuring economic development because it extends beyond the traditional scope of conventional economic indices.

Following the introduction, we structured this chapter as thus; Section 2 briefly reviewed some related literatures by providing some conceptual issues necessary to understand more fundamental critiques of development and theoretical underpinning, together with the empirical literature. Section 3 provides the research methods while Section 4 presents and discusses the results. Section 5 provides the conclusion and policy recommendation.

2. Review of related literature and theoretical underpinning

2.1 Conceptual issues

2.1.1 Economic development

Economic development is a multifaceted concept with diverse perspectives, lacking a widely embraced definition. Over time, scholars have offered diverse definitions, with perspectives evolving from a narrow focus on GDP growth in the 1950s and 1960s to broader views considering social, political, and environmental factors. Scholars like Sen [25] emphasize the inadequacy of income measures alone, proposing a capability approach that emphasized expanding people's freedom and well-being. He sees the ability to access education, healthcare, and unemployment insurance as central elements that expand people's capabilities [26]. According to Sen [27], furthermore, "the main purpose of development is to spread freedom and its 'thousand charms' to the unfree citizens" implying that freedom is not only valuable in itself but also leads to a multitude of other positive outcomes, such as economic prosperity, social harmony, and personal fulfilment. Todaro and Smith [28, 29] viewed development as enhancing human lives and capabilities by raising people's level of living, self-esteem, and freedom while Sachs [10] ties economic development to the goal of eradicating poverty and promoting sustainability. This reflects a global perspective that considers not only individual well-being but also broader issues of equity and environmental sustainability.

Consequently, the emphasis on multi-dimensional approaches has led to the development of alternative frameworks for measuring economic development known as the Human Development Index (HDI) constructed with inputs from Amartya Sen by the United Nation Development Program (UNDP) [30]. This incorporates a single composite index measures of three equally weighted indicators: longevity (a proxy for health measured by life expectancy at birth and Nutrition); Education- (composite of the adult literacy rate and the combined gross enrolment ratio for primary, secondary, and post-secondary schools); and standard of living measured by GNI per capita [31]. The Human Development Index (HDI) is a globally accepted measure. Unfortunately, it does not reflect the true developmental situation in the developing countries such as Nigeria. Critics argue it falls short in capturing the complexities of development, where issues such as gender disparity, poverty, unemployment and inequality persist. The HDI, though valuable, does not fully reflect recent policy changes or address aspects like human security, empowerment and inequality ([32] by UNDP) (hdr.undp.org/data-center).

Seers [33] advocated a comprehensive approach to development, emphasizing poverty reduction, employment generation, and reduction in inequality, improvement in health, education and living standard in addition to topline measures like increase in GDP per capita growth. He argued that a narrow focus on economic growth, without considering its impact on poverty, inequality and unemployment reduction (social welfare) could lead to skewed development. The ideas put forth by these scholars [26, 33] significantly influenced the shift towards a broader understanding of poverty and development. However, Dudley Seers, a British economist, provided a comprehensive framework for understanding economic development, a concept that replaced the growth fetishism with social development, a theory he propounded known as Seers' Three-Pillar Model. In 1969, he signaled this shift about the meaning of development succinctly emphasizing that genuine economic development transcends mere increase in per capita income, requiring a simultaneous improvement in all three critical dimensions. World Bank [34] aligned with Seers' development concepts, defining development as progress in the quality of life encompassing higher income, quality education, improved health and nutrition, poverty reduction, a hygienic environment, equal opportunities, enhanced personal freedom, and an enriched cultural life. This perspective from the World Bank implies that development is a multi-dimensional process characterized by significant transformations in social structure, national institutions, and the acceleration of economic growth.

2.1.2 Public health expenditure

Public health expenditure refers to the financial resources invested by the government to promote and maintain the health of its citizens. World Bank [35] defines public health expenditure as covering the provision of health services (preventive and curative), family planning activities, nutrition activities and emergency aid designated for health but does not include provision of water and sanitation. All can be financed through domestic funds or through external resources. Ndedi et al. [36] in Olayiwola et al. [37] argued that health expenditure means investment in health sector and infrastructure, spending on medical care, community health activities, prevention, rehabilitation, health administration and regulation, and capital formation which indirectly means investment in human capital and leads to human capital accumulation.

Health status is a crucial determinant of the quality of human capital resources, which helps to promote economic growth and development of a nation [38]. Health is recognized as an essential component of human development. According to Gyimah-Brempong and Wilson [39] health is a crucially important economic asset for many poor people and their livelihoods depend upon it.

2.1.3 Global health security (GHS)

WHO [4] defines global health security as "the activities required, both proactive and reactive, to minimize vulnerability to acute public health events that endanger the collective health of the populations living across geographical regions and international boundaries." It focuses on preparing, preventing, detecting, and responding to infectious disease threat that have the potentials to cross borders and spread rapidly, endangering human health and economies worldwide. This includes efforts to strengthen healthcare systems, improve surveillance and response capabilities, and promote international collaboration to address health emergencies effectively. However, strong healthcare systems are foundational to effective global health security. This involves investments in healthcare infrastructure, workforce development, and access to essential medical supplies and treatments [40].

2.2 Theoretical underpinning

2.2.1 Theories of public expenditure

Adolph Wagner, a German economist, in his Law of "increasing state Activities" states that, there are inherent tendencies for the activities of the government to increase both extensively and intensively. He postulates that during the process of economic development the share of public spending in national income tends to expand [41]. Hence, there is a functional relationship between the growth of an economy and government expenditure. The expansion in government activities leads to the increase in public expenditure which automatically leads to the growth in the economy [42–45]. Thus, the expansion of public expenditure can be seen as a product of the economic development and not vice versa (Bird [46] in [47]).

2.2.2 Dudley Seers theory of development: Seers Three-Pillars Model

Development theorist and practitioner such as Dudley Seers and Denis Goulet championed the notion that development entails much more than economic growth or increase in income per capita, but should encompass broader social and human aspects. The Dudley Seers theory of development, also known as the Seers' Three-Pillar Model, was proposed by Dudley Seers, a British economist, in the 1960s. According to Seers [33] the purpose of development is to reduce poverty, inequality and unemployment. Seers shifted away from such believe by asking the following questions about a country's development: What has been happening to poverty? What has been happening to unemployment? What has been happening to inequality? If all three of these have been less severe, then beyond doubt this has been a period of development for the country concerned. If one or two of these central problems have been growing worse, especially if all three have, it would be strange to call the result "development", even if per capita income has soared [33]. Thus, Seers propounded a theory on economic development which emphasized the necessity of addressing poverty, inequality and unemployment as key imperatives for development.

2.3 Profile of health budgetary allocation in Nigeria

FG budgetary allocations to health sector (in ₦ billion) and health budget expenditure breakdown (2001–2021) have been presented in both **Figures 1** and **2** respectively.

Figure 1 reveals the variations in the health sector budgetary allocation between 2001 and 2021.

The graph illustrates the allocation of funds to the health sector as a percentage of the total federal budget in Nigeria, considering other funding in the service-wide vote. In 2012, the highest allocation was 6.08% of $29,276.71 (N4, 648,849), and subsequent years (2016–2021) saw marginal increases, with percentages ranging from

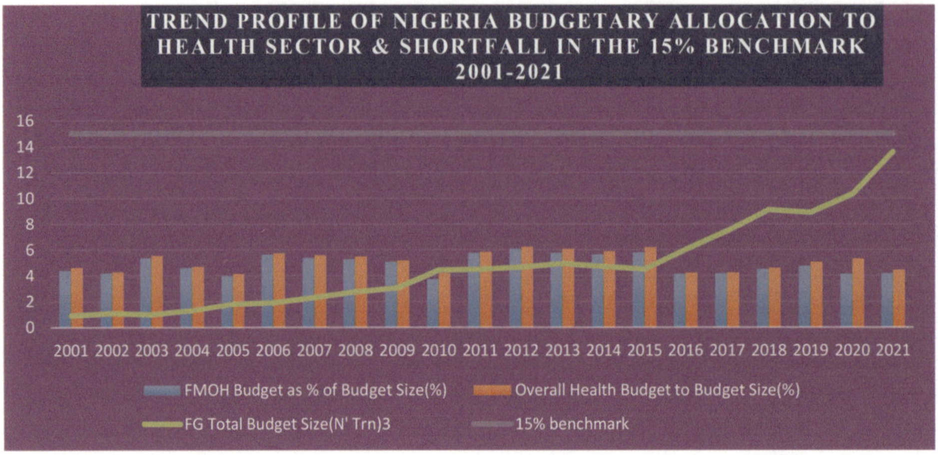

Figure 1.
Trend of Nigeria budgetary allocation to health sector with shortfall in the 15% Benchmark (2001–2021).

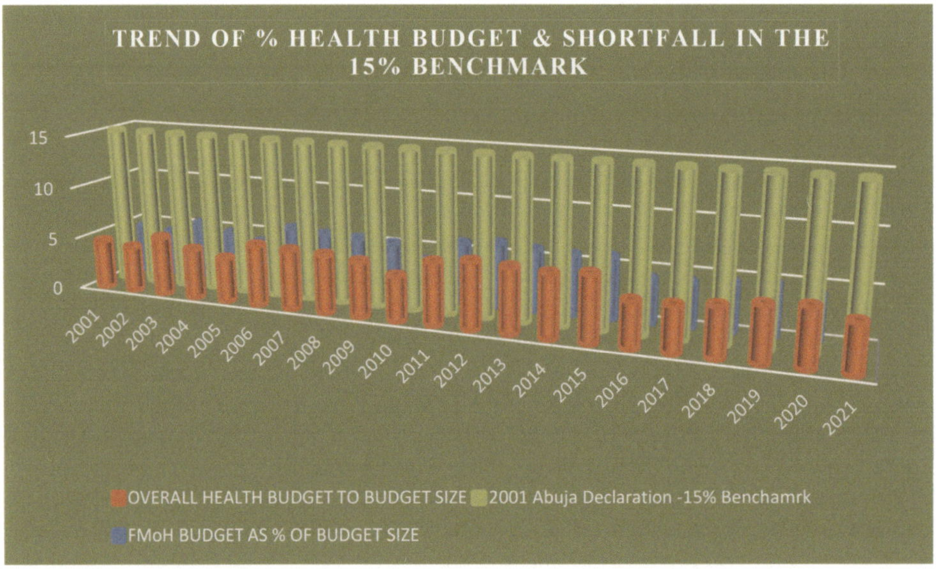

Figure 2.
Trend of health budget shortfall in the 15% Benchmark in Nigeria (2001–2021). Source: [20], (PACFaH Scale) 2021.

4.13%, 4.17%, 4.51%, 4.75%, 4.14% and 4.18% respectively. This slow upward trend reflects a deviation from the Abuja Declarations of 15% benchmark, indicating insufficient commitment of FG to prioritizing health.

Despite the COVID-19 pandemic, there was no substantial increase in health budget allocation either to meet African Union's 15% or the WHO's 11% benchmark. This suggests a notable gap between budgetary allocations and the healthcare needs of the population, potentially hindering economic development. The persistently low health expenditures may be a contributing factor to Nigeria's sluggish economic growth and development. Consequently, understanding the impact of public health expenditure on economic development in Nigeria becomes a crucial area for investigation. The aim of this study is to inspire a new perspective among policymakers, urging them to adopt strategies that simultaneously enhance public health, improve health status/outcomes, and foster economic development, thereby creating a more robust and resilient global health security framework. However, **Figure 2** shows a clearer trend of the overall health budget to budget size, budget as a percentage of budget size and 2001 Abuja declaration of 15% funding benchmark.

Figure 2 is a clear indication that the FG budgetary allocations which fell far below the 15% Abuja benchmark were abysmally low and grossly inadequate. Even the COVID-19 pandemic that causes a wide scare among Nigerians did not provide desired stimulus to the FG to prioritize health by increasing budgetary allocation to the health sector. Overall health budget to budget to budget size was 4.45% as at 2021 while Budget as % of budget size was 4.18 in 2021.

2.4 Empirical literature review

Previous studies examining the relationship between public health expenditure and economic growth have generally emphasized the importance of sufficient investment in healthcare for achieving positive health outcomes and fostering economic growth. However, studies specific to Nigeria have shown mixed results, with challenges such as inefficient resource allocation, weak health infrastructure, and high disease burden hindering the effectiveness of health investments. Moreover, the interplay between health status indicators and economic development in Nigeria has been a subject of debate, with some scholars arguing for a causal relationship and others suggesting a more complex interaction. Understanding these dynamics is crucial for designing evidence-based policies to strengthen Nigeria's health system and enhance its contribution to global health security. Therefore, exploring the intricate connection among public health expenditure, health status, and economic development in Nigeria, alongside the innovative concept of introducing a composite economic development index (EDI) as a metric, is imperative for informing strategies to improve healthcare, enhance well-being, and bolster global health security.

Makuta and O'Hare [15] investigated the relationship between public health spending (PSH), quality of governance (QoG), and health outcomes in Sub-Saharan Africa from 1996 to 2011. Using a two-staged least square (2SLS) regression technique on panel data from 43 countries, the study found that improving the quality of governance positively impacted health outcomes. Additionally, the research revealed that the same increase in public health spending is twice as effective in reducing under-five mortality and increasing life expectancy in countries with higher quality of governance compared to those with poor governance. In summary, the study emphasizes the significant role of governance quality in enhancing the effectiveness of public health spending on health outcomes in Sub-Saharan Africa.

2.5 Review of Literature

Ibe and Olulu-Briggs [48] examined the impact of public health expenditure on economic growth in Nigeria from 1981 to 2013. The results showed that increasing public health expenditure in Nigeria positively and significantly impacts economic growth, and a unidirectional causality was observed between GDP and all public health expenditure variables, including gross capital formation, total education, and total health expenditure, as indicated by various analytical techniques including OLS regression, co-integration, and Granger causality used in the study. Their results suggest a need for policymakers to prioritize healthcare budget allocations for sustained economic development, despite the study's limitations, such as the inclusion of non-associative variables like total education expenditure.

Boachie and Ramu [49] studied the effect of public health expenditure and health status in Ghana. The study covered the period, 1990–2012. Study employed standard OLS and Newey-white estimation technique. After controlling for real per capita income, literacy level and female participation in the labour market, results indicate evidence that the declining infant mortality rate in Ghana is explained by public health spending among other factors. Thus, they concluded that public healthcare expenditure is associated with improvement in health status through reduction in infant mortality. The study constitutes suitable reference materials for the present study.

Piabuo and Tieguhong [50] conducted a comparative analysis on the impact of health expenditure on economic growth in Central African State (CEMAC) countries and other selected African nations. They used three panel regression models and found that health expenditure positively influenced economic growth in both groups. Additionally, a negative significant relationship existed between household expenditure and GDP per capita for five African countries, while CEMAC countries showed a negative non-significant relationship. The study highlighted a bidirectional causal relationship between GDP per capita and health expenditure in CEMAC, contributing valuable techniques for comparative analysis.

Boachie et al. [51] re-examined the relationship between government health expenditure and health outcomes in Ghana from 1980 to 2014. Using life expectancy, infant, and under-five mortality rates as health outcome measures, the research employed both OLS and 2SLS estimators. The findings indicated that, apart from income, an increase in public health expenditure was associated with improvements in health outcomes in Ghana. Specifically, higher public health expenditure correlated with reduced infant and under-five mortality rates per 1000 live births and an increase in life expectancy at birth. This study provides valuable reference material for a detailed analysis in the present dissertation.

Udeorah et al. [52] studied the impact of health care expenditure on economic growth in Nigeria from 1980 to 2016. The study used descriptive statistics and Generalized Method of Moments (GMM) test for data analysis. Findings indicate that, healthcare expenditure had no significant impact on economic growth; and education expenditure had positive significant impact on economic growth. Policy implication of findings is the need for government to embark on massive health education of citizens to foster economic growth. Its analytical framework is robust. It has relevance as a guide in the conduct and advancement of the present study.

Obienyi et al. [53] examined the effects of health outcomes, measured by life expectancy, on labor productivity and industrial output in Nigeria. The study spanned across 1981–2015. Using a simultaneous regression model with the aid of three-stage least square (3SLS) estimation, the study indicate the significant positive impact of health outcomes on labor productivity and subsequent effects on industrial output. However, health outcomes are not significantly influenced by health expenditure, emphasizing the need for increased funding in the health sector.

Dhrifi [54] carried out a study titled, "Health-care expenditure, economic growth and infant mortality: evidence from 93 developed and developing Countries". The study spanned across 1995–2013. Study employed three-stage least square techniques for data analysis. Results indicate that health expenditure has a positive effect on reducing child mortality only for upper-middle income and high income countries, whereas for low-income and lower-middle income countries, health spending does not have a significant impact on child health status. Furthermore, public health spending has a greater effect on mortality rates than private expenditure at lower development levels. At high development levels private health expenditure has a positive impact on child mortality. This study is relevant to the present study as it has yielded suitable reference materials for a detailed analysis.

Ibikunle [55] studied life expectancy, public health spending and economic growth in Nigeria. The study covered the period, 1995–2017. Situational analysis, ordinary least square and the granger causality test were employed for data analysis. Results from situational analysis indicate that the trend of GDP and life expectancy were upward while health expenditure had an irregular trend. The OLS results indicate that both government spending on health and life expectancy had positive significant effect on GDP. Furthermore, the results indicate unidirectional relationship between life expectancy and GDP and; a bidirectional relationship between life expectancy and healthcare spending. There is no causal relationship between health expenditure and GDP. Policy implication of the findings is the need for government to increase spending on health so as to improve the health status of individuals. The major weakness of the study is the application of multiple regression and ordinary least square analysis in a study involving small sample and reporting economic development instead of economic growth. However, the study was considered relevant as its findings would be useful for accommodating findings from the present study.

Nwani and Kelikume [56] studied "public health expenditure, health status and economic growth: New evidence from Toda-Yamamoto approach for Nigeria". Study spanned across 1981–2018. The study employed Toda-Yamamoto techniques for data analysis. The result based on the co-integration showed that public health expenditure, health status and economic growth have long run association. Toda-Yamamoto causality test result revealed the absence of causality between health expenditure and health status. Similarly, health status and economic growth are not causally interdependent. On the basis of the findings, the study vehemently concludes that efforts to stimulate economic growth by targeting health outcomes improvement through public expenditure will be futile.

Edeme and Olisakwe [57] linked public health expenditure, economic growth, and health outcomes in Nigeria, employing pairwise Granger causality. The study reveals that increased public health expenditure decreases infant mortality rates, with a unidirectional causality from public health expenditure to economic growth.

Anowor et al. [58] explored the nexus between healthcare financing and economic performance in ECOWAS countries from 1985 to 2017. Using Panel autoregressive distributed lag (PARDL), they found both private and public expenditures had a significant positive effect on economic performance. The study emphasized the importance of involving private healthcare institutions in health policy formulation for coordinated health professional activities. The study has its strength in its use of panel data and a strong analytical framework that supported the extensive estimation of variables included in the model. It has relevance to the present study in the sense that its findings were found useful for the purpose of comparison.

Ndaguba and Hlotywa [59] examined the impact of public health expenditure on economic development in South Africa. Study spanned across 1996 and 2016. Time series data were used for the study. The study applied VECM, VARS, OLS, and ADRL and Phillips-Perron (PP) for data analysis. Findings indicate that there is no cause-effect relationship between public health expenditure and economic development in South Africa. There is positive significant relationship between public health expenditure and HDI. There is inverse relationship between unemployment and economic development. There is a direct relationship between population growth and economic development; and there is a direct relationship between public health expenditure and HDI. The major weaknesses of this study are the use of HDI as a proxy for economic development and the application of multiple regression techniques in a study involving small sample. However, the study has yielded variables which were considered relevant for inclusion in the present study.

Khalid and Qayyum [60] analyzed the growth-health relationship in Pakistan from 1990 to 2020 using ARDL. They found strong short-term ties among GDP, foreign direct investment, fertility, and life expectancy, with fertility rate having a significant long-term effect on GDP. Despite a deviation from the study's objectives, the findings provided suitable reference material for the present study.

Olayiwola et al. [37] examined the connection between public health expenditure and economic growth in Nigeria within the context of Wagner's Theory. The study covered the period, 2000–2016. Using granger causality test, they concluded that there was a long-run relationship between public health expenditure and economic growth but a unidirectional causal relationship, challenging Wagner's theory. Despite the weakness, the results of the study have provided insight into the possible outcomes of the present study.

Ewurum [6] examined the nexus among public health expenditure, environmental pollution, governance and health status in Nigeria. The study covered the period 1981–2020. Using ARDL and 2SLS, results revealed a negative and significant effect of public health expenditure on health outcome (IMR and U5MR). Also that increase in economic growth is associated with an improvement in the health status of the population in Nigeria.

Canbay and Kirca [61] conducted a review of the bidirectional causal relationship between health expenditures and per capita income in BRICS+T countries from 2000 to 2018. Applying bootstrap, they found uni-directional causal relationships from per capita income to total and public health expenditures in various countries, providing valuable insights and analysis techniques for the present study.

3. Research methods

3.1 Theoretical framework

The chapter is anchored on Wagner's law of increasing state activities" which states that during the process of economic development, the share of public spending in national income expands, that is, public expenditure is endogenous to economic development. Hence, there is a functional relationship between the growth of an economy and government expenditure [41]. Also, this chapter utilizes Seers' Three-Pillar model—examining poverty, inequality, and unemployment—to assess the development of a nation like Nigeria, emphasizing that genuine economic development transcends mere increases in per capita income, requiring a simultaneous improvement in all three critical dimensions.

3.2 Model specification

To evaluate the relationship among public health expenditure, health status and economic development in Nigeria: global health security, the works of Dhrifi [54] simultaneous equation model was adopted with some modifications. Hence, three key variables namely, public health expenditure, health status and economic development were modeled within simultaneous equation framework and these three variables are endogenous.

The primary objective of this paper is to examine whether increased public health expenditure has the potential to reduce key components of the composite economic development index (EDI), namely poverty, inequality, and unemployment. This is to be achieved by examining how such expenditure positively impacts on the health status of the population through reduction in mortality rates, with a subsequent analysis of the significance of any observed effects on these economic and health-related indicators. Thus, the study has three equations to estimate the objective of this chapter. The three equation models are specified as follows:

$$EDI = f\ (PHExp, HS, RGDPpc, LR, WATER, PHY, LEXP, Upop, QoG, PvHE) \quad (1)$$

$$PHExp = f\ (EDI, HS, RGDPpc, LR, WATER, PHY, LEXP, Pov, Upop, QoG) \quad (2)$$

$$HS = f\ (EDI, PHExp, RGDPpc, LR, W/ELECT, PHY, Pov, LEXP, Upop, QoG, PvHE) \quad (3)$$

Building upon the extant literature that explores the relationship among public health expenditure, health status and economic development, this chapter seeks to elucidate the nuanced relationships within this triadic framework by explaining the set of the explanatory variables which includes public health expenditure (PHExp) measures by domestic general government health expenditure per capita, representing health financing; health status index (HS) is a composite health status index constructed as a linear combination of infant mortality (IMR), under-five mortality (U5MR), maternal mortality (MMR) and crude death rate (CDR); real gross domestic product per capita (RGDPpc); literacy rates (LR) representing female education; water/electricity representing health infrastructure and sanitation; Doc/Physician density (PHY) representing human resource for health: life expectancy (LEXP) is included as a covariate and the rationale for selecting life expectancy stems from the intention to investigate if enhancing the health status of the citizens, as reflected in increased life expectancy, correlates with and potentially contributes to the attainment of sustained economic development. Poverty (Pov); Urbanization (Upop) captured by urban population; quality of governance (QoG) measured by control corruption; and private health expenditure (PvHE) represented by domestic general private health expenditure per capita. Also, composite economic development index (EDI) is a measure that combines multiples of indicators such as poverty, inequality and unemployment to assess the overall economic development of mostly the developing countries. However, this EDI was developed by the researcher to assess the economic development of Nigeria.

Given the measures for composite economic development index represented as EDI, a composite index function was computed with the use of principal component analysis. This composite index is a combination of three (3) components—Poverty, Inequality and Unemployment as defined by Dudley Seers [33]; Public Health Expenditure and health outcomes (HS), the above general models are stated in a structural form as follows:

3.3 Structural forms of the model

Equation 1: Impact of public health expenditures and other covariates variables on economic development.

$$\begin{aligned} EDI = {} & \ltimes o + \ltimes_1 PHExp + \ltimes_2 HS + \ltimes_3 RGDPpc + \ltimes_4 LR + \ltimes_5 W/ELECT \\ & + \ltimes_6 PHY + \ltimes 7LExp + \ltimes_8 Upop + \ltimes_9 QoG + \ltimes_{10} PvHE + V_1 t \end{aligned} \quad (4)$$

Equation 2: Impact of economic development on public health expenditure.

$$PHExp = \leftthreetimes o + \leftthreetimes_1 EDI + \leftthreetimes_2 HS + \leftthreetimes_3 RGDPpc + \leftthreetimes_4 PHY + \leftthreetimes_5 POV + \leftthreetimes_6 Upop + \leftthreetimes_7 QoG + V_2 t \quad (5)$$

Equation 3: Impact of economic development and public health expenditure on health outcomes.

$$\begin{aligned} HS = {} & \beta o + \beta_1 EDI + \beta_2 PHExp + \beta_3 RGDPpc + \beta_4 LR + \beta_5 W/ELECT + \beta_6 PHY + \beta_7 Pov \\ & + \beta_8 LEXP + \beta_9 Upop + \beta_{10} QoG + \beta_{11} PvHE + V_3 t \end{aligned} \quad (6)$$

There are only three structural relationships. Thus, EDI, PHExp and HS are endogenous variables and the models are over-identified. Hence, OLS is not the preferred method for estimating the structural equations. Given that the model is over-identified, instrumental variables (IV) estimation techniques (3SLS) is more appropriate. IV methods help address endogeneity and measurement error in the independent variables, providing more reliable estimates in over-identified models. The error terms V_1t, V_2t, and V_3t are called structural disturbances. The coefficients are $\ltimes o$-$\ltimes_{10}$, $\leftthreetimes o$- and βo-β_{11}.

This chapter sourced its data from the World Bank, World development indicators, Central Bank of Nigeria, National Bureau of Statistic, series of health issues publication, Global Statistical books, African Research Review, World Health Organization (WHO). Study used annual time series data for Nigeria spanning over the period, 1981–2020. The study employed interpolation, where necessary, to fill missing data. This gave us a larger sample size.

4. Data presentation, analysis and discussion of results

4.1 Summary of descriptive statistics

In order to gain insight into the nature and characteristics of the data, the descriptive statistics of all the variables over the period, 1981–2020 are reported in **Table 1**.

4.2 Three stage least squares (3SLS) results for public expenditure, health status and economic development interrelationships

Table 2 presents the results for the system estimation of the simultaneous equations based on the three-stage least squares (3SLS) procedure for the composite health status index, public health expenditure and economic development equations. For the system estimation, the first two lags of each of the composite health status index, public health expenditure and composite economic development index are used as instruments.

It is important to note that for the composite health status, higher values would signify worsening health status while low values would indicate improving health

Variables	Mean	Median	Maximum	Minimum	Std. dev.	Obs.
HS	694.903	750.708	774.505	543.412	88.199	40
PHEXP	108.690	20.581	1477.700	0.041	244.253	40
PHY	0.255	0.192	0.449	0.050	0.099	40
EDI	59.724	60.023	74.509	49.589	7.721	40
POV	52.226	54.836	64.900	38.033	8.270	40
PvHE	52.850	65.556	80.138	23.848	23.012	40
QOG	16.013	16.000	28.000	4.000	8.177	40
RGDPpc	1874.181	1671.740	2688.267	1388.535	468.832	40
LR	46.389	43.882	64.254	41.387	4.893	40
UPOP	36.581	35.255	51.958	22.671	8.631	40
W/ELECT	104.412	76.104	310.415	37.602	59.528	40
LEXP	48.445	46.388	55.018	45.637	3.171	40

Source: Author's Computation using E-views 12.

Table 1.
Descriptive statistics.

status due to reduction in mortality rates. Similarly, the composite economic development index is constructed in the same fashion as the health status where higher (lower) values indicate deteriorating (improving) development outcomes. Higher inequality, poverty and unemployment are suggestive of poor development outcomes.

In **Table 2**, result for the health status (HS) equation, indicates that the composite economic development index (EDI) which depicts deteriorating development conditions has the tendency to worsen the composite health status due to its positive effect. This is also true for the poverty rate which has a positive effect as well. On the other hand, higher income level is associated with an improvement in the composite health outcome due to its negative effect; the negative effect also holds for literacy rate, health infrastructure proxied by the composite indicator from water and electricity, physician density, life expectancy and the corruption index. However, these variables are not statistically significant. This is contrary to the findings by Dhrifi [54] and Boachie et al. [51].

Meanwhile, the variables with statistically significant effect are both the public and private health expenditure. Public health expenditure has a negative effect on overall health status with a 1% increase corresponding to a 0.022 percentage point decline in health status. This means that public health expenditure is vital and very important for improving the overall health status and conditions in the country. Moreover, health is an important component of public service delivery of which its provision is the responsibility of government. Through effective and efficient utilization of public resources towards the provision of quality and efficient healthcare service delivery, the health conditions of the teeming populace can be significantly enhanced with increased accessibility and affordability. Hence, public health spending in providing the requisite health infrastructures, equipment and medicines, and as well a well-qualified healthcare personnel is an indispensable factor. Similar result has been found by Boachie, et al. [51].

	HS equation			PHEXP equation			PIU equation		
	Coefficient	**Std. error**	**Prob.**	**Coefficient**	**Std. error**	**Prob.**	**Coefficient**	**Std. error**	**Prob.**
Constant	**6.446****	2.674	0.018	125.983	43.226	0.005	3.665	2.777	0.018
EDI	0.217	0.372	0.561	−12.854	10.749	0.235	—	—	—
PHEXP	**−0.022*****	0.008	0.007	—	—		0.009	0.009	0.284
HS	—	—	—	**−25.709*****	5.980	0.000	**0.688*****	0.216	0.002
RGDPC	−0.069	0.069	0.320	**−5.751****	2.528	0.026	**−0.221*****	0.058	0.000
LR	−0.018	0.020	0.362	—	—		0.031	0.030	0.303
W/ELECT	−0.007	0.013	0.588	—	—		0.016**	0.007	0.037
PHY	−0.024	0.011	0.033	**−0.854***	0.457	0.065	0.009	0.009	0.119
POV	0.222	0.414	0.594	**22.572*****	7.532	0.004	—	—	—
LEXP	−0.421	0.572	0.465	—	—		**−0.899****	0.338	0.009
UPOP	0.119	0.167	0.479	**13.261*****	3.771	0.001	**0.369****	0.144	0.012
PVHE	**0.049*****	0.018	0.006	0.863	0.792	0.279	**−0.096*****	0.014	0.000
QOG	−0.007	0.010	0.436	−0.436	0.394	0.271	−0.015	0.009	0.108
Obs	38			38			38		
R-squared	0.988			0.966			0.987		
Adj. R-squared	0.983			0.957			0.982		
Durbin-Watson	1.762			2.117			1.653		

Embolden are variables with statistical significance. All variables are expressed on their natural logarithmic transformation. Source: Author's Computation using Eviews 12.
**Significance level for 10%. **Significance level for 5%. ***Significance level for 1%.*

Table 2.
3SLS results for public heath expenditure, health status and economic development global health security.

Meanwhile, private health expenditure has a positive effect with a coefficient elasticity of 0.049 implying that private health expenditure is associated with deteriorating overall health status. While this may be counterintuitive, one possible explanation is that there is limit to which private spending can contribute to improved health conditions. The saying that "money can buy medicine, but it cannot buy health" suffices for this evidence especially in the context of Nigeria where "medical tourism" has been on the increase especially among the elites and public officials due to the dysfunctional nature of the country's healthcare system. Thus, for others that cannot patronize foreign medical services, they are limited to what is available locally which is mostly inadequate for treating life-threatening ailments.

Result for public health expenditure (PHExp) equation, indicates that the composite economic development index, private health expenditure and corruption index are unimportant due to their statistical insignificance. Meanwhile, the effect of composite health status is significant at 1% with a coefficient elasticity of −25.71 percentage point. In other words, it implies that worsening health status leads to a reduction in public health expenditure. While this result is counterintuitive as deterioration in health conditions should stimulate more public health spending to curb the trend, the evidence is suggestive of the dilemma in the Nigerian case where public expenditure is insufficient to provide adequate healthcare service delivery to the teeming population. As already known, the budgetary allocation for the health sector in Nigeria is grossly inadequate to cater for the ever-expanding demand for healthcare services.

The impact of income level is associated with a reduction in public health expenditure. Specifically, 1% increase in the income level leads to −5.75 percentage point reduction in public health expenditure. This effect is statistically significant at the 10% level. Again, the result is counterintuitive because it suggests that as income increases, government's effort towards providing affordable healthcare service delivery through its health spending might decline. Interestingly too, with expansion in the income level, the individuals may substitute the patronage of public for private healthcare services given the low quality of public healthcare delivery. Further, the impact of physician density has a negative effect on public health expenditure. In this case, a 1% increase in the physician density will result in a 0.854 percentage point reduction in the public health expenditure. The crux of this result boils down to the quality of the physicians. If the skills of the physicians are high, then government spending for training and re-training may reduce overtime with increased effectiveness and efficiency. On the other hand, if the physicians are poorly trained and less skilled, government will have to spend significant resources either for re-training or recruitment of better qualified health personnel. This result is in line with the findings by [55].

The impact of poverty and urban population on public health expenditure are positive and statistically significant at the 1% level. For instance, a 1% increase in the poverty level and urbanization rate will lead to 22.57 and 13.26 percentage point increase in public health expenditure. By implication, high poverty level will entail less accessibility and affordability of healthcare service delivery, of which a possible remedy would be for government to subsidize health services which in turn will mean an increase in health spending. Similarly, an expansion in urbanization will create higher demand pressure on existing healthcare services and facilities, and in turn, government will have to increase health spending in other to expand such facilities through the construction of new healthcare centres, employment of new healthcare personnel, and provision of medical equipment and drugs etc. In a nutshell, the overall result show that public health expenditure in Nigeria is more responsive to existing health conditions (status), the income level of the citizens, the number and density of physician or medical practitioners, the existing poverty level and the state of urbanization in the country. This is similar to the findings by Nwani and Kelikume [56].

Lastly, for the economic development index (EDI) equation, the impact of public health expenditure and health status on the composite economic development index is examined. The impact of public health expenditure is positive though statistically insignificant. This means that public health expenditure may not be a strong determinant of economic development through lowering inequality and poverty as well as unemployment. This result clearly describes the Nigerian situation where budgetary allocations for public health expenditure are significantly small and insufficient to facilitate effective and efficient public health service delivery. Other variables which are relatively non-significant in the economic development equation include literacy rate, physician density and corruption level. On the other hand, the impact of composite health status is positive with an elasticity of 0.688 and significant at the 1% level. This means that a 1% increase in the health status variable which signifies deteriorating health conditions lead to 0.688 percentage points deterioration in the development outcomes. Put differently, an improvement in health status is associated with better development outcomes which enhance productivity due to healthy living and access to quality healthcare services. Similarly, the impact of income level has a negative effect with an elasticity of −0.221 and statistical significance at the 1% level. Thus, a 1% increase in the income level reduces the composite economic development variable by −0.22 percentage points. This means that higher income will result in better development outcomes as it will reduce the inequality and poverty gaps and by implication unemployment as more people become employed due to an expansion in economic activities. This is in line with the findings by Eneji et al. [9]; Deluna and Peralta [62].

The impact of water and electricity infrastructure on composite economic development index is positive with an elasticity of 0.016 and statistical significance at the 5% level. The significance of this variable underscores the important of water accessibility and adequate and stable power supply for rapid economic development. Both variables are indispensable in all facets of human activities, and so, contribute to sustainable development. Further, the impact life expectancy on the composite economic development index is negative with a coefficient of −0.899 and statistical significance at the 5% level. Higher life expectancy can contribute to economic development through a larger proportion of active labour which can be harnessed to boost productivity growth. In the same vein, private healthcare expenditure also leads to better development outcomes. An increase in private healthcare expenditure by 1% leads −0.096 percentage point reduction in the composite development measure which signifies better development outcomes. Meanwhile, the effect of urban population is positive with a coefficient elasticity of 0.369 and statistical significance at 5% level. In other words, a 1% increase in urbanization rate is associated with 0.369 percentage points deterioration in economic development. This can be explained by the fact that greater urbanization without corresponding surge in job opportunities and employment nor adequate infrastructural provisions can lead to poor living conditions, urban sprawl, negative externalities, which ultimately would tend to worsen or retard sustainable development. Similar findings can be seen in Edeme and Olisakwe, [57].

In summary, the results clearly provide evidence on the significant effect of public health expenditure on the composite health status in the health status equation, and also a reverse significant effect of the composite health status on public health expenditure in the health expenditure equation. This means that there is a bi-directional relationship between public health expenditure and the composite health status. Meanwhile, in the economic development index equation, the direct impact of public health expenditure is non-significant whereas the composite health status is significant. Judging from the foregoing, it can be inferred that the impact of public health expenditure on economic development works through the health status channel. This is because public health expenditure affects the composite economic development index indirectly through its effect on composite health status. Importantly, such development enhances the nation's capacity to effectively respond to global health security challenges, reducing vulnerability to diseases, and fortifying overall health security.

4.3 Discussion of empirical results

Results from the three-stage least squares (3SLS) estimation indicates that public health expenditure contributes to reducing the composite measure of health status.

The effect is negative and statistically significant, and supported by studies such as Eneji et al. [9] and Dhrifi [54]. On the other hand, composite health status index affects public health expenditure negatively and significantly. This means that there is a bi-directional causal relationship between public health expenditure and health status. This evidence is similar to Ibikunle [55] who found a bidirectional relationship between life expectancy as a measure of health outcomes and healthcare spending; but it's in contrast to some other studies such as Obienyi et al., [53]; Nwani and Kelikume [56].

Also, the composite measure of health status affects positively and significantly the composite measure of economic development; whereas there is a positive reverse effect from the composite economic development index to the composite health status though the relationship is statistically insignificant. This implies that there is a uni-directional causal relationship from health status to economic development. In other words, improving health conditions can be catalytic to economic progress and development. Lastly, there is no causal relationship between public health expenditure and the composite measure of economic development. This evidence is support by the study of Ibikunle [55] that found no causality between health expenditure and economic growth in Nigeria.

Overall, the results suggest that public health expenditure affects the composite economic development index indirectly by reduction in poverty, income inequality and unemployment through its effect on composite health status. In other words, an increased public health spending channeled towards providing the requisite health care infrastructures, healthcare subsidies, medical personnel, and effective healthcare service delivery fosters a healthy, vibrant and energetic population and labour force, which in turn, boost labour productivity which is essential for achieving sustainable economic development. Thus, the development initiatives not only improve the health and well-being of the population but also create a foundation for a resilient and secure nation that can effectively respond to and mitigate global health security challenges.

In summary, a resilient and well-functioning national health system is not only a fundamental component of a healthier nation but also a cornerstone for global health security and cooperation. It represents a commitment to the well-being of citizens and contributes to the stability and prosperity of the global community. It suggests that they are actively participating in and promoting activities that foster economic development, reduced poverty, and enhance the overall welfare of their population.

5. Conclusion

This study evaluates the interrelationship among public health expenditure, health status and economic development in Nigeria. The study applied Dudley Seers' 'Three-Pillar Model' of development on Nigeria economy. This was achieved by developing a composite economic development index (EDI) as measure for economic development. The overarching conclusion derived from this study is that public health expenditure exert significantly and positively on health status to foster economic development through the instruments of income, health education, development of health infrastructure, poverty reduction, employment creation, reduction in income inequality which shows the better income and wealth distribution, physician density, urbanization, quality of governance and reduction in healthcare costs. What this implies is that health status of the citizens is a critical medium through which public health expenditure impact positively on economic development, but government must ensure adequate allocation of resources to health sector, reliable power generation and distribution, reduction in mortality rates, reduction in poverty, unemployment rates, income inequality and corruption. When Nigeria invests in healthcare, improves the health of its citizens, and experiences economic development, it not only benefits its own population but also contributes to global health security by reducing the risk of diseases spreading beyond its borders. It's a way of creating a healthier and safer world for everyone.

Author details

Ngozi Chioma Ewurum[1*] and Samuel Oseloka Okafor[2]

1 Department of Economics, Michael Okpara University of Agriculture, Umudike, Nigeria

2 Department of Economics, Nnamdi Azikiwe University, Awka, Nigeria

*Address all correspondence to: ewurum.ngozi@mouau.edu.ng

References

[1] Eboh IA, Aduku EB, Onwughalu UB. Health Expenditure, Chikd mortality and economic growth in Nigeria. International Journal of economic Development Research (IJEDR). 2022;**3** (3):198-216

[2] Foreign, Commonwealth & Development Office and Wendy Morton MP. Health Systems Strengthening for Global Health Security and Universal Health Coverage: FCDO Position Paper. Policy Paper; 14 Dec 2021

[3] Sustainable Development Goals and Goal 3. Available from: https://sustainabledevelopment.un.org/SDG3

[4] World Health Organization. The World Health Report 2007 - A Safer Future: Global Public Health Security in the 21st Century. 2007. Available from: https://www.who.int/whr/2007/whr07_en.pdf

[5] Duff JH, Liu A, Saavedra J, Batycki JN, Morancy K, Stocking B, et al. A global Public Health Convention for the 21st Century. The Lancet Public Health. 2021;**6**(6):e428-e433

[6] Ewurum NC. Nexus among public health expenditure, environmental pollution, governance and health status: Empirical perspective from Nigeria. International Journal for Humanities and Social Sciences (IJHS): Open-Access Journal. 2022;**2**(2):1-9

[7] Policy Brief First Quarter. Nigeria: Health budget analysis. Budgit. 2018. Available from: www.yourbudgit.com

[8] Foreign, Commonwealth & Development Office and Wendy Morton MP. Health Systems Strengthening for Global Health Security and Universal Health Coverage: FCDO Position Paper. Policy Paper; 2021

[9] Eneji AM, Dickson VJ, Onabe BJ. Health care expenditure, health status and National Productivity in Nigeria (1999–2012). Journal of Economics and International Finance. 2013;**5**(7):258-272. DOI: 10.5897/JEIF2013.0523

[10] Sachs J. The End of Poverty: Economic Possibilities for our Time. New York: The Penguin Press; 2005

[11] Sen A. Development as Freedom. New York: Alfred A. Knopf; 1999

[12] Solow RM. A contribution to the theory of economic growth. The Quarterly Journal of Economics. 1956;**70** (1):65-94. DOI: 10.2307/1884513

[13] Todaro MP. A model of labour migration and urban unemployment in less developed countries. The American Economic Review. 1969;**59**(1): 138-148. American Economic Association

[14] Health in the Post-2015 Agenda. Report of the Global Thematic Consultation on Health. The World We Want. Apr 2013. pp. 1-108. Available from: http://ww.worldwewant2015.org/health

[15] Makuta I, O'Hare B. Quality of governance, public spending on health status in Sub-Saharan Africa: A Panel Data Regression Analysis. BMC Public Health. 2015;**15**:932. DOI: 10.1186/s12889-015.228

[16] United Nations, Department of Economic and Social Affairs, Population Division. World Population Prospects 2019: Highlights (ST/ESA/SER.A/423). 2019

[17] Sirag A, Adamu P, Nor NM. An assessment of health care and economics

growth in Sudan: An ARDL bound testing approach. Journal of Economics and Sustainable Development. 2013;**4** (16):5-13

[18] Okafor SO, Jegbefumwen K, Maduka OD, Okeke AC. A three-factor model of inclusive, sustainable and resilient economic development for developing countries. Applied Economics and Finance. 2016;**3**(4):57-72. Available from: http:/aef.redfame.com

[19] Amiri A, Gerdtham U. Impact of maternal and child health on economic growth: New evidence based granger causality and DEA analysis. Study commissioned by the Partnership for Maternal, Newborn & Child Health (PMNCH). Final version. 2013

[20] FMOH. Nigerian National Health Insurance Scheme and Improvement of the Health Status of Nigerians. Abuja; 2021

[21] WDI. 2014, 2015, 2017, 2018. International Data for Countries. 2024

[22] Ministry of Budget and National Planning of Nigeria. 4 Mar 2021. Available from: https://nationalplanning.gov.ng/bagudu-seeks-improved

[23] Cortes M, Valliant J, Zottel S, Vishwanath T, Kojima M, Balch O, et al. Nigeria in Times of COVID-19: Laying Foundations for a Strong Recovery (English). Washington DC: World Bank Group; 2020

[24] Ejiogu A, Okechukwu O, Ejiogu C. Nigerian budgetary response to the COVID-19 pandemic and its shrinking fiscal space: Financial sustainability, employment, social inequality and business implications. Journal of Public Budgeting, Accounting & Financial Management. 2020;**32**(5):919-928. DOI: 10.1108/JPBAFM-07-2020-0101

[25] Sen A. In: Chenery H, Srinivasan TN, editors. The Concept of Development: Handbook of Development Economics. Vol. 1. Elsevier Science Publishers B. V; 1988. pp. 9-26

[26] Haslam PA. What is development? From economic growth to the sustainable development goals. In: Haslam P, Schafer J, Beaudet P, editors. Introduction to International Development: Approaches, Actors, Issues, and Practice. 4th ed. Don Mills: Oxford University Press; 2021. 23 p

[27] Sen A. Development as Freedom. 2nd ed. Oxford New York: Oxford University Press; 2001

[28] Todaro MP, Smith SC. Economic Development. 12th ed. Library of Congress Cataloging-in-Publication Data. The George Washington University. United State of America: Pearson; 2015. pp. 1-891. ISBN 978-0-13-340678-8. ISBN 0-13-340678-41

[29] Todaro MP, Smith SC. Economic Development. 12th ed. Library of Congress Cataloging-in-Publication Data. The George Washington University. Pearson; 2015. pp. 1-891. ISBN 978-0-13-340678-8 – ISBN 0-13-340678-4 1

[30] United Nations Development Program. Human Development Report 1990. New York: Oxford University Press; 1990

[31] Nafziger WE. From Seers to Sen: The Meaning of Economic Development. WIDER Working Paper Series Research Paper No. 2006-20, World Institute for Development Economic Research (UNU-WIDER). 2006

[32] Human Development Report. UNDP. 2023. Available from: hdr.undp.org/data-center

[33] Seers D. The Meaning of Development, IDS Communication 44. Brighton: IDS; 1969

[34] World Bank Report. World Development REPORT 1991. The Challenge of Development. 1991. pp. 1–11. DOI: 10.1596/978-0-1952-0868-9

[35] World Bank. 2014. The World Bank Annual Report 2014. Washington, DC. Available from: http://hdl.handle.net/10986/20093. License: CC BY-NC-ND 3.0 IGO

[36] Ndedi AA, Metha A, Nisabwe F. The impact of Health expenditures on Economic Growth of Cameroon: A literature Review perspective. 2017. Available from: https://ssrn.com/abstract=3036510. 10.2139/ssrn.3036510

[37] Olayiwola SO, Bakare-Aremu TA, Abiodun SO. Public health expenditure and economic growth in Nigeria: Testing of Wagner's Hypothesis. African Journal of economic Review (AJER). 2021;**IX** (II):130-150

[38] Kelani FA, Odunaya HA, Ozegbe AE, Nwani S. Health status, labour productivity and economic growth in Nigeria. Journal of Economics, Management and Trade. 2019;**23**(1):1-12. Article no. JEMT.46997. DOI: 10.9734/jemt/2019/v23i130116. ISSN: 2456-9216

[39] Gyimah-Brempong K, Wilson M. Human capital and economic growth: Is Africa different? Journal of Africa Development. 2005;**7**(1):73-109

[40] World Health Organization Definition of Health Security. Available from: https://www.who.int/health-topics/health-security#tab=tab_1

[41] Wagner AH. Finanzwissenschaft. Leipzig: C. F. Winter; 1883

[42] Agiobenebo TJ. Public Sector Economics: Theories, Issues and Applications. 5th ed. Port Harcourt, Nigeria: KB&1 Casco/Services Nigeria; 2019

[43] Ahuja HL. Modern Economics: An Analytical Study. 16th ed. New Delhi, India: S. Chand & Co., Ltd; 2012

[44] Bhatia HL. Public Finance. 22nd Revised ed. New Delhi, India: Vikas Publishing House PVT Ltd; 2001

[45] Musgrave RA, Musgrave PB. Public Finance in Theory and Practice. 5th ed. Delhi, India: Tata McGraw-Hill; 2011

[46] Bird RM. Wagner's law: A pooled time series and cross section comparison. National Tax Journal. 1971;**38**:209-218

[47] Magazzino C, Giolli L, Mele M. Wagner's Law and Peacock and Wiseman's displacement effect in European Union Countries: A Panel Data Study. International Journal of Economics and Financial Issues. 2015;**5** (3):812-819

[48] Ibe RC, Olulu-Briggs OV. Any Nexus between Public Health Expenditure and Economic Growth in Nigeria? IIARD International Journal of Banking and Finance Research. 2015;**1**(8):1-12. Available from: www.iiardpub.org

[49] Boachie MK, Ramu K. Effect of public health expenditure on health status in Ghana. International Journal of Health. 2016;**4**(1):6-11

[50] Piabuo SM, Tieguhong JC. Health Expenditure and Economic Growth – A review of the literature and an analysis between the economic community for central African states (CEMAC) and selected African countries. Piabuo and Tieguhong Health Economics Review. 2017;7:23. DOI: 10.1186/s13561-017-0159

[51] Boachie MK, Ramu K, Polajeva T. Public health expenditures and health outcomes: New evidence from Ghana. Economic Development of Africa. 2018; **6**(4):58 Available from: www.mpdi.com/journal/economies

[52] Udeorah SAF, Obayori JB, Onuchuku O. Health care expenditure and economic growth in Nigeria. International Journal of Research and Innovation in Social Science (IJRISS). 2018;**II**(III):33-36

[53] Obienyi P, Yuni DN, Ojike O, Uwajumogu NR. Health, labour productivity and industrialization in Nigeria, Public Health Expenditure, Health status and Economic Growth: New Evidence from Toda-Yamamoto approach for Nigeria. World Applied Sciences Journal. 2018;**38**(2):353-360

[54] Dhrifi A. Health-care expenditure, economic growth and infant mortality: Evidence from developed and developing countries. CEPAL Review No 125. August 2018. JEL Classification. H51, O47, 112

[55] Ibikunle JA. Life expectancy, public health spending and economic growth in Nigeria. Social Sciences. 2019;**8**(6): 369-376. DOI: 10.11648/j.ss.21090806.20

[56] Nwani SE, Kelikume I. Public Health Expenditure, Health status and Economic Growth: New Evidence from Toda-Yamamoto approach for Nigeria. Journal of Scientific Research and Reports. 2019;**2019**:1-13. DOI: 10.9734/jsrr/2019/v24/330155

[57] Edeme RK, Olisakwe O. Public health expenditure, economic growth and health outcomes in Nigeria. International Journal of Public Policy and Administration Research. 2019;**6**(1):23-32

[58] Anowor OF, Ichoku HE, Onodugo VA. Nexus between healthcare financing and output per capita: Analysis of countries in ECOWAS sub-region. Cogent Economics & Finance. 2020;**8**(1):1-14

[59] Ndaguba EA, Hlotywa A. Public health expenditure on economic development: The case of South Africa between 1996 and 2016. Cogent Economics & Finance. 2021;**9**(1):1-13

[60] Khalid N, Qayyum A. An empirical analysis of the growth-health relationship in Pakistan. Quantitative Economics and Management Studies (QEMS). 2021;**2**(3):182-191. DOI: 10.35877/454RI.qems272

[61] Canbay S, Kirca S. Health expenditure (total, public and private) and per capita income in the BRICS+T: Panel Bootstrap Causality Analysis. Journal of Economics, Finance and Administrative Science. 2022;**27**(1):52-67. DOI: 10.1108/JEFAS-06-2021-0105

[62] Deluna RS, Peralta TF. Public health expenditure, income and health outcomes in the Philippines. MPRA.Ub. Uni-Muenchen.De.Corpus ID: 56210506. 2014. Economics Medicine

Chapter 10

Commodity Security: The Role of Drug Revolving Fund Scheme in Low- and Middle-Income Countries

Jibrailu L. Maliyogbinda

Abstract

The purpose of the study is to establish the role of Drug Revolving Fund (DRF) Scheme in achieving commodity security in LMICs. DRF scheme is a self-sustaining health financing strategy that charges "user fees" just enough to recover the cost of health commodities and aims to ensure that quality lifesaving health commodities are available, affordable, and accessible to all irrespective of one's financial status, thereby contributing to achieving universal health coverage, especially through the primary health care system. The study, using a literature review approach, aimed to establish that commodity security can be realized through functional DRF scheme as a component of a sustainable health financing strategy in the face of foreign aid donor fatigue and dwindling government investment in public health care due to other competing demands. The study finds that a functional DRF scheme requires a strong political and financial commitment, robust management, and technical systems, and involves stakeholder and community participation, and use of operational guidelines and that going to scale are best achieved when done in a phased, and incremental manner. The contribution to knowledge of the study is that the DRF scheme is a feasible pathway to attaining commodity security without exerting enormous demands on already scarce resources of LMICs.

Keywords: commodity security, supply chain management, universal health coverage, global health security, global aid donor fatigue, health financing, drug revolving fund system

1. Introduction

Universal health coverage (UHC) means that all people have access to the full range of quality health services they need, when and where they need them, without financial hardship [1]. Therefore, access to affordable and acceptable quality medicines is perhaps the most crucial element in achieving UHC among citizens as indicated by target 3.8 of the UNSDGs, which specifically states to "Achieve UHC, including financial risk protection, access to quality essential health care services and access to safe, effective, quality and affordable essential medicines and vaccines for all," [1] making commodity security, therefore, a critical component of achieving UHC.

The ability of every person to obtain and use quality lifesaving medicines whenever and wherever he or she needs them is known as commodity security [2, 3]. Several governments in developing countries, especially in sub-Saharan Africa, provide drugs free of charge to certain segments of the population that are considered most vulnerable, for example, pregnant, and lactating women and children under the age of five, mostly for the treatment of malaria and diarrhea and other related childhood diseases. Furthermore, most of the free drug interventions in low- and-middle-income countries (LMICs) are financed by foreign aid donors, and therefore, may not be sustainable in the long run, for reasons that include scarce resources and many competing demands and global aid donor fatigue among other issues [4].

Therefore, there is an urgent need for LMICs, where health care services for the majority of citizens are through the public health facilities, to develop a sustainable approach to achieving commodity security, and UHC thereby, for their citizens, especially the most vulnerable that can be further affected and impoverished by huge out-of-pocket expenditure to access health care services, including affordable and quality lifesaving medicines [5]. A sustainable pathway for LMICs to achieve quality health commodity availability, accessibility, and affordability, thereby gaining commodity security for citizens, is arguably the drug revolving fund (DRF) scheme.

The DRF scheme within Bamako initiative was adopted as the initial approach for sustainable financing of drug supply, especially at the primary health care level [6]. The DRF scheme is a concept that should promote access and ensure the availability and affordability of drugs in public health facilities. It guarantees the sustainability of drug supplies and services. The focus of the scheme is to ensure the sustainability and continuity of the essential drugs program [7, 8].

After the launch of Bamako Initiative in the 1980s, there were several failed attempts to establish drug-revolving schemes in the country from the 1980s to 1990s [7, 8]. The drug-revolving scheme still exists in most states in Nigeria but only in principle with no substance on the ground. In 2008, Partnership for Transforming Health Systems Phase 2 (PATH2) establishes sustainable drug supply system (SDSS), which incorporated the principles of Bamako Initiative-DRF system. Pilot states in this intervention include Enugu, Jigawa, Kaduna, Kano, and Lagos. Other states that received "light touch" were Bauchi, Borno, Nasarawa, and Zamfara states.

Challenges included inadequate or lack of capitalization, ambiguous management structures, lack of financial sustainability plan, inadequate human resources for health in quantity and training, lack of responsible procurement practice, and poor accountability among others. In the two states that were considered successful, some of the reasons attributed to that include responsible procurement, establishment of framework agreements between the drug management agencies and suppliers, "ring-fencing" of funds for health commodity, financial sustainability plans, including diversification of income, and operating in line with established guidelines [9–12].

Recently, donors like TGF, USAID, and BMGF have launched fresh efforts to help sub-national entities in Nigeria revitalize their DRF scheme, though with differing approaches. BMGF had between 2016 and 2021 supported the supply chain transformation program in Niger and Kaduna states through its technical partner, Pamela Steel Associates. The intervention focused on supporting drug management agencies to revitalize the DRF scheme. Currently, BMGF through African Resource Centre (ARC) as a technical partner is supporting some states to establish a public private partnership (PPP) with Pharma industries ("Suppliers") with the aim to create market for the manufacturers and availed states with a dependable source of health commodities through establishment of MoU. In addition, the Pharma industries are encouraged, as part of their Corporate Social Responsibility (CSR), to embark on some interventions like upgrading warehouses, etc., for the states. Lastly, TGF is investing in building resilient and sustainable systems for health (RSSH) across Nigeria through National Agency for the Control of Aids (NACA) as Principal Recipient (PR) with the National Product and Supply Chain Management Programme (NPSCMP) as Sub-Recipient (SR) focusing on strengthening the Logistics Management Coordinating Units (LMCU) and proposed infrastructural projects especially upgrading of state central medical stores to pharma grade. It is yet to be seen what these renewed interventions will be.

Lastly, the study is organized under the following major sections:

1. **Commodity security**-Drivers of commodity security (supply chain and related functions), commodity security as a component of global health security.

2. **Universal health coverage**-Concept and principles, primary health care as the road to UHC, commodity security as a critical component of UHC.

3. **Foreign aid donor fatigue**-Potential drivers, impact of foreign aid donor fatigue on the ability of LMICs to achieve UHC.

4. **Health financing strategies**-Types of health financing strategies, sustainable health financing options for LMICs.

5. **DRF scheme**-Concepts and principles, the history of DRF scheme, how DRF scheme can achieve commodity security, examples of successful implementation of DRF scheme in Kano-Nigeria and Khartoum-Sudan.

6. **Results and discussions**-Lessons learnt from successful implementation of DRF scheme in LMICs.

7. **Conclusion**

2. Methodology

This study, using a literature review approach, aims to establish the role of DRF scheme in LMICs toward achieving commodity security. An assessment of specific DRF scheme, its design, or implementation is beyond the scope of this study. Nonetheless, some cases of a functional DRF scheme were mentioned. Furthermore, this study also establishes connections between commodity security and DRF scheme with themes like UHC, global aid donor fatigue, and sustainable health financing for LMICs. A literature review is a piece of academic writing demonstrating knowledge and understanding of the academic literature on a specific topic placed in context. It includes a critical evaluation of the material with the aim to build an argument. In conducting a review of related literature, electronic search of peer-reviewed journal articles, edited academic books, articles in professional journals, statistical data from government websites, and technical reports were carried out for specific keywords either alone or in combination, including commodity security, universal health coverage, foreign aid donor fatigue, health financing strategies, and drug revolving fund.

The criteria for the selection of materials or studies to be reviewed was based on if the materials were published in English language, if the study population are in LMICs, and whether the studies have defined inclusion criteria and/or ethical clearance. The study was conducted between March 2023 and June 2023. The information generated was analyzed qualitatively leading to findings and conclusions.

3. Commodity security

Commodity security is defined as the ability of every person to obtain and use quality lifesaving health commodities whenever and wherever he or she may need them [2, 3]. In other words, the ultimate goal of commodity security from a customer perspective is the satisfaction of clients or customers seeking health care services by ensuring that lifesaving health commodities are available when needed. Therefore, commodity security will remain a mirage without a functional supply chain system.

3.1 Drivers of commodity security: logistics and supply chain management

"A supply chain is a set of 3 or more organisations linked directly by one or more of the upstream or downstream flows of products, services, funds and information from a source to a customer" [13]. The three basic or minimum organizations linked in a supply chain are manufacturers, transportation companies, and the buyer. Logistics which is the operational component of a supply chain is defined as "the flow of material, information and funds between consumers and suppliers" [14].

Positive health outcomes are highly dependent on how well the health delivery system, including information, financing, personnel, and supply chain (including supplies)—is performing. From a logistics perspective, we can say that the success of any health intervention program depends on a strong, functional, and resilient logistics system. The importance of having lifesaving health commodities at health facilities whenever and wherever they are needed cannot be overemphasized. However, the availability of these health commodities will not be possible without a well-functioning supply chain system. The supply chain system and logistics system both need to be managed systematically for effectiveness and efficiency in order to achieve the ultimate goal of the logistics system, which is to satisfy its "six rights + 1" and that is ensuring that the right goods, in the right quantities, in the right condition, are delivered to the right place, at the right time, for the right cost, and to the right customer. Therefore, "Supply chain management is defined as management of the 2-way linkages and coordination of activities and flows (of goods, services, information and funds) from raw materials through to the end user both within and outside the organisation" [13].

A functional logistics and supply chain system depends on the availability of trained and well-motivated health personnel that ultimately drive such a system. Human beings are at the heart of every successful logistics system. Supply chain management of lifesaving health commodities, including high-value medicines like antiretroviral (ARV) drugs, vaccines, and cancer drugs, involves a series of activities to guarantee their continuous flow from the point of manufacture to the point where they are used by consumers.

3.2 Supply chain and related functions

The supply chain or its functions operate within a management system that provides decision-makers with relevant information to help determine what types of products are needed, where and when they are needed, and in what quantities. Commodity security can only be guaranteed if the supply chain and related functions are functioning at optimal levels. The supply chain and related functions are broadly classified into core supply chain functions, which include product selection and rational use, quantification, procurement, warehousing and distribution, and data management, while the supply chain-related functions otherwise known as institutional enabling environment enabling areas include governance and leadership, staffing and training, financial management, and quality management system. The institutional enabling environment areas create a conducive operating landscape for the core supply chain to thrive.

3.2.1 Core supply chain functions

Core supply chain functions are critical to achieving commodity security as these are activities that directly influence the identification of lifesaving health commodities to their ultimate use by clients. Put differently, core supply chain functions, or activities are at the heart of fulfilling the six "rights" of the logistics system and thereby achieving commodity security as demonstrated below:

- The RIGHT **product** is possible through **product selection.**
- In the RIGHT **quantity** is possible through **quantification.**
- And the RIGHT **condition** is possible through **warehousing.**
- To the RIGHT **place** is possible through **warehousing and distribution.**
- At the RIGHT **time** is possible through **distribution.**
- For the RIGHT **cost** is possible through **procurement.**

The purpose of the logistics system is to provide the six "rights" as earlier explained; and by doing so it ensures that the customer, for which the whole system exists to satisfy, achieves commodity security. Therefore, it can be concluded that the purpose of the logistics system is to achieve commodity security. Hence, commodity security is not possible without a functional supply chain system and its core functions, which include product selection, data management, quantification, procurement, warehousing, and distribution as illustrated in **Figure 1**.

3.2.2 Institutional enabling environment functions

The institutional enabling environment functions or areas make it possible for effective and efficient implementation of core supply chain functions. Every functional system, including the logistics and supply chain system, needs well-qualified and trained personnel to be successful because systems are manned by humans. Also, to establish and sustain any system requires funding and efficient management of those funds. Lastly, without sound governance and leadership, the right vision and support to make a success of the logistics and supply chain system will be lacking. Lastly, there must be a system of quality assurance and control which together establishes a quality management system to ensure the supply chain system

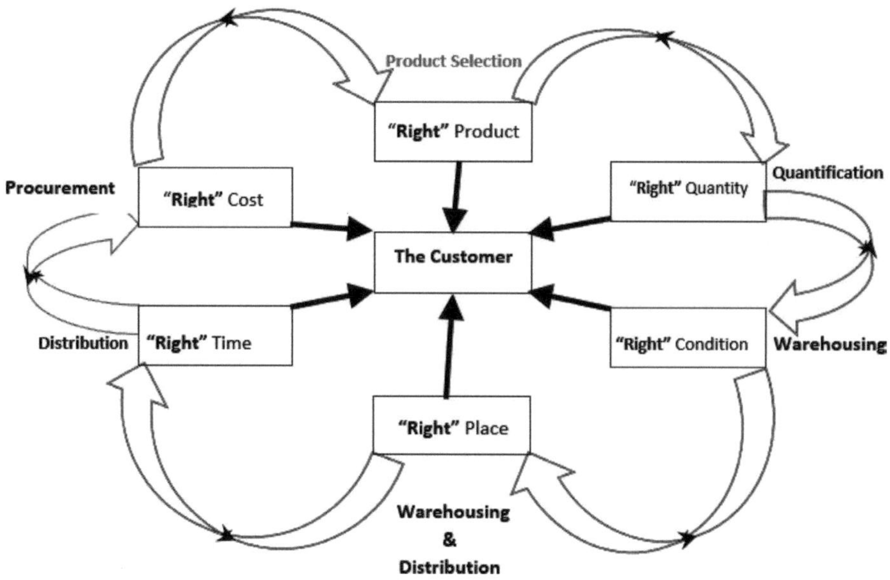

Figure 1.
Schematic diagram showing a relationship between supply chain functions and the six "rights".

and its core functions are functioning properly and progressing toward achieving its desired goal. The quality management system also incorporates continuous improvement elements to ensure resilience in a dynamic operating environment.

3.3 Commodity security as a component of global health security

"Global health security is the existence of strong and resilient public health systems that can prevent, detect, and respond to infectious disease threats, wherever they occur in the world" [15, 16]. The strategic vision of the global health security agenda focuses on three basic priority areas namely to prevent avoidable outbreaks, to detect threats to global health early, and to respond rapidly and effectively [15, 16]. In these three focus areas, lifesaving health commodities are a critical component. For instance, vaccines play a critical and central role in preventing deadly disease outbreaks in children and adults alike. Equally true is the role of laboratory commodities in detecting and diagnosing strange diseases early, thereby limiting the spread of such diseases to a pandemic level. Lastly, if and when these diseases are detected and diagnosed, drugs against them are needed to treat those affected and thereby improving their quality of life and reducing morbidity. Therefore, commodity security is critical to achieving the global health security agenda.

4. Universal health coverage: concepts and principles

Universal health coverage means that all people and communities receive health services, including access to treatment with quality and affordable lifesaving health commodities, whenever and wherever they need it without constituting undue financial burden to citizens [1]. The principle of universality forms a core component of UHC. Simply put, the mandate of the UHC is to reach everyone with quality health care irrespective of their social status. True universality means that some interventions or practices in LMICs where some segments of the population are considered most vulnerable, for instance, children and pregnant women, and therefore qualify for free health care are discriminatory and do not ensure equity for all citizens. Unfortunately, such discriminatory practices are being funded by the global aid donors by their choice for which segment of the population they want to focus upon; and arguably, it could be as a result of scarce resources or global aid donor fatigue. This again is one reason why the LMICs must find a sustainable way to achieve commodity security for their citizens rather than relying on global aid to meet the health care needs of their citizens, and worst, only some segments for that matter, thereby making it difficult to realize the mandate of UHC.

4.1 Primary health care as the road to universal health coverage

Primary health care (PHC) is fundamental to achieving UHC and represents a pathway to move toward UHC, especially in LMICs. It is a critical milestone along the road to achieving UHC targets. It enables universal, integrated access to quality health care services and products people need for health and well-being, thereby improving universal coverage and financial protection. According to WHO projections, about 75% of the projected health gains from the SDGs could be achieved through PHC and 90% of essential UHC interventions can be delivered through PHC with significant cost efficiencies, especially when an integrative PHC approach is used [17, 18].

PHC remains the most cost-effective way to address comprehensive health needs close to people's homes and communities [18]. In low- and middle-income countries, more than half the 15.6 million excess deaths are amenable to health care and 42% of them are due to not using health services [19]. Geographic access—the distance people must travel to access health services—is a common barrier, and PHC is the most viable solution to removing that barrier to accessing health care in most if not all LMICs.

PHC is the most efficient way of using available resources to deliver services. It ensures that effective interventions are delivered at the place with the lowest cost within the service delivery system [18]. This critical role that the PHC plays is closely augmented by the DRF scheme's core principle of ensuring that the most effective interventions allocated a lower mark-up to protect the poor from undue financial hardship [...]. Therefore, PHC contributes to financial protection for individuals and households, which can be caused by both rare events of expensive treatments and cumulated expenditure of more frequently needed services. Through PHC, people can avoid unnecessary expensive treatments and deteriorations in health conditions that require more expensive treatment from a lack of early intervention. PHC is also the most equitable way for delivering needed services. It is the most frequently used service by everyone, and with the service being closer to the people and community, it improves service coverage and quality [18].

4.2 Commodity security as a critical component of universal health coverage

Universal health coverage (UHC) mandate seeks to accomplish three related objectives: equity in access—where everyone who needs health services should get them, including those who cannot pay for them; quality of health services—good enough to improve the health of those receiving the services; and financial-risk protection—ensuring that the cost of health care, including the cost of lifesaving health commodities, does not put people at risk of financial hardship [20, 21]. Commodity security equally entails that lifesaving health commodities are available everywhere they may be needed by those who need to use them. This, however, does not guarantee usage but only that it assures seekers of health care services that if need arises, the health commodities that will save their lives will be available at every health facility. This is very important, especially for LMICs, where the majority of the populace resides in rural and in some cases hard-to-reach locations. Therefore, commodity security helps to build confidence among citizens that when they go to health facilities to seek care, which in most cases will require the need for lifesaving health commodities, they are assured that those commodities will be available. Also, commodity security promotes health-seeking behavior among citizens because of the confidence in the health care system to be able to make available health commodities that will restore their health again. Hence, commodity security has in these ways contributed to access to UHC among the most vulnerable populace in the society. Secondly, commodity security envisages that lifesaving health commodities will be available to those who need them at an affordable price, without having to put health care services seekers under financial hardship. Therefore, knowing that there will be health commodities a client needs at the health facility and that they are not out of reach financially becomes a motivation to seek health care at the nearest health facility. Until those who seek health care services can afford the cost of their medications, then one cannot say that commodity security exists. However, because majority of the population in LMICs is poor, the issue of affordability seems to hinder the pace at which the quest for UHC is being achieved and the more reason for LMICs to find a sustainable health financing strategy of option [22].

5. Foreign aid donor fatigue

Foreign aid is defined as "the international transfer of capital, goods, or services from a country or international organization for the benefit of the recipient country or its population. Aid can be economic, military, or emergency humanitarian" [23]. Foreign aid may be given for different purposes both as a diplomatic tool or in pursuance of foreign policy. Whatever the purpose is, the aid is given more to serve the interest of the donor country or institution first and second to benefit the recipient country.

Foreign aid donor fatigue or simply "donor fatigue" is defined as "a phenomenon in which people no longer donate to charities, although they have in the past" [24]. Expressed differently, it can also mean the hesitancy of the international community (either nations, private organizations, or individuals) to respond to a call for action toward a humanitarian crisis, be it a natural disaster (earthquakes, tsunamis/floods, wildfires, etc.) or man-made (e.g., wars, conflicts, terrorism). On a larger scale, it can also refer to a slowness to act on the part of the international community or any other donor base in response to a humanitarian crisis or call-to-action. Foreign aid seems to be at a crossroads when it is needed the most in LMICs. Since the early 1990s, there has been a pronounced fall in the real amount of foreign aid provided by donors for developing countries [25–27].

The term "donor fatigue" was espoused by donors and development aid agencies in the late 70s to convey their frustration at the slow pace of change in their recipient countries and communities, despite their huge investments. They were frustrated with the slow progress and impact of their technical and financial investments.

Many donors described this phenomenon as the "leaking basket" which dissipates invested resources [25]. It is also true, especially in Africa, which has relied heavily on aid flows, and has witnessed little, if any reduction in poverty. Indeed, the number of people living in poverty worldwide is likely to rise in the remaining years of the twentieth century [24–27]. On the face of it aid is being withdrawn when it is still desperately needed [25]. However, the question is: why should not it? Is foreign aid effective in alleviating poverty? If not, reducing it may be the sensible thing to do. If there are no developmental returns, why incur the cost? [25–27].

5.1 Potential drivers of foreign aid donor fatigue

There are several reasons why foreign aid donors are showing signs of fatigue or reducing the amount of aid they give to LMICs. The debate on potential drivers of foreign aid donor fatigue is as varied as the individuals or institutions you are dealing with. Simply put, differing reasons exist based on individual perspectives and may be a result of social constructs, rather than reality. The following potential drivers of donor fatigue are examined, though briefly:

5.1.1 Policy shift

What seems to be like "donor fatigue" may actually be a shift in the policy of the donor country for strategic reasons. And because policies are most times aligned with political leadership at the helm of affairs, there may be changes with every incoming administration that can have negative or positive effects on the country's foreign aid policy. This change will either manifest as an increase in the volume of foreign aid or as a decrease to it. For instance, the Trump administration in pursuance of its "America First" agenda pursued changes to foreign aid funding, desiring to reduce federal spending, including ending the need for foreign assistance. Some initiatives built on the work of previous administrations, while others conflicted with, and in some instances sought to dismantle, long-standing U.S. programs and policies [28].

5.1.2 Negative perception

There are some many opinions out there in the public about how foreign aid is administered in beneficiary countries. True or not, this negative publicity tends to raise internal tension and heat up the polity in donor countries with the resultant effect being more scrutiny about the volume of aid leaving donor countries to LMICs. National budgets are a trade-off between many competing demands, hence public support or otherwise by taxpayers and voters is considered critical to the sustenance, decline, or total removal of foreign aid programs. In addition, the legitimacy of any aid program as expressed by citizens can determine the quality of foreign aid. Therefore, public opinion is a critical factor in the continued flow of foreign aid from donor countries [29–31]. Some of these negative perceptions are related to corruption associated with aid administration in recipient countries, with little progress recorded despite a huge volume of aid flowing into those countries for specific interventions, etc.

5.1.3 Corruption

The perception of corruption in aid-recipient countries has been shown to cause donor fatigue. However, it is also true that corrupt countries are the ones with the highest need for foreign aid [25]. This is contradictory, yet true and represents a dilemma to donor countries and their citizens in that the reason for donor fatigue is the same reason why more aid is channeled into those countries either because it is a moral burden to support the vulnerable poor, or in the hope of bringing good governance and development or simply because it serves a strategic national interest of the donor country [25].

5.1.4 Economic recession

"Economic crises generally lead to reductions in foreign aid. However, the widely held view that budgetary constraints caused by economic crises reduce aid is inaccurate because donor government outlays actually tend to increase" [32]. When recession hit donor countries especially in such a way that it takes a huge toll on the banking sector, then it becomes difficult for foreign aid to flow out of those countries because of the fiscal cost associated with the banking sector.

Economic recession that hit hard on financial institutions of donor countries makes it less likely for politicians to show willingness or have the ability to provide foreign aid in this situation. It is common practice for banks to provide credit facilities to offset the cost and effect of economic recession in LMICs through development and economic recovery funds, but when the toll is heavy on financial institutions in donor countries, it results in donor fatigue and less flow of aid to help development agenda of LMICs. Also, voters place a lower priority on aid during economic downturns and politicians respond by cutting aid. Therefore, economic downturns lead to reduced public support for helping the poor abroad [32].

5.1.5 Increased demand for aid

Before now, there were problems in just a few places in the world, however, these days there seem to be many problems in many countries at the same time, including countries where foreign aid flow out from. Today, the whole of Europe is engulfed in a proxy war with Russia over the invasion of Ukraine. This is the case of your house on fire, likewise your neighbor's house; which are you supposed to focus on first? Therefore, it may not literally mean that foreign aid has been reduced, but that there are so many demands placed on the available budget which consequently reduces the volume of aid to LMICs. Hence, when foreign aid is not flowing toward countries that need it as expected, it is tagged as foreign aid donor fatigue without considering the enormous pressure on donor countries. And the fact that nontraditional recipients are beginning to require aid.

5.1.6 Internal crisis

As quoted somewhere above, the fact that there are so many problems in so many places all at the same seems to be weighing heavily on the ability of developed nations to keep up with their commitment to foreign aid. Most recently, the world was plagued with the Covid-19 pandemic of 2020, which hit the hardest developed, traditional donor nations. As if that was not enough, the Russia war on Ukraine erupted, which has involved almost all of Europe and the USA. And multiplied regional antagonism among friendly nations. Lastly, the effect of climate change and its consequence on energy has all gotten the "plate" of the developed nations full. The resultant effect is that LMICs are receiving less attention and foreign aid from developed nations to help deal with their developmental problems.

5.2 Impact of foreign aid donor fatigue on the ability of LMICs to achieve UHC

In summary, the issue of foreign aid donor fatigue which is causing a decrease in the volume of funds donor countries are prepared to commit to tackle developmental issues in LMICs is no longer in doubt while LMICs are more desperately in need of more aid to be able to meet their obligations to their citizens. There is the foreign debt servicing burden, low internally generated revenues, constant budgetary deficits, and increasing demand for scarce resources due to population growth. Therefore, if foreign aid continues to dwindle, it will constitute a risk to meeting the target of UHC by 2030, as envisioned by the UNSDGs. Therefore, there is a need for careful transitioning from foreign aid so as not to reverse the gains achieved in public health programs, such as HIV/AIDS, immunization, malaria, tuberculosis, nutrition, maternal and child health. Already, aid flows for HIV programs have stagnated in recent years, likely as a result of foreign aid donor fatigue. Estimates of future funding requirements needed to sustain present gains and to achieve universal treatment coverage to sustain existing programs and achieve universal treatment coverage suggest indicates that the current funding is less than sufficient, and more is being required [32–34]. Inferentially, there is almost a 100% chance that if the current trend in foreign aid donor fatigue should continue, LMICs will not be able to close the funding gap, and the vision for UHC will be compromised. For instance, when donor commitment toward malaria and childhood vaccination programs decreased due to foreign donor aid fatigue, there was a reversal of the gains already recorded in those public health programs [35, 36]. Therefore, if LMICs are not to be caught napping, there is an urgent need to search for a sustainable health financing strategy that can sustain the present gains being recorded through foreign aid inflows into the health sector. It is obvious that foreign withdrawal is a matter of when and not if.

6. Health financing strategies

Health commodities can save lives and have the ability to improve health outcomes and reduce mortality and morbidity due to diseases. It is also true that these lifesaving health commodities come at a cost and this cost is sometimes beyond the reach of the poor in the society. Simply put, health commodities are needed to save lives and improve health, but at what cost?

Health financing is a strategy to make health care services, including lifesaving health commodities, accessible to citizens whenever and wherever they may need it without unnecessary financial burden. According to the Ref. [37], health financing is a core function of health systems that can enable progress to attain UHC through ensuring there is commodity security and effective health care service as envisioned by SDG 3.8. Sadly, there are still many people in society that cannot afford the cost of health care, including the cost of obtaining lifesaving health commodities. There are also situations where people pay out-of-pocket but do not get quality and therefore value for their money.

6.1 Types of health financing strategies

There are five functional health care financing strategies identified and practiced globally. These strategies are listed and represented by a schematic diagram in **Figure 2**.

1. General tax revenues,

2. Social insurance,

3. Private/voluntary insurance,

4. Financial aid (by donors, NGOs),

5. Community-based insurance and

6. "User Fees" or individual out-of-pocket payment.

6.1.1 General tax revenues

Health financing with general tax revenues is a common practice in the developed nations of the West and is feasible because of their economic stability; however, that is not the case in LMICs as revenues so generated through general taxes are small and inadequate in light of other competing demands. There are three ways revenues can be generated through general taxes—direct, indirect, or excise taxes [38, 39].

6.1.2 Social insurance

Here, health care services are paid for through contributions by the employee and their employer. The health fund is usually independent of the government but works within a tight framework of regulations. Premiums are linked to the average cost of treatment for the group as a whole, as against an individual, which results in cross-subsidies from the healthy to the less healthy [38, 39].

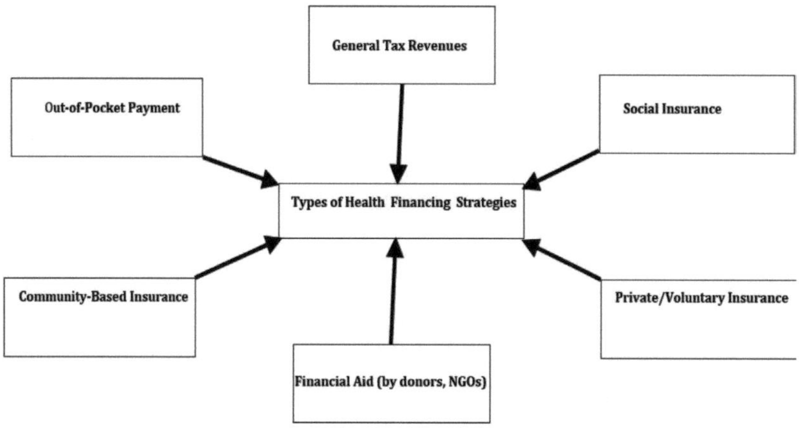

Figure 2.
Types of health financing strategies.

DOI: http://dx.doi.org/10.5772/intechopen.112790

6.1.3 Private insurance

This is also referred to as voluntary insurance. People pay premiums related to the expected cost of providing services to them. This occurs when employers and/or individuals choose to purchase insurance from private firms so as to mitigate the potential loss of income associated with illness or the costs of health care consumption. Thus, people who are in high health risk groups pay more, and those at low risk pay less. Cross-subsidy between people with different risks of ill health is limited. Membership of a private insurance scheme is usually voluntary. The insurance fund is held by a private (frequently for-profit) company [38, 39].

6.1.4 Financial aid

Financial aid, also known as charitable donations, comes from the developed nations and private organizations channeled through NGOs. The work of non-profit organizations in the development and financing of public health cannot be understated. The activities of the organizations are mostly for specific interventions, such as the treatment of HIV/AIDS, tuberculosis, malaria, immunization against targeted childhood illnesses, maternal neonatal, and child health. Financial aid has become a major source of health financing in LMICs. Furthermore, financial aid goes beyond intervention in health and comprises several technical assistances, including in areas of democracy, food sufficiency, and humanitarian interventions during natural or man-made disasters, for example, during internal or external conflicts [39].

6.1.5 User fees

User fees, also known as individual, out-of-pocket payments, is another form of health financing where individuals seeking health care services pay for those services out of their personal funds. Even in the developed countries with universal health coverage, individual out-of-pocket payments represent an important mechanism of health care financing. These payments, at times, are made as payment-in-full for a particular service received, or as cost-sharing instituted by insurance or government plans in the form of deductibles, co-payments, and coinsurance [38, 39].

6.1.6 Community-based health insurance

Community-based health insurance is a form of private health insurance where individuals, families, or community groups finance or cofinance the costs of their health care services. It is intended for people living in the rural area as well as for people in the informal sector who cannot get adequate public, private, or employer-sponsored insurance. Here, premiums are commonly set according to the risk faced by the average member of the community; that is, there is no distinction in premiums between high and low-risk groups. However, unlike social health insurance schemes, enrolment is generally voluntary and not linked to employment status. Funds are held by a private nonprofit entity [38, 39].

6.2 Sustainable health financing option for LMICs

Recently, there have been more discussions on ways for nations to achieve sustainable health financing toward realizing the goals of UHC, including ensuring commodity security to citizens. According to the Ref. [37], "experience demonstrates that real progress is possible in countries at all income levels. However, each country's pathway will differ depending on the local context." The WHO is of the opinion that health financing reforms should not simply be imported from one country to another, but the unique context of each country and its starting point in terms of health financing arrangements must be considered. It goes on to state that the underlying causes of performance problems differ in each country, and it is these causes that the reforms proposed in a health financing strategy must address. It is also true that there may not be just one way or health financing strategy for countries to achieve UHC; however, some strategies may be more feasible, based on the context and level of development of a country. This is true for LMICs, where almost all the health-financing strategies discussed above play a part.

But the question to ask is—are all these strategies sustainable? And if the answer is no, then what is the most sustainable strategy for LMICs to achieve commodity security, which is a critical component of UHC? According to Ref. [37], country experience should be looked at through the lens of the health financing functions, rather than labels, and can provide valuable lessons. Labels such as "social health insurance," "community insurance," or "tax-funded systems" mean little by themselves and hide the complex choices and options available to countries as they raise, pool, and use funds to ensure the availability and use of quality services. Three core health-financing functions as identified by the WHO are:

- Revenue raising (sources of funds, including government budgets, compulsory or voluntary prepaid insurance schemes, direct out-of-pocket payments by users, and external aid)

- Pooling of funds (the accumulation of prepaid funds on behalf of some or all of the population)

- Purchasing of services (the payment or allocation of resources to health service providers)

For LMICs, whose majority of the population resides in rural settings far away from urban health centers where revenues from the tax are mostly invested; and other forms of health financing make more sense. For those people in rural settings, available, quality, and affordable lifesaving health commodities to treat their basic illnesses are most important to them. The DRF scheme, as we shall see later, guarantees quality and affordable lifesaving health commodities to the poorest of the poor through design that incorporates "exemption and deferral." Secondly, because the DRF scheme is expected to be financed once, thereafter, it is self-sustaining through the principle of user fees for cost recovery and sustainability. Therefore, it is not designed for profit, but to bring health care services closer and more accessible to the people.

7. Drug revolving fund scheme: concepts and principles

The provision of access to quality and affordable essential medicines is a critical element of the UHC; however, most people, especially the most vulnerable in society, lack access to these commodities that their lives depend upon most of the leading causes of mortality and morbidity in LMICs are preventable or treatable with lifesaving health commodities [40, 41]. Drug Revolving Fund (DRF) is a scheme where medicines are sold at a light mark-up on the cost-price, and the revenue generated is used to replenish stocks, with the aim to provide safe and quality drugs at affordable prices and is usually part of the wider user fee model of sustainable health financing [41, 42].

The core concepts and principles of the DRF scheme as derived from the Bamako Initiative include but are not limited to:

- Promote additional investment and attract resources that citizens spent on accessing health care services in the private and informal sectors back to the public system.

- Increase in access to primary health care by raising effectiveness, efficiency, financial viability, and equity to health services.

- Meet basic community health needs through increased access to quality lifesaving health commodities and technologies.

- Improve regular contact between health care providers and the communities they serve.

- That communities should participate directly in the management and funding of lifesaving health commodities and technologies.

- Capture a fraction of the funds' households were already spending in the informal sector and combine them with government and donor funding to revitalize health services and improve their quality through community participation.

- Community participation in the management and control of resources at the health facility will ensure ownership and accountability of public health services to users.

- The pricing mechanism guarantees that basic services are priced below what is obtainable in the private sector and cross-subsidized with higher mark-ups on lower priority interventions.

- Develop local criteria for exemption and deferral for the poor so that no one is denied access to care because of their financial status.

- Autonomy from central administrative interference, and in the use of revenue accruing from the sales of health commodities and ensuring that procurement funds are "ring fenced" from access and use other than as outlined in the guidelines for the scheme.

In summary, the DRF scheme is designed to be self-sustaining and to ensure the availability, affordability, and accessibility of quality health commodities and technologies at facilities after initial investment either by the government or donors thereby reducing the burden of regular or annual budgetary allocations.

7.1 The history of drug revolving fund scheme

The DRF has its origin in the Bamako Initiative, which was adopted to tackle the poor availability of medicines in sub-Saharan Africa, especially at the primary health care level. The Bamako Initiative was the brainchild of UNICEF and WHO and was adopted by African ministers of health in 1987. The initiative was based on the realization that many of the LMICs especially those of sub-Saharan Africa faced issues of resources and the practicality to implement successfully comprehensive primary health care (PHC) which is critical to achieving UHC. Most of the PHC centers, including public hospitals in urban settings, were merely consulting clinics where clients come to get a diagnosis and prescription and then go the private drug outlets, which are mostly unlicensed and unsupervised, to fill their prescriptions at an exorbitant price. This situation has resulted in loss of confidence in the public health care system in LMICs. Africa's ministers of health believed that the Bamako Initiative can reverse this ugly trend. The Initiative proposed the use of an essential drug list and the development of realistic national drug policies to support the provision of essential drugs. Among other provisions that included community participation in the implementation of the scheme to promote accountability and ownership [6].

7.2 How drug revolving fund scheme can achieve commodity security

It has been established in Sections 3.2 and 3.3, respectively, that achieving UHC is only possible through functional primary health care and that when commodity security exists at primary health care, it restores confidence in public health care and encourages health-seeking behavior among citizens especially the vulnerable masses in rural settings which form the majority of the population in LMICs. Furthermore, the concepts and principles of the DRF scheme enumerated above, if implemented carefully will lead to commodity security for citizens. In this section, it will be further discussed as to how DRF scheme through some of its concepts and principles can bring about commodity security.

7.2.1 Ownership through community participation

The concept of community participation not only promotes ownership of the DRF scheme internally (for the staff that runs the scheme in the health facilities) and externally (for the clients from the catchment area of the health facility and beyond), but it also helps to enlighten community members about the existence of the scheme and mobilize community patronage. As quoted earlier, the impression about public health facilities to the ordinary citizen is that they are just "mere consulting clinics," which further worsens the poor health-seeking behavior of average community members. Therefore, the concept of community participation in the DRF scheme ensures that citizens have regular contact with their health care providers, where quality health commodities can be accessed whenever and wherever the need may arise.

7.2.2 Autonomy and ring: Fencing of procurement funds

The DRF scheme principles envisaged that funds for procurement of health commodities are "ring-fenced" from interference by authorities not involved with the operation of the scheme in any health facility. Simply put, the funds for procurement cannot and should not be used for any other purpose other than for the purpose of procurement of health commodities for the health facility where they are domiciled. Secondly, autonomy in the discretionary of revenue accruing from sales of health commodities is the sole prerogative of the members of the DRF committee; therefore, it is expected that such funds should be used to ensure the availability of health commodities at the health facility, which is one of the components of commodity security is therefore guaranteed under a functional DRF scheme.

7.2.3 Differential pricing mechanism

In the DRF scheme, the most effective interventions were priced below private sector charges and cross-subsidized through higher markup and higher co-payments on lower priority interventions [6]. Simply put, health conditions that are considered to be of high impact on citizens, such as malaria and common infections, and may be associated with the poorest of the poor are applied a lower "mark-up" so that community members within that social bracket are not exposed to unnecessary financial hardship while accessing health care services. Equally, interventions that are sought by community members in the upper social class are priced higher in a bit to offset the subsidy for the most effective interventions. This concept ensures that those with life-threatening conditions are not prevented from accessing acre because of their financial status, thereby making sure every person is able to obtain and use quality, affordable lifesaving health commodities whenever and wherever the need arises.

7.2.4 Use of "mark-up" for sustainability purposes

The DRF scheme was designed to be self-sustaining through the application of "user fees" not for profit but as a strategy for "cost recovery" to ensure the sustainability of the scheme such that the revenue from sales of health commodities is reinvested to procure and make them available and affordable. The concept of "cost recovery" and "user fees" in DRF scheme has attracted a lot of debate for and against. Those argue that "user fees" promotes responsible use of health care services as people tend to abuse and not value anything tagged as free. On the other hand, the opponents of "user fees" insist that charging the poor fees to access health care services will only drive them away from visiting health care centers even when they are very sick [5–8]. However, those who oppose "user fees" do not yet understand that the unbearable out-of-pocket expenditure, which they fear will further impoverish the poor is a result of the fact that those purchases are made from for-profit, private drug stores and private clinics occasioned by lack of availability of health commodities at the public health facilities ab initio.

7.2.5 Exemptions and deferrals

The DRF scheme in its provision envisaged that even at "cost recovery" mark-up, still there may be people in the communities that due to one reason or the other may not be able to afford the cost of the health commodities they need to save their lives and has provided an escape route or solace for such individuals so that no one is denied access to treatment because of their financial status. The DRF scheme has two ways to ensure everyone is able to obtain and use quality health commodities whenever and wherever the need arises. The first is known as "exemption"-which means individuals are exempted from paying 'user fees' because they have been assessed to be poor and cannot afford the cost of their treatment. The second is known as "deferral" which means that some individuals may not afford the cost of their treatment at the moment that they need it because of a temporal bad financial situation but could be able to pay in the future when their situation improves. In such a case, the payment for the cost of their treatment is deferred to a future date. Therefore, the DRF scheme is able to guarantee that every person is able to obtain and use quality health commodities whenever and wherever he or she needs it—this is called commodity security.

7.3 Example of successful implementation of drug revolving fund scheme

The DRF scheme is not without challenges, yet there are examples of successful implementation in several LMICs, which serve as best practices to other countries or sub-national entities within a country to borrow a leaf from. Some of the challenges experienced and are being experienced include but are not limited to weak political and financial commitment, poor leadership and managerial competence, resistance to change, and poor management of receivables, in the operations of the scheme [2, 6, 41]. Below are selected examples of successfully managed DRF schemes.

7.3.1 Drugs and medical consumables supply agency, Kano, Nigeria

Kano state is the most populous state in Nigeria with a population of 940,128 according to the census data of 2006 and was projected to be 14,253,549 in 2019 by the National Bureau of Statistics of the Federal Republic of Nigeria.

Before the support by Department for International Development (DFID), UK, in 2008, through the Partnership for Transforming Health Systems Phase 2 (PATHS 2), health facilities in Kano have lost patronage of the citizens and health workers were not working in the best environment because of lack of needed basic structures and systems [43]. As part of the key objective of the intervention, the focus was to improve the sustainable availability of health commodities at the health facilities, at the same time looking into other health system strengthening objectives [43]. Prior to the DFID-PATHS2 intervention, the total amount used for procurement of health commodities by the Kano state government was a meager N32million, as a result, most public health facilities resorted to self-help to source their supplies from the open market, which inculcated the prevalence of "parallel DRF" (a situation where health workers exploit clients by selling health commodities, usually brought in by them and hidden in their drawers and under their consulting tables, to them at exorbitant prices) [9]. The support by the UK government under PATHS2 will later continue with the Maternal, Newborn and Child health Program (MNCH2).

Between 2008 and 2013, procurement increased exponentially from N133 million in 2008 to N1 billion in 2013 with an increased number of sales transactions from a mere 402 to 2081 in the same period and with just 183 health facilities being supported by the DRF scheme to a whooping 699 [9]. This is an indication of an increased confidence in public health facilities and their patronage as well. Furthermore, the availability of health commodities rose from 6.5% to 84.95% in 657 primary health centers (PHC) while it rose at the secondary health centers (SHC) from 36% to 92.31% between 2008 and 2013 [41] and cumulatively, availability of health commodities on request rose from 25% in 2007 to 93% in 2015 [44]. Therefore, there was increased availability of health commodities, which is one of the core tenets of the DRF scheme.

On affordability, three successive annual drug price surveys carried out between 2008 and 2013 revealed that prices of health commodities in public health facilities are lower by about 63% than what they cost at private pharmacies and drug stores. In addition, in an attempt not to deny any person health care because of their financial status, Kano State DRF also incorporated a "deferral and exemption" policy, whereby the poor can access health care services free of charge or with deferred payment [9].

On accessibility, the increase in revenue from a mere N133 million to about N1 billion, representing a percentage increase of about 800%, from 2008 to 2013 showed that more people are having access to health commodities than when the DRF scheme came in place [9]. This is further confirmed under the MNCH2 when it reported that the Agency went from supplying 20 PHC facilities, and 10 SHC facilities across the state as of November 2015, to supplying over 700 health facilities across Kano (661 PHCs, and 39 SHCs) from two central medical stores and four zonal stores [44].

To conclude, a look at success factors toward the successful implementation of DRF scheme by the DMCSA, Kano, is worth highlighting here. Firstly, there is strong political buy-in in the scheme, which ensured that vested personal interests in the procurement process and contracting for supplies of health commodities, and operation of parallel DRF in health facility workers does not derail the scheme. Political buy-in also ensured that enabling policy guidelines are in place to regulate the conduct of bureaucrats and power play between different departments and units within the Ministry of Health and other relevant stakeholders [43]. Secondly, clarity in the implementation model has been identified as one of the success factors for the successful implementation of DRF by the DMCSA, Kano-Nigeria. Whereas others approach the implementation of the DRF scheme either as free, partial subsidy or full cost recovery or a mixture of all; DMCSA Kano-Nigeria chose a full cost recovery (for the cost of health commodities) approach excluding personnel overhead cost, infrastructure, cost of equipment [43]. Thirdly, the DMCSA Kano-Nigeria implemented a competitive pricing approach for determining the mark-up on the cost of health commodities which makes the selling price of the items affordable to clients. Also, DMCSA-supported facilities do not charge consultation fees to clients, which in other facilities account for a substantial part of the out-of-pocket expenses born by clients. Furthermore, the mark-up elements adopted in DMCSA are just for sustainability to cover the cost of potential expiries, inflation, monitoring and evaluation, exemptions, and deferrals all of which is not more than 20% added to the cost of health commodities [43]. Fourthly, capacity development and system strengthening are one of the success factors observed in the successful implementation of DRF scheme by the DMCSA. Activities being implemented include training for various staff involved in the running of the scheme at state, local government, facility, and community levels. These trainings are segmented to match the knowledge need and role of the staff being trained such as forecasting and quantification and procurement at the state level, monitoring and supportive supervision, and reporting [43, 44]. Lastly, community engagement and participation have been critical to the successful implementation of DRF scheme by the DMCSA by ensuring that there is local ownership, which leads to community members canvassing for support for the development of infrastructure, funding by political leadership, accountability of the scheme to the community it serves among other roles [43].

7.3.2 National medical supplies fund, Khartoum, Sudan

The National Medical Supplies Fund (NMSF), created by an act in 2015, is the government's main store responsible for securing medicines, consumables, and medical equipment for the public sector. Before this time, it was called the Central Stores for Sudan Medical Supplies since 1935. It became a public corporation in 1991 with the adoption of "user fees" and "cost recovery" system policy to finance health services. In 2002, NMSF established states revolving drug funds aiming to expand the coverage for safe, effective, and acceptable quality medicines [45].

The impact of DRF through the NMSF, Khartoum-Sudan has been reported in two separate studies indicating that the availability of key items on average was greater than 93% in DRF-supported health facilities compared to 86% in those not supported by the DRF scheme [46]; however, these studies revealed that availability of essential medicines in DRF-supported health facilities ranged from 95 to 100% [46, 47]. Consequently, increased attendance and utilization of health services at public health facilities saw a steady rise with only a small number of the public attributing their lack of visit to lack of availability or affordability of essential medicines [46, 47]. Hence, sustained availability of low-cost medicines at primary health care centers closer to the people who are most vulnerable and disadvantaged can be achieved through the DRF scheme [46].

Success factors to the DRF scheme of the NMSF, Khartoum-Sudan was first, identified as due to substantial initial financial investment through capital seed stock of medicines that was provided by Save the Children International to the scheme to kick off at the onset [47]. Secondly, political commitment, in providing a legal framework for NMSF to operate, and allowing it to maintain a separate account so that its managers have a free hand in keeping generated revenues out of public treasury regulation, was instrumental to its success to this day [47]. Therefore, it is important that DRF scheme be provided with initial capital to set out and be allowed freedom to manage proceeds of sales of health commodities for the purpose of the scheme and excluded from the Ministry of Finance. Thirdly, the NMSF Khartoum-Sudan was given a free hand to apply private sector management style in running its business affairs and focusing on performance and results within the public sector [47]. The private sector approach entrenched the culture of accountability and transparency in financial management and allows measures that recruit staff based on competency and reduce risk to the operations of the organization. Fourthly, applying the principle of pooled procurement helped to price discounts due to economies of scale and keep the cost of health commodities as low as possible and contributed to responsiveness to stock-out situations in DRF-supported health facilities by not restricting purchase by health facilities to a cash-and-carry basis at the time of purchase [47]. Fifthly, the NMSF Khartoum-Sudan ensured that expensive drugs remain continuously available, subsidized, and affordable through the sale of cheaper essential medicines at low cost with a focus on high turnover instead [47]. This principle ensures that potential losses from the sale of expensive medicines are covered through the expected high turnover from sales of cheaper essential medicines and guarantees continued funding and subsidy for others. Lastly, monitoring, evaluation, and reporting of DRF activities at the health facilities by the supervision teams helped to ensure visibility, financial accountability, transfer of skills, and redistribution of health commodities from overstocked facilities to where they may be most needed, thereby leading to prevention of loses through potential expiry and damage [47].

8. Results and discussions

The results and discussions are structured as lessons learnt from implementation of successful Drug Revolving Fund Scheme in LMICs as synthesized from the review of the literature and from specific examples of successful implementation of DRF schemes in LMICs as mentioned above under Section 7.3 and are presented below. Indeed, very useful lessons have been learned from implementation of DRF scheme at national and sub-national levels that can provide good guidance for intending implementers. Below are some of the most critical lessons learned.

8.1 Political commitment

This is the most crucial and rate-determining step in establishing a successful DRF scheme. First, a DRF scheme must need to be empowered by a legal framework in order to succeed and as well as not to be easily affected when there is a change in political leadership. The act establishing the DRF scheme must envisage likely challenges and tackle them. For instance, the procurement funds and revenue from the sales of health commodities must be "ring-fenced" and shielded from external interference. It is equally important that revenue from the DRF scheme should not be subjected to any form of tax and import duties so as to avoid passing the burden on clients.

8.2 Initial capital investment

"Medicines safe lives and improve health, but they are costly" [40]. Following next to political commitment is a financial commitment from the government or donors to help supply the initial capital investment necessary to kick start the DRF scheme without which the concept of a DRF scheme will just be a mere wish. The failure of many DRF schemes in LMICs is due to a lack of financial commitment and the release of the needed initial capital investment. This initial capital investment could be in the provision of "seed stock" or funds to procure "seed stock" that will then be sold and revolve to generate more revenue and the circle continues leading asset growth of the DRF scheme. It is important that this initial capital investment be adequate and done once, as the idea of DRF scheme is to be self-sustaining and free the government from making recurrent annual budgets and releases. If this is happening, then the DRF scheme is not being run professionally.

8.3 Stakeholder engagement and buy-in

The health care sector is multidisciplinary with varied interests that differ one from another. Secondly, there are different revenue generation points or service delivery points such as the laboratory unit, theater unit, maternity unit, radiology unit, nursing unit, and pharmacy unit, within any health facility especially if it is a secondary of tertiary health facility. These different units or departments are being supervised by their parent professional bodies or departments in the Ministry of Health. It is therefore natural for different sections of the health facility to be apprehensive about what the concept of the DRF scheme entails for them. Thirdly, there is also the fact that health workers in LMICs are known to bring private business dealings into public health facilities because of lack of adequate funding by the government to provide all the necessary support for a conducive working environment. For instance, when there is no funding for procurement, it is easy for the pharmacist to buy their personal drugs and sale to clients. Likewise, when doctors and nurses realize that there are no health commodities at the pharmacy, they too are known to sale medicines to their patients in the consulting rooms. The same goes for the laboratory scientist who runs diagnostic tests who also buy all the necessary reagents and run the laboratory as their personal business premises. However, the concept of the DRF scheme will change all these unethical practices that seem to be a "new normal" and are bound to be resisted for personal interest. Therefore, all these stakeholders must be carried along in the initial consultation and design of the DRF scheme, otherwise, it will be frustrated.

8.4 Phased implementation approach

Establishing a DRF scheme, just like any other change program, requires an incremental approach so that successes or milestones can be reached and celebrated at intervals, which serve to build trust and provide the basis for motivation and more effort. The incremental approach also enables the system to monitor and evaluate progress and develop lessons learned for continuous improvement. For instance, the scheme can kick off with a number of limited health facilities onboarded and thereafter they can be increased when the system has fully stabilized in terms of adequately meeting the expectations of stakeholders, for example, in meeting the health commodity requirements of health facilities since the DRF scheme envisaged that all health facilities must source their commodities centrally. If "going to scale" was done too quickly the system may not be able to withstand the shock in increased demand from health facilities and this can create the impression that the scheme is not able to meet their health commodity requirements, which may result in health facilities "seeking self-help." Similarly, some concepts like "exemption and deferral" can be delayed until the scheme has matured and accumulated reasonable revenue to absorb such costs.

8.5 Robust management and technical systems

There are three critical systems that have contributed to the success of DRF schemes in places the scheme has been launched-these are financial management and accountability system, functional supply chain system, and strong monitoring evaluation. For any DRF scheme to succeed, these three different but complementary systems must work in harmony. A strong financial and accountability system is required to ensure that there are no revenue leakages in the system that will starve it of needed funds.

Equally critical is the need for a functional supply chain system especially in the use of data for demand and supply planning such that procurement is guided by the use of data to avoid stuffing the supply chain pipeline that could lead to potential expiry and waste. Also, procurement should be "pooled" to maximize economies of scale and drive prices lower. However, even more critical is the need for a transparent and responsible procurement devoid of corruption, otherwise, the final prices to the consumers will be high, which will defeat the concept of affordability and access. Finally, on functional supply chain systems, most successful DRF schemes incorporate last-mile distribution to deliver health commodities to the doorsteps of the health facilities. This is a good practice that allows health care workers to focus on providing health care services to their clients rather than being engulfed in logistics matters.

Lastly, monitoring and evaluation is another system that must be in place to ensure that the scheme does not derail from its set goals and targets. Hence, there should be periodic supportive supervision of supported health facilities as well as regular performance review meetings to review the operation of the scheme and to proffer solutions to issues and to encourage continuous improvement.

8.6 Availability of, and compliance to operational guidelines

Strict compliance with operational guidelines of the DRF scheme is very critical to the success of the scheme. Systems like the DRF scheme must have operational guidelines or standard operating procedures (SOPs) that define roles and responsibilities, processes, procedures, list forms of records and job aids describing how tasks should be completed successfully. The lack of robust operational guidelines or lack of strict compliance with it is probably the major reason for failed DRF schemes.

8.7 Stakeholder participation and collaboration

Earlier we have seen the role of stakeholder engagement, and buy-in, which is very critical from the onset to bring key opinion leaders (KOLs) to the table to accept the new changes in administration and control with respect to running the DRF scheme and this need to continue all through the life of the scheme. This is different from stakeholder participation and collaboration, which comes to bear during the actual implementation of the scheme. This applies to the front-line staff of different departments and units in the health facility or sector and the community it serves. Every person should be seen to be participating in the running of the DRF scheme, including the members of the communities it serves. This fosters ownership and local support that is needed for the successful implementation of the scheme.

9. Conclusion

Commodity security guarantees a situation where every person is able to obtain and use quality lifesaving health commodities whenever and wherever he or she may need them, which is a critical component to achieving universal health coverage. The need to achieve universal health coverage through building and strengthening primary health care closer to the people is needed now than ever before. But even more critical is to ensure that the primary health care system is equipped with necessary tools, including lifesaving health commodities and technologies that are qualitative, available, affordable, and accessible to all irrespective of their financial status. The increased demand for foreign aid donors among other reasons has led to a situation where donors who hitherto responded to call to assist LMICs are either not forthcoming or the volume of such donations have drastically reduced, a situation that has now come to be known as foreign aid donor fatigue. Therefore, there is a need for LMICs to fashion out a sustainable health financing strategy that will recognize the competition on the already scarce resources available to LMICs governments so that the gains obtained by donor-supported public health interventions, such as HIV/AIDS, malaria, tuberculosis, and childhood vaccinations programs, are not reversed when foreign aid becomes unavailable or too little to make any reasonable difference to the myriad of existing and new public health challenges bedeviling LMICs. The DRF scheme is one of the recognized strategies for health financing that is self-sustaining, where "user fees" are charged to clients just enough to cover the cost of health commodities through individual out-of-pocket payments and community co-payments. Therefore, political leaders and stakeholders in the health sector need to show renewed commitment to supporting the establishment and reengineering of DRF scheme to ensure commodity security to their citizens, thereby contributing to realizing the UNSDGs of achieving UHC for all.

Conflict of interest

The author declares no conflict of interest.

Author details

Jibrailu L. Maliyogbinda
Texila American University, Zambia

*Address all correspondence to: jibrailu@outlook.com; jibrailu.lot@gmail.com

References

[1] The World Health Report 2010–Health Systems Financing: The Path to Universal Coverage. Geneva: World Health Organization; 2010. Available from: http://www.who.int/whr/2010/whr10_en.pdf [Accessed: May 26, 2023]

[2] Raja R. Commodity Security for Essential Medicines: Challenges and Opportunities. Arlington, VA: USAID|DELIVER PROJECT; 2008. Available from: https://www.rhsupplies.org/uploads/tx_rhscpublications/CSEssMedChall.pdf [Accessed: May 26, 2023]

[3] USAID. The Logistics Handbook: A Practical Guide for the Supply Chain Management of Health Commodities. 2nd ed. Arlington, VA: USAID|DELIVER PROJECT; 2011. (First edition 1998). Available from: http://ghsupplychain.org/sites/default/files/2019-07/Logistics%20Handbook.pdf [Accessed: May 26, 2023]

[4] WHO. Arguing for Universal Health Coverage. 2013. Available from: http://www.who.int/health_financing/UHC_ENvs_BD.PDF [Accessed: May 26, 2023]

[5] Bedado D, Kaso AW, Hailu A. Magnitude and determinants of out-of-pocket health expenditure among patients visiting outpatients in public hospitals in East Shoa zone, Ethiopia. Clinical Epidemiology and Global Health. 2022;**15**:101066

[6] Garner PA. The Bamako initiative. BMJ Clinical Research. 1989;**299**(6694):277-278. DOI: 10.1136/bmj.299.6694.277

[7] Ogbonna BO, Nwako CN. Essential drugs revolving fund scheme in Nigeria; from the edge of a precipice towards sustainability. Journal of Advances in Medical and Pharmaceutical Sciences. JAMPS. 2016;**8**(2):1-8. Article no. JAMPS.259502

[8] Ohaju-Obodo JO, Ighehosa SU, Asalu AE, Okoli RI, Omokhafe AA. An evaluation of the drug revolving fund (DRF) scheme in Nigeria: Two decades after its adoption. ACR. 2006;**1**:20-24

[9] PATHS 2 Logistics Report. A technical brief. In: Increasing Efficiency in the Drug Supply System in Nigeria. 2014. Available from: https://www.cabrisbo.org/uploads/files/Documents/case_study_2016_cabri_health_dialogue_increasing_efficiency_in_the_drug_supply_system_in_nigeria_engl.pdf [Accessed: June 08, 2023]

[10] Sambo MN, Lewis I, Sabitu K. Essential drugs in primary health centers of north Central Nigeria: Where is Bamako initiative? Nigeria Journal of Clinical Practice. 2008;**11**(1):9-13

[11] Chukwuani CM, Olugboji A, Ugbene E. Improving access to essential drugs for rural communities in Nigeria: The Bamako initiative re-visited. Pharmacy World & Science. 2006;**28**(2):91-95

[12] Sule YZ, Mora AT, Dagogot CN. Lessons from the Kaduna sustainable drug supply intervention initiative. West African Journal of Pharmacy. 2016;**27**(2):53-64

[13] Monczka RM, Handfield RB, Giunipero LC, Patterson JL. Purchasing and Supply Management. 4th ed. USA: South-Western; 2009. p. 10

[14] Frazelle E. World-Class Warehousing and Material Handling.

New York: McGraw-Hill; 2002. p. 5. DOI: 10.1036/0071418172

[15] Global Health-CDC and the Global Health Security Agenda. Available from: https://www.cdc.gov/globalhealth/security/what.htm [Accessed: June 03, 2023]

[16] CDC. Advancing the Global Health Security Agenda. Available from: https://www.cdc.gov›pdf›GHSA Report final [Accessed: June 03, 2023]

[17] WHO. Universal Health Coverage. 2022. Available from: https://www.who.int/news-room/fact-sheets/detail/universal-health-coverage-(uhc) [Accessed: May 29, 2023]

[18] WHO. Primary Health Care on the Road to Universal Health Coverage: 2019 Monitoring Report. Geneva: World Health Organization; 2020. License: CC BY-NC-SA 3.0 IGO. Available from: https://www.who.int/publications-detail-redirect/9789240004276 [Accessed: May 29, 2023]

[19] Kruk ME, Gage AD, Joseph NT, Goodarz D, Garcia-Saiso S, Salomon JA. Mortality due to low-quality health systems in the universal coverage era: A systematic review of amenable deaths in 137 countries. The Lancet. 2018;**392**(10160):2203-2221. Available from: https://pubmed.ncbi.nlm.nih.gov/30195398/ [Accessed: May 29, 2023]

[20] The World Health Report 2010–Health Systems Financing: The Path to Universal Coverage. Geneva: World Health Organization; 2010. Available from: http://www.who.int/whr/2010/whr10_en.pdf [Accessed: June 03, 2023]

[21] Penchansky R, Thomas JW. The concept of access: Definition and relationship to consumer satisfaction. Medical Care. 1981;**19**:127-140. DOI: 10.1097/00005650-198102000-00001

[22] Ahuja A, Peungchanchaikul C, Piyagarn N. On Monetary and Fiscal Policy Mix over Thailand's Business Cycles. Bank of Thailand Discussion Paper DP/09/2004. Bangkok: Bank of Thailand; 2004

[23] Victoria Williams. Foreign Aid. Encyclopedia Britannica. Available from: https://www.britannica.com/topic/foreign-aid [Accessed: June 05, 2023]

[24] SE Smith. What Is Donor Fatigue? Available from: https://www.smartcapitalmind.com/what-is-donor-fatigue.htm [Accessed: June 05, 2023]

[25] Bauhr M, Charron N, Nasiritousi N. Does corruption cause aid fatigue? Public opinion and the aid-corruption paradox. International Studies Quarterly. 2013;**57**:568-579. DOI: 10.1111/isqu.12025

[26] Elongué CCN, VanDyck CK. Overcoming Development Aid Fatigue, Deciding Together and Shifting Power to Communities in Africa, WACSeries, Issue Paper. Vol. 7. Issue 2. Accra, Ghana: West Africa Civil Society Institute; 2021

[27] Bird G. The political economy of foreign aid: Fatigue or regeneration? In: International Finance and the Developing Economies. London: Palgrave Macmillan; 2004. DOI: 10.1057/9780230599840_13

[28] Congressional Research Service. Selected Trump Administration Foreign Aid Priorities: A Wrap-Up. 2021. Available from: https://crsreports.congress.gov/product/pdf/R/R46656 [Accessed: June 05, 2023]

[29] Lumsdaine DH. Moral Vision in International Politics. Princeton: Princeton University Press; 1993

[30] Paxton P, Knack S. Individual and country level factors affecting support for foreign aid. International Political Science Review. 2012;**33**(2):171-192

[31] Collier P. The Bottom Billion. New York: Oxford University Press; 2007. p. 183

[32] Heinrich T, Kobayashi Y, Bryant KA. Public opinion and foreign aid cuts in economic crises. World Development. 2016;**77**:66-79. DOI: 10.1016/j.worlddev.2015.08.005

[33] Mao W, McDade KK, Huffstetler HE, Dodoo J, Abankwah DNY, Coleman N, et al. Transitioning from donor aid for health: Perspectives of national stakeholders in Ghana. BMJ Global Health. 2021;**6**:e003896. DOI: 10.1136/bmjgh-2020-003896

[34] Grépin KA. Efficiency considerations of donor fatigue, universal access to ARTs and health systems. Sexually Transmitted Infections. 2012;**88**:75-78. DOI: 10.1136/sextrans-2011-050148. Available from: https://pubmed.ncbi.nlm.nih.gov/22345022/ [Accessed: June 05, 2023]

[35] Hardon A, Blume S. Shifts in global immunisation goals (1984-2004): Unfinished agendas and mixed results. Social Science & Medicine. 2005;**60**:345e56

[36] Sachs J, Malaney P. The economic and social burden of malaria. Nature. 2002;**415**:680e5

[37] WHO. Health Financing. Available from: https://www.who.int/health-topics/health-financing#tab=tab_1 [Accessed: June 04, 2023]

[38] Bennett S, Gilson L. Health Financing: Designing and Implementing Pro-Poor Policies. DFID Health Systems Resource Centre; 2001. Available from: http://www.heart-resources.org/wp-content/uploads/2012/10/Health-financing.pdf [Accessed: June 04, 2023]

[39] Drouin A. Methods of Financing Health Care-a Rational Use of Financing Mechanisms to Achieve Universal Coverage. International Social Security Association; 2008. Available from: http://www.issa.int/Resources [Accessed: June 04, 2023]

[40] Management Sciences for Health. MDS-3. Managing Access to Medicines and Health Technologies. Arlington, VA: MSH; 2012. Available from: https://msh.org/resources/mds-3-managing-access-to-medicines-and-health-technologies/ [Accessed: June 06, 2023]

[41] C Anyakora, O Odibeli. BusinessDay. Drug Revolving Fund in Africa: A Step towards Health Security. 2022. Available from: https://businessday.ng/opinion/article/drug-revolving-fund-in-africa-a-step-towards-health-security/ [Accessed: June 06, 2023]

[42] Yadav P, Smith L. Pharmaceuticals and national health systems. In: Encyclopedia of Health Economics. 2014. pp. 37-48. Available from: https://www.tandfonline.com/doi/full/10.4161/23288604.2014.968005 [Accessed: June 06, 2023]

[43] CABRI. Increasing Efficiency in the Drug Supply System in Nigeria. Available from: https://www.cabrisbo.org/uploads/files/Documents/case_study_2016_cabri_health_dialogue_increasing_efficiency_in_the_drug_supply_system_in_nigeria_engl.pdf [Accessed: June 08, 2023]

[44] MNCH2. Improving Reliability of Drugs and Medical Supplies Through Integrated Supply Chain Management. Case Study No. 2|September 2016. 2016.

Available from: https://www.mnch2.com/wp-content/uploads/2014/12/Case-Study DMCSA-MNCH2_2016.pdf [Accessed: June 08, 2023]

[45] Ali GKM. Integration in medicines supply Sudan experience. In: GHSC Summit 2016. Dar es Salaam, Tanzania; 2016. Available from: http://ghscs.com/wp-content/uploads/2017/01/T1-6_Integration-in-Medicines-Supply-Sudan-experience.pdf [Accessed: July 01, 2023]

[46] Ali GKM. Accessibility of medicines and primary health care: The impact of the revolving drug fund in Khartoum state. International Journal of Public Health and Epidemiology. 2019;**8**(5):001-008. Available from: https://www.internationalscholarsjournals.com/articles/accessibility-of-medicines-and-primary-health-care-theimpact-of-the-revolving-drug-fund-in-khartoum-state.pdf

[47] Ali GKM. How to establish a successful revolving drug fund: The experience of Khartoum state in the Sudan. Bulletin of the World Health Organization. 2009;**87**(2):139-142. World Health Organization. DOI: 10.2471/BLT.07.048561

Chapter 11

The Road to Universal Healthcare Coverage in the Face of COVID-19: South Africa's Struggles and Prospects

Nelly Sharpley

Abstract

The COVID-19 pandemic has exposed the fragility of healthcare systems worldwide, especially in developing countries like South Africa. The country has been grappling with a long-standing struggle to achieve universal healthcare coverage, and the pandemic has brought to the fore the urgent need to address the disparities in healthcare access and outcomes. This paper explores South Africa's journey towards universal healthcare and the challenges and solutions it has encountered in the face of the COVID-19 pandemic. It discusses the impact of the pandemic on the country's healthcare system and highlights the inequities in access to care, especially among vulnerable populations. It also examines the policy responses implemented by the government to address these challenges, including the use of digital technology and community-based care. The paper concludes by emphasizing the need for sustained efforts to achieve universal healthcare in South Africa beyond the pandemic and the importance of global solidarity in this pursuit.

Keywords: universal healthcare, COVID-19, South Africa, healthcare disparities, policy responses

1. Introduction

Universal healthcare, also referred to as universal health coverage (UHC), has been advocated by the World Health Organization (WHO) as the primary framework for healthcare provision [1]. UHC aims to ensure that individuals and communities have access to essential health services without facing financial hardships. It encompasses a wide range of high-quality healthcare services, including health promotion, prevention, treatment, rehabilitation, and palliative care.

The foundation of UHC can be traced back to the WHO's declaration in 1948, which recognized health as a fundamental human right and stressed the importance of affordable and timely access to comprehensive healthcare services for all individuals [2]. The ultimate goal of UHC is to remove financial barriers and guarantee universal access to healthcare, irrespective of an individual's socioeconomic status or geographic location. However, despite this declaration, South Africa currently lacks UHC and operates with two parallel healthcare systems: the private and public sectors, which coexist with each other.

Ensuring accessibility to healthcare remains a significant challenge in South Africa, particularly in rural areas where healthcare services are inadequate. Moreover, the public healthcare system faces difficulties in retaining healthcare professionals, exacerbating the existing disparities in care. Approximately 80% of the population relies on the public system, which receives government subsidies but suffers from underfunding and poor management. The country boasts over 400 public hospitals, managed at different levels by provincial health departments and municipal authorities, including regional hospitals and primary care clinics.

The healthcare system in South Africa is divided into two unequal parts: private and public. The private sector is renowned for its high-quality services, advanced medical technology, and well-equipped facilities, but is only accessible to those who can afford private health insurance or out-of-pocket payments. Private healthcare providers prioritize patients' satisfaction by providing shorter wait times and a higher standard of care due to better infrastructure and resources available in these facilities. However, the high cost of private healthcare in South Africa makes it inaccessible to a large portion of the population. On the other hand, the government-funded public healthcare system provides services either for free or at significantly subsidized rates, catering to the majority of South Africa's population who cannot afford private healthcare. Public healthcare facilities, including hospitals, clinics, and health centres, are widely available but often face challenges related to resource shortages, infrastructure deficiencies, and staff shortages. The public healthcare system serves a larger portion of the population, especially those without private health insurance, and is more accessible in rural and underserved areas. However, it also faces numerous challenges, including underfunding, overcrowding, and shortages of medical staff, equipment, and essential medicines resulting in longer waiting times, inadequate services, and sometimes compromised quality of care [3, 4]. According to Netshiswinzhe et al. [5], apartheid has had a significant impact on access to and utilization of healthcare services in South Africa. They discuss this in their article "Understanding the Influence of apartheid on Access and Utilization of healthcare services in South Africa" [6]. On the same view [7] also presents the challenges noted on SA public health system.

The significant disparities in healthcare quality between the private and public sectors contribute to unequal healthcare access based on socioeconomic status. Addressing these disparities requires comprehensive reforms, increased funding, improved management, and equitable distribution of resources to bridge the gap between the two systems, aiming for more equitable healthcare access and quality for all South Africans. It is imperative that the government takes immediate action to address the challenges faced by the public healthcare system to ensure that all South Africans have access to high-quality healthcare services, regardless of their socioeconomic status [8, 9]. Currently, moving closer to achieving UHC, South Africa is currently implementing healthcare system reforms through the establishment of a national health insurance (NHI) program. In parallel, South Africa introduced the Ideal Clinic framework in 2020 as a step towards UHC, with a focus on infrastructure, staffing, medication and supplies, administrative processes, and bulk supplies. The framework also emphasizes the adoption of relevant clinical policies, protocols, and guidelines, as well as collaboration with partners and stakeholders. These initiatives aim to enhance healthcare delivery and bring South Africa closer to achieving UHC, although challenges and disparities between the two healthcare systems persist [10, 11].

Public healthcare system is discussed by Rispel et al. [12] in their article "Analysis of the ideal clinic programme as a platform for the delivery of quality health services in South Africa: Case study of primary healthcare in KwaZulu-Natal and as noted above, the study highlights prospects and problem.

When the COVID-19 pandemic engulfed the world, the healthcare system in South Africa was already overwhelmed due to the burden of diseases and its direct impact on socioeconomic inequalities within the country [13]. This situation exacerbated the challenges faced by the majority of disadvantaged populations residing in rural areas. Although the country has made efforts to provide accessible primary healthcare through community-based clinics and centers, there has been a failure to effectively address the underlying socioeconomic inequalities within the system [14].

Consequently, in many areas, the process of healthcare coverage became superficial, resulting in a lack of access to necessary services and treatment. Even though the physical infrastructure of the healthcare system may be visible, in some cases, it does not meet the requirements for effective healthcare provision. As a consequence, the expansion of healthcare coverage became an unattainable goal, further widening health inequalities [14]. The COVID-19 pandemic has starkly highlighted and exacerbated the pre-existing inequalities in South Africa, particularly in rural areas. As Bank and Sharpley [15] have pointed out, the rural poor have been subjected to what they call "Ukuvala ISango"—a total closure of the gate to healthcare access and basic services. In the face of this crisis, rural populations have been left to fend for themselves, with no screening or testing available to them. Clinics have been closed, rendering primary healthcare an illusory prospect for most rural residents, especially those with chronic conditions. Only the affluent working class could afford medical protection against the pandemic, pushing the rural poor even further to the margins. This is a dire situation that the pandemic exposed that demands immediate attention and action. At the time of vaccination, there was a significant mobilization of resources to get the rural population vaccinated. Mobile clinics and temporary stations were erected to ensure that everyone had access to the vaccine. However, it is concerning that many rural people reported feeling coerced into taking the vaccine. This is unacceptable as every individual has the right to make their own informed decisions about their health without any undue pressure. No one should be threatened with being denied access to essential services, basic necessities, or social grants for choosing not to take the vaccine [15].

2. Literature

2.1 South African health care system during COVID-19

Gebremeskel et al. [16] asserted that health system resilience was defined as the ability of health actors, institutions, and populations to establish absorption, adaptation, accessibility, and transformation capabilities to prepare for surprises in the health system and respond effectively to disruptions. Health system resilience is openly related to health system governance, that is, resilience depends on the decisions of groups and individuals as they make change, monitor, and enforce the rules that direct the health system. The COVID-19 pandemic has exposed the long-standing structural causes of health inequalities. There are anxieties that public health policies could amplify the harmful effects of these inequalities unless vigilant efforts are made to mainstream these social weaknesses into public health systems [16].

Masuku et al. [17] displays that child and youth caregivers were exposed to poor mental health because they experienced anxiety, insecurity, and stress. Moreover, these workers have faced challenges when working under the so-called new normal, which was introduced as part of a non-pharmaceutical response to contain the spread of COVID-19 [17].

According to Banda Chitsamatanga and Malinga [18], the hasty spread of the COVID-19 leads to panic around the world and calling into question the preparedness of public health systems to deal with it. This has undoubtedly made the word COVID-19 a new slogan. Banda Chitsamatanga and Malinga [18] distinguished that despite economic inequality and differential income status, the pandemic has exposed that there are ingrained problems in overburdened public health systems. In addition, the situation is further projected and exacerbated by primary socioeconomic issues identical to poverty, unemployment, inequality, slow economic development, inadequate water and sanitation, and food insecurity, which have made it challenging to cope with the pandemic.

Access to contraception became a challenge due to lockdown, reduced mobility, reduced availability of public transport, and the closure of non-essential retail outlets and youth centers also limited young people's access to contraception. Hence, a lack of these goods can lead to risky sexual practices and unwanted pregnancies [19], both of which were long-standing problems before lockdowns were imposed in response to COVID-19 [20]. For people living with HIV, condom shortages can increase the likelihood of HIV transmission. Additionally, fear of contracting SARS-CoV-2 discourages individuals from attending public clinics [21]. Therefore, there is a need to strike a balance between directly responding to the COVID-19 pandemic and respecting human rights and supporting children and young people, mainly vulnerable groups, to ensure that food, education, and counseling services are available. More generally, the COVID-19 public health crisis highlights the importance of offering fiscal support to improve healthcare systems.

Consequently, there is vigorous evidence of medical plants in the use of both traditional and biomedical products and services in South Africa [22], and traditional health practitioners are regularly the first healthcare approach for patients when they become ill. Some people feel that the solution to COVID-19 would come through traditional health practitioners rather than biomedical interventions [23], while others fear infection of COVID-19 in healthcare settings, suggesting that the focus on safe access to healthcare services is crucial.

2.2 Challenges in coping with COVID

Gebremeskel et al. [16] asserted that health system resilience was defined as the ability of health actors, institutions, and populations to establish absorption, adaptation, accessibility, and transformation capabilities to prepare for surprises in the health system and respond effectively to disruptions. Health system resilience is openly related to health system governance, that is, resilience depends on the decisions of groups and individuals as they make changes, monitor, and enforce the rules that direct the health system. The COVID-19 pandemic has exposed the long-standing structural causes of health inequalities. There are anxieties that public health policies could amplify the harmful effects of these inequalities unless vigilant efforts are made to mainstream these social weaknesses into public health systems [16].

Furthermore, Masuku et al. [17] specified that child and youth caregivers were exposed to poor mental health because they experienced anxiety, insecurity, and stress. Moreover, these workers have faced challenges when working under the so-called new normal, which was introduced as part of a non-pharmaceutical response to contain the spread of COVID-19 [17].

According to Banda Chitsamatanga and Malinga [18], the hasty spread of COVID-19 leads to panic around the world and calls into question the preparedness of public health systems to deal with it. This has undoubtedly made the word COVID-19 a new slogan. Banda Chitsamatanga and Malinga [18] distinguished that despite economic inequality and differential income status, the pandemic has exposed that there are ingrained problems in overburdened public health systems. In addition, the situation is further projected and exacerbated by primary socioeconomic issues identical to poverty, unemployment, inequality, slow economic development, inadequate water and sanitation, and food insecurity, which have made it challenging to cope with the pandemic.

While countries implement public health measures to lessen transmission of SARS-CoV-2, young girls and women, people who identify as LGBTI, people engaged in sex work are more likely to become victims of police brutality [24]. Access to contraception became a challenge due to lockdown, reduced mobility, reduced availability of public transport, and the closure of non-essential retail outlets and youth centers also limited young people's access to contraception. Hence, a lack of these goods can lead to risky sexual practices and unwanted pregnancies [19], both of which were long-standing problems before lockdowns were imposed in response to COVID-19 [20]. For people living with HIV, condom shortages can increase the likelihood of HIV transmission. Additionally, fear of contracting SARS-CoV-2 discourages individuals from attending public clinics [21]. Therefore, there is a need to strike a balance between directly responding to the COVID-19 pandemic and respecting human rights and supporting children and young people, mainly vulnerable groups, to ensure that food, education, and counseling services are available. More generally, the COVID-19 public health crisis highlights the importance of offering fiscal support to improve healthcare systems.

Consequently, there is vigorous evidence of medical plants in the use of both traditional and biomedical products and services in South Africa [22], and traditional health practitioners are regularly the first healthcare approach for patients when they become ill. Some people felt that the solution to COVID-19 would come through traditional health practitioners rather than biomedical interventions [23], others fear infection of COVID-19 in healthcare settings, suggesting that the focus on safe access to healthcare services is crucial.

3. Methodology

The methodology was partly an ethnographic mixed methods approach with both qualitative and quantitative data tools used. Data was collected through situational observations, dialogs and the use of a semi-structured questionnaire processed through the use of epicollect5 data collection software, for 1800 households from 10 rural local municipalities in the rural Eastern Cape from the former Transkei side. Quantitative Data was analyzed through the use of SPSS and the qualitative data was coded and thematically arranged cross-tabularised and matched to/against the quantitative data. The Eastern Cape is a province that is predominantly rural and most of its population depends on public healthcare provisioning. The map below shows the areas that were covered in the study we conducted on COVID-19 and vaccine hesitancy, which was a built-up study from the same rural municipalities that participated in the EC study on Covid and rural South Africa, both utilized in this paper. The red dots represent rural settlements in the study under the selected local municipalities mentioned (**Figure 1**).

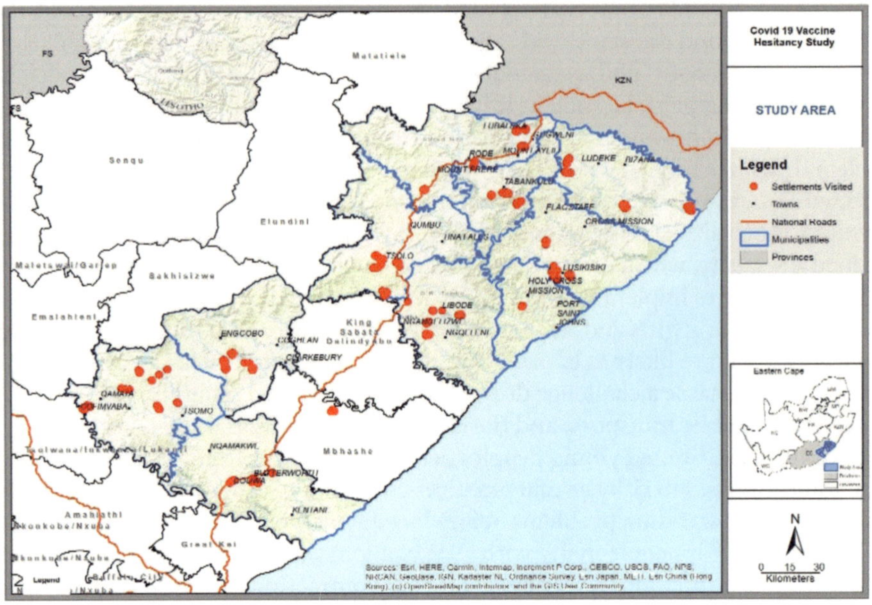

Figure 1.
Rural settlements where participants were drawn.

4. Data presentation

The data is presented to reflect the demographic characteristics as well as the below is the presentation of data drawn from the three phases of the COVID-19 research study project conducted in the same local municipalities concurrently. The selected data speaks to the objectives of this paper, which is to reflect on the road to universal healthcare in the face of COVID-19 and SA.

Figures 2–4 represent the population profile of the participants in the study, their gender, education and employment.

Figure 2 shows most of the participants from some settlements being females, even though male representation is relatively fair. The explanation for this is that although the research was open for both males and females to participate, since the participants were captured from their homes, predominantly it was noticed that women were the ones mostly available in the homes. The reason for that can be listed among others, as the prevalence of female-headed households, the flexibility that women have in participating in research studies as this research observed voluntary participation and females being the highest population group in the areas.

Figure 3 shows that the majority of the participants in the COVID and vaccination study we did in rural South Africa had none to minimum education, which does not guarantee any significant employment or income.

Figure 4, the text describes the employment status of the participants and highlights that the majority of people in rural settlements are not employed. As explained in the background, the rural population, which makes up the highest proportion of the South African population, relies on public resources for healthcare.

Data Presenting COVID-19 Experience in EC—closure of clinics and long queues of people looking to be severed for their health needs and only to be turned back home without any assistance (see **Figures 5–7**).

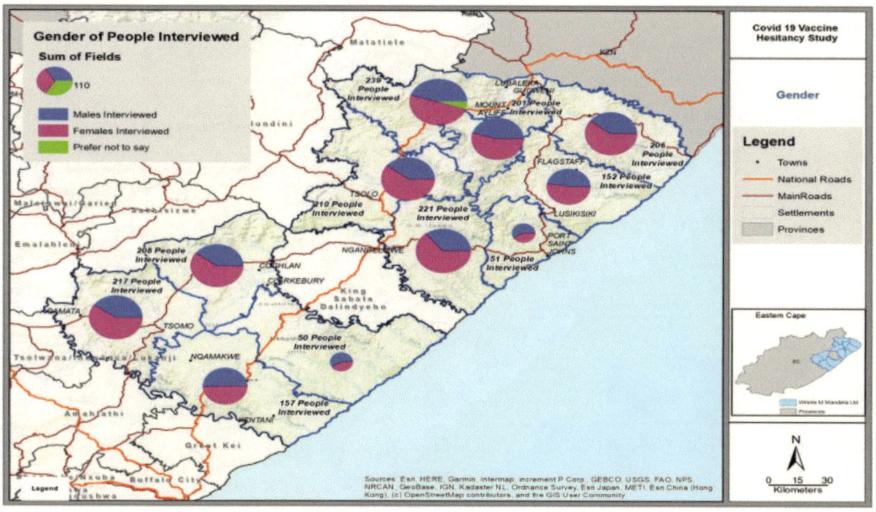

Figure 2.
Population profile.

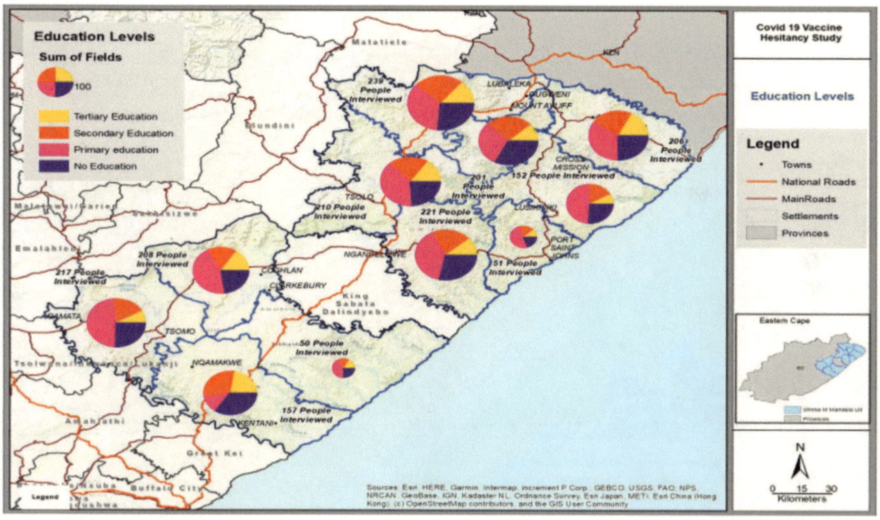

Figure 3.
Educational level of participants.

5. Discussion

South Africa has grappled with challenges in achieving universal healthcare, primarily due to the stark disparities between its private and public healthcare sectors [11]. The emergence of the COVID-19 pandemic exacerbated existing health disparities, disproportionately affecting the rural poor and underserved communities, further hindering their access to quality healthcare services [15]. The reality of healthcare provision in South Africa, especially in rural areas, falls short of the envisioned standards of universal healthcare [15]. The COVID-19 pandemic exacerbated existing healthcare inequalities, particularly in terms of affordability, accessibility,

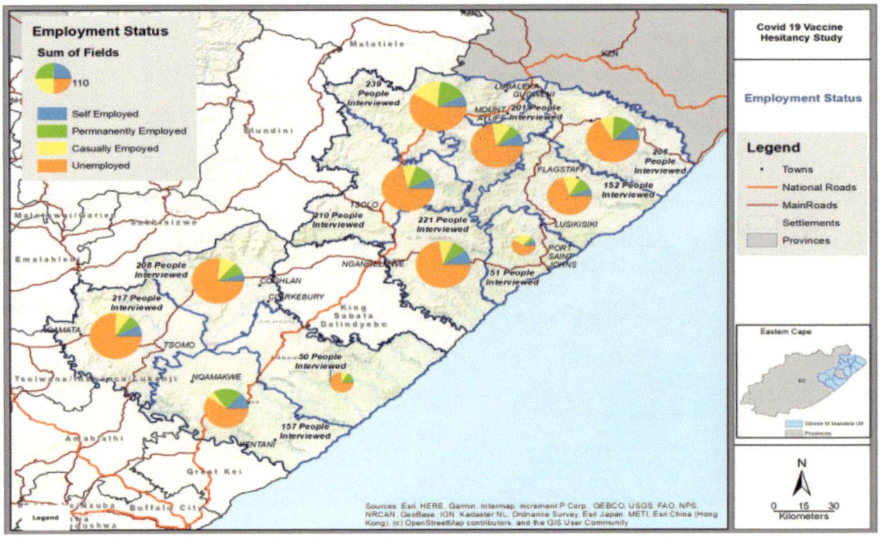

Figure 4.
Employment status of participants.

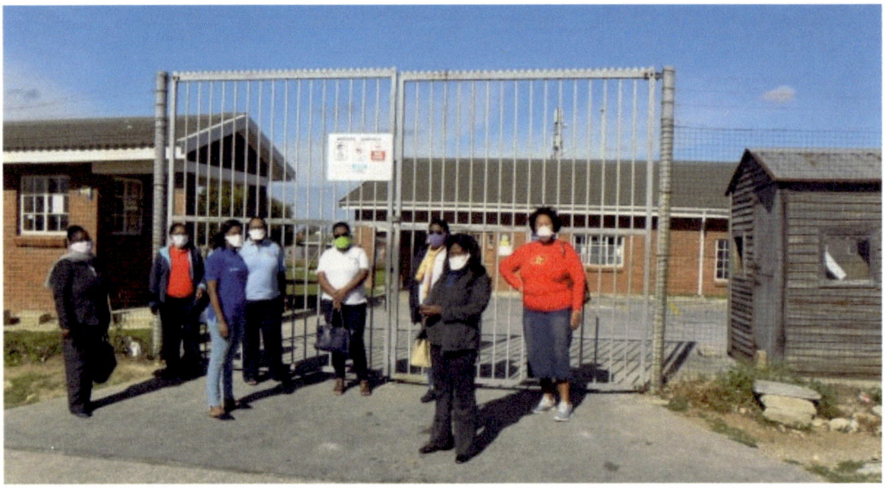

Figure 5.
Clinic closed after staff tested positive with COVID-19. Nursing staff at Motherwell NU2 clinic stand outside the main gate. The clinic was closed after staff members tested positive for COVID-19. Photo: Joseph Chirume, GroundUp. Accessed 17.07.23. http://www.hsrc.ac.za/en/review/hsrc-review-nov-2020/health-care-during-covid19.

and inadequate infrastructure [15]. During the pandemic, rural clinics and healthcare centres were shuttered, resulting in limited access and inadequate compliance with COVID-19 regulations [15]. Nurses lacked adequate training to handle COVID-19 cases, leading to referrals to larger hospitals [15]. The dual healthcare system in South Africa, comprising private and public sectors, poses challenges in achieving equitable healthcare access, especially for rural communities [4, 11]. Access to quality healthcare resources during the pandemic favored those with financial means for private

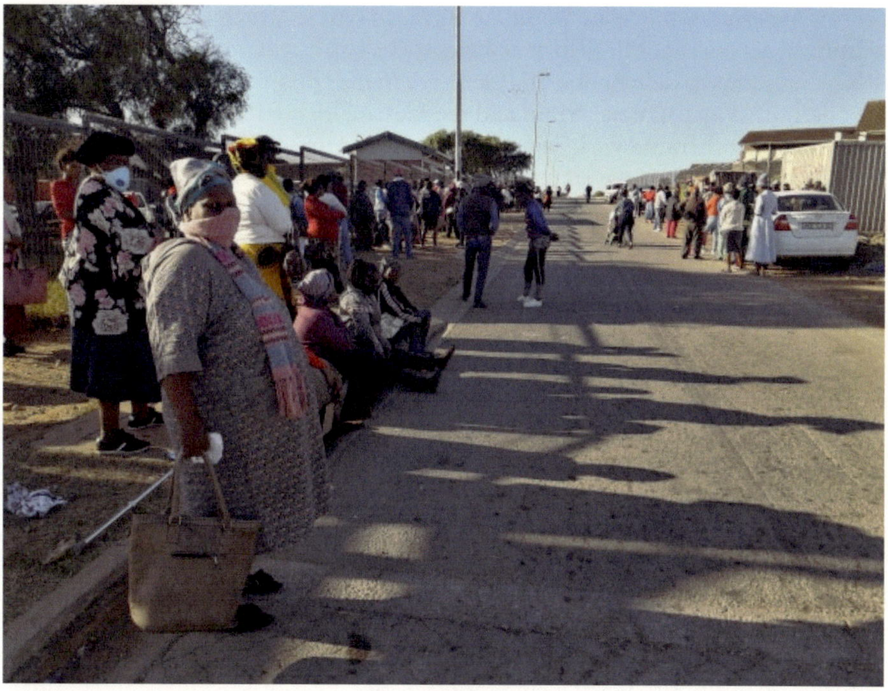

Figure 6.
Patients sent away due to clinic closure after 11 nurses died of COVID-19 infection. Dozens of patients were sent away in May 2020 after the eastern cape Department of Health shut down Zwide Clinic in Port Elizabeth following the death of a nurse and 11 other staff members testing positive for the coronavirus. Photo: Mkhuseli Sizani, GroundUp. Accessed 17.07.23. http://www.hsrc.ac.za/en/review/hsrc-review-nov-2020/health-care-during-covid19.

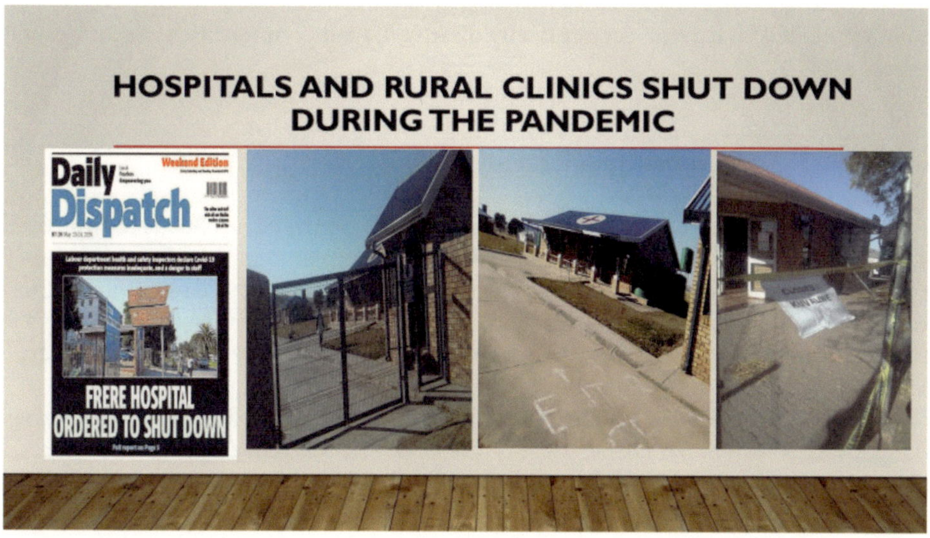
HOSPITALS AND RURAL CLINICS SHUT DOWN DURING THE PANDEMIC
Daily Dispatch
Weekend Edition
FRERE HOSPITAL ORDERED TO SHUT DOWN

Figure 7.
Picture showing most clinics and community healthcare centres in the rural areas closed as well as one major district hospital ordered to close.

healthcare services, while rural populations faced barriers such as affordability and geographical access [12, 22]. Efforts to bridge this gap have introduced primary healthcare systems to deliver essential services to marginalized communities but have been constrained by financial strain and inadequate infrastructure [3, 25]. Initiatives like the "ideal clinic framework" aimed to establish high-quality primary healthcare services but faced limited coverage and implementation challenges [12, 26].

Discourse on a national health insurance system has been ongoing to provide affordable healthcare access to all citizens, but actualization remains elusive, leaving economically disadvantaged communities vulnerable [7, 9].

South Africa has yet to achieve universal healthcare coverage, and the existing dual healthcare in the country system perpetuates healthcare disparities. The COVID-19 pandemic highlighted the unequal access to quality healthcare, especially for marginalized communities. Policy reforms and a comprehensive approach are necessary to address these challenges and move towards equitable healthcare access for all South Africans [27]. The COVID-19 pandemic exacerbated these existing disparities, particularly impacting the rural poor's access to healthcare services [15]. The closure of rural clinics and healthcare centres during the pandemic worsened the situation, leaving vulnerable communities without essential healthcare services [15]. Nurses lacked proper training to manage COVID-19 cases, resulting in referrals to urban hospitals and further limiting rural populations' access to adequate care [15]. Rural communities faced multifaceted challenges during the pandemic, including limited transportation options to reach healthcare facilities, non-operational clinics, and a lack of adherence to COVID-19 regulations due to inadequate infrastructure [22]. These challenges disproportionately affected the rural poor, hindering their ability to seek timely healthcare, including COVID-19 screening and essential medical services [28]. Despite efforts to bridge the gap between private and public healthcare sectors, initiatives such as the "ideal clinic framework" faced implementation challenges and limited coverage, especially in rural areas [12, 26]. Discussions around a national health insurance system aimed at providing affordable healthcare for all citizens remain unresolved, leaving economically disadvantaged communities without proper coverage [9].

6. Conclusion and recommendations

In order to advance towards universal healthcare, South Africa needs to conduct a thorough policy review to evaluate the feasibility of implementation. Reforms aimed at providing equitable healthcare are crucial to ensure that the fundamental right to health is upheld for the entire population. Universal health coverage (UHC) plays a critical role in global health security. It can improve the capacity for health security, including preventing and controlling emerging diseases. Inadequate UHC in one country may cause population movements across borders to seek care in neighboring countries. UHC is a major cornerstone of the UN Sustainable Development Goals. It is vital for strengthening health systems and enhancing countries' future health security. Although the relationship between UHC and global health security is complex, it is widely recognized that they are interdependent and mutually reinforcing. Strengthening health systems is the most promising mechanism for benefiting both UHC and global health security. This exposition emphasized in this conclusion has been expressed by several scholars [29, 30]. Therefore, achieving UHC is not only a matter of health equity but also a critical component of global health security.

Author details

Nelly Sharpley
The University of KwaZulu-Natal, Durban, South Africa

*Address all correspondence to: sharpleyn@ukzn.ac.za

References

[1] World Health Organization. Universal Health Coverage (UHC). 2021. Retrieved from Tracking Universal Health Coverage: 2021 Global monitoring report (who.int), 27 June 2022

[2] World Health Organization. Constitution of the World Health Organization. 1948. Retrieved from Universal health coverage (UHC) (who.int), 29 June 2023

[3] Mayosi BM, Lawn JE, van Niekerk A, Bradshaw D, Abdool Karim SS, Coovadia HM, et al. Health in South Africa: Changes and challenges since 2009. The Lancet. 2012;**380**(9858):2029-2043

[4] Goudge J, Gilson L, Russell S, Gumede T, Mills A. The household costs of health care in rural South Africa with free public primary care and hospital exemptions for the poor. Tropical Medicine & International Health. 2019;**24**(2):200-206

[5] Netshiswinzhe MD, Ramathuba DU, Lebese TR, Makhado L. A model to prevent substance use/abuse by student nurses at Limpopo College of Nursing, South Africa. Healthcare. 2023;**11**(16):2285

[6] National Institutes of Health. African Journal of Primary Health Care & Family Medicine. 2009

[7] McIntyre D, Thiede M, Padarath A. How to do (or not to do) ... conducting a stakeholder analysis. Health Systems Trust. 2019. Available from: http://www.hst.org.za

[8] Shisana O, Hall E, Maluleke KR, et al. The Impact of HIV/AIDS on the Health Sector, National Survey of Health Personnel, Ambulatory and Hospitalised Patients and Health Facilities 2002. Cape Town: HSRC, MEDUNSA & MRC; 2003. ISBN 10: 1-875017-85-2. ISBN 13: 978-18750-1785-0

[9] Nxumalo N, Goudge J, Manderson L. Community-based health insurance in South Africa: Exploring the implications of choice for policy and regulation. Health Policy and Planning. 2020;**35**(5):590-597. DOI: 10.1093/heapol/czaa021

[10] Bresick G, von Pressentin KB, Mash R. Evaluating the performance of south African primary care: A cross-sectional descriptive survey. South African Family Practice. 2019;**61**(3):109-116. DOI: 10.1080/20786190.2019.1596666

[11] World Health Organization. Health Systems in Transition: South Africa. South Africa: World Health Organization; 2018

[12] Rispel LC, Moorman J, Nkosi M, Dikweni L, Twalo T, Goldstein SJ. Analysis of the ideal clinic programme as a platform for the delivery of quality health services in South Africa: Case study of primary healthcare in KwaZulu-Natal. South African Health Review. 2019;**2019**(1):57-67

[13] Tessema GA, Kinfu Y, Dachew BA, Tesema AG, Assefa Y, Alene KA, et al. The COVID-19 pandemic and healthcare systems in Africa: A scoping review of preparedness, impact and response. BMJ Global Health. 2021;**6**(12):e007179

[14] Ndivhuwo Mukwevho. COVID-19 has widened South Africa's inequality, leaving black women worse off – Health News. 2021. [Accessed July 13, 2023]

[15] Bank L, Sharpley N. Covid and Custom in Rural South Africa: Culture, Healthcare and the State. Vol. 2. Durban, South Africa: UKZN Press; 2023. p. 275

[16] Gebremeskel TG, Kiros K, Gesesew HA, et al. Awareness, perceptions, and preventive practices of COVID-19 among health workers in Tigray, North Ethiopia. Journal of Public Health (Berlin). 2022;**30**:2253-2260. DOI: 10.1007/s10389-021-01595-x

[17] Masuku AS, Hlengwa RT, Mkhize LV, Sibiya MN. Vulnerability and agency in the time of COVID-19: The narratives of child and youth care workers in South Africa. International Journal of Environmental Research and Public Health. 2023;**20**(6):5010

[18] Banda Chitsamatanga B, Malinga W. 'A tale of two paradoxes in response to COVID-19': Public health system and socio-economic implications of the pandemic in South Africa and Zimbabwe. Cogent Social Sciences. 2021;**7**(1):1869368

[19] World Health Organization. Trends in Maternal Mortality 2000 to 2020: Estimates by WHO, UNICEF, UNFPA, World Bank Group and UNDESA/ Population Division: Executive Summary. 2023

[20] Marlais M, Wlodkowski T, Vivarelli M, Pape L, Tönshoff B, Schaefer F, et al. The severity of COVID-19 in children on immunosuppressive medication. The Lancet Child & Adolescent Health. 2020;**4**(7):e17-e18

[21] Matsilele T, Tshuma L, Msimanga M. Reconstruction and adaptation in times of a contagious crisis: A case of African newsrooms' response to the Covid-19 pandemic. Journal of Communication Inquiry. 2022;**46**(3):268-288

[22] Moshabela M, Schneider H, Silal SP, Cleary SM, Gale NK. Factors associated with patterns of plural healthcare utilization among patients taking antiretroviral therapy in rural and urban South Africa: A cross-sectional study. BMC Health Services Research. 2020;**20**(1):1-11

[23] Gittings L, Toska E, Medley S, Cluver L, Logie CH, Ralayo N, et al. 'Now my life is stuck!': Experiences of adolescents and young people during COVID-19 lockdown in South Africa. Global Public Health. 2021;**16**(6):947-963

[24] Govender K, Cowden RG, Nyamaruze P, Armstrong RM, Hatane L. Beyond the disease: Contextualized implications of the COVID-19 pandemic for children and young people living in Eastern and Southern Africa. Frontiers in Public Health. 2020;**8**:504. DOI: 10.3389/fpubh.2020.00504

[25] Harris B, Eyles J, Penn-Kekana L, Thomas L. Revisiting health insurance and access to healthcare in South Africa. Social Science & Medicine. 2019;**236**:112447

[26] National Department of Health. Ideal Clinic Manual: A guide for implementing the Ideal Clinic Initiative in South Africa. 2016

[27] Fusheini A, Eyles J. Achieving universal health coverage in South Africa through a district health system approach: Conflicting ideologies of health care provision. BMC Health Services Research. 2016;**16**:1-11. DOI: 10.1186/s12913-016-1797-4

[28] Siedner MJ, Gostin LO, Cranmer HH, Kraemer JD. Strengthening the detection of and early response to public health emergencies: Lessons from the COVID-19 pandemic. Journal of Infectious Diseases. 2020;**222**(2):170-172

[29] Assefa Y, Hill PS, Gilks CF, Damme WV, Pas RV, Woldeyohannes S, et al. Global health security and universal health coverage: Understanding convergences and divergences for a synergistic response. PLoS One. 2020;**15**(12):e0244555. DOI: 10.1371/journal.pone.0244555

[30] Wenham C, Katz R, Birungi C, Boden L, Eccleston-Turner M, Gostin L, et al. Global health security and universal health coverage: From a marriage of convenience to a strategic, effective partnership. BMJ Global Health. 2019;**4**(1):e001145. Available from: https://pubmed.ncbi.nlm.nih.gov/30713747/

Chapter 12

Perspective Chapter: Global Health Security through Psychoeducation and Microfinance with At-Need Groups

Sara Spowart

Abstract

This chapter discusses and explores the relevance of microfinance with psychoeducation for the improvement of global health security. It specifically discusses the importance of microfinance interventions for vulnerable populations, with an accompanying emphasis on mental health. Depression is one of the greatest issues worldwide and currently causes the largest number of days of disability. Depression hinders health and development and is currently considered one of the most important health issues by the World Health Organization. Microfinance is a mechanism that can be directed towards low-income, at-need populations and address mental illness through group support and small loans.

Keywords: microfinance, psychoeducation, Global Health, vulnerable populations, prevention

1. Introduction

An estimated 250 million individuals suffer from anxiety disorders and 300 million experience depression worldwide. In addition to this, more than 80% of those suffering from anxiety and depression disorders live in low and middle-income countries. Moreover, those that live in low and middle-income countries are exposed to higher levels of hunger, food insecurity, social prejudice and marginalization, violence, trauma, stress, and poorer quality of life and psychosocial status. Generally, individuals living in poverty or extreme poverty have any underlying mental health disorders exasperated and are exposed to many severe stressors [1]. According to the World Bank, extreme poverty occurs when a person is living on $1.90 a day or less and it is estimated that almost 770 million people live at this level. Economic growth is a critical factor in poverty reduction. Micro-credit to those living in extreme poverty, and low-income women and children in rural areas reduces poverty, increases empowerment and improves positive mental health outcomes [2].

Microfinance was popularized in 1976 by the Grameen Bank in Bangladesh. The original intention with microfinance was to provide small quantities of money to low-income, at-need populations. These individuals worked as farmers or lived in village-type environments. The purpose was for them to use loan money to purchase essential items like food, or to grow and expand their businesses to improve their economic situations [2]. Since this time, the evidence has shown that providing increased access to food and ways to increase money-growing activities through microfinance loans, helps people increase their individual agency, well-being and empowerment [2] (The Association des Femmes du Mali pour la Solidarite el le Developpement, personal communication, July 15, 2023; Espoir des Femmes et des Enfants du Mali (EFEM), personal communication, July 15, 2023).

Microfinance loans, especially when accompanied with group support, not only empower individuals but can reduce depression by helping borrowers have hope for a better life. Hopelessness and disempowerment are key components of depression and low-levels of well-being. Therefore, microfinance when accompanied with group support and targeted towards impoverished female borrowers, has a very strong multiplying positive impact on some of the most disadvantaged regions of the world. However, the amount of money needed for microloans varies depending on the environment and local economy. For example, a microloan of $500 in Mexico may not go as far as a $500 loan in Mali, Africa. The economic situations of every country, and within various regions and places in countries differ, and so the most suitable loans for individuals are largely circumstance-specific and also related to the purpose of each loan [2] (The Association des Femmes du Mali pour la Solidarite el le Developpement, personal communication, July 15, 2023; Espoir des Femmes et des Enfants du Mali (EFEM), personal communication, July 15, 2023).

Cash transfer programs can also reduce trauma and depression by creating a safety net that help protect individuals from worsening depression and stress due to poverty. Wollburg et al. [1] identified the connection between poverty and poor mental health through an investigation of cash transfers on low and middle-income countries for mental health. This was done through an assessment of 4000 studies on cash transfers for the impact of stress, anxiety and depression and looked at adolescents and adults in poverty. A total of 26,794 participants and 17 studies were evaluated in sub-Saharan Africa, Latin America and South Asia were assessed. Cash transfers were found to positively impact depression and anxiety disorders, and this is very significant for overall global health security [1].

2. Microfinance and global health security

The landscape of global health security has changed in the last decades. In the past there was a major emphasis in the World Health Organization and in development initiatives on infectious disease, vaccinations and medical treatments. However, in the last decade there has been a shift towards chronic disease issues such as heart disease, cancer, diabetes, addiction and contributing factors such as obesity, age, lifestyle and well-being. In the most recent years, there has been a shift from physical disease to the importance of mental health issues. Right before the COVID-19 pandemic the WHO identified depression, suicidal ideation and isolation as some of the most pressing overall health concerns worldwide. However, COVID-19 only helped to exasperate and worsen the levels of every type of mental illness and contributing factors such as addiction, obesity, domestic violence, isolation, stress and economic instability. Although it is not properly documented to this day, it is estimated that the worst levels and highest prevalence of mental illness, (specifically anxiety and depression disorders) exist in low and middle-income countries. These regions also have a paucity of mental health literacy, knowledge, access and availability of treatment [3, 4].

Microfinance initiatives play an important role in empowering impoverished populations and vulnerable or disadvantaged groups such as women in rural areas. Empowerment here refers to in-need populations increasing their authority, status, agency and living standards. Since the 1990s, microfinance has demonstrated an ability to empower at need women to increase their quality of life and overall well-being. In addition to this, microfinance has created the development of micro-entrepreneurship. Micro-entrepreneurship refers to the creation and maintenance of small businesses for the poor to improve their economic circumstances. Micro-entrepreneurship through microfinance can reduce unemployment and its associated social and health problems [5] (The Association des Femmes du Mali pour la Solidarite el le Developpement, personal communication, July 15, 2023; Espoir des Femmes et des Enfants du Mali (EFEM), personal communication, July 15, 2023).

Core components of microfinance include that borrowers are from low-income groups, the loans do not have collateral, they are short in duration and given in small quantities. Microfinance loans are used for income generation and there is a high repayment rate, particularly among female borrowers. The role of women and microfinance in India has been transformational in eradicating poverty over the last 30 years. This is particularly true of women that lived in rural India in relative isolation and who lacked basic services. Microfinance groups help provide support women in these rural areas and empower them to improve their economic status. These groups also help support women in their household decision-making, welfare, improvement of gender-based norms, family's health, individual health and access to non-formal education. However, in spite of the benefits, there is a major gap in supply and demand of microfinance loans and programs for those most in need [5] (The Association des Femmes du Mali pour la Solidarite el le Developpement, personal communication, July 15, 2023; Espoir des Femmes et des Enfants du Mali (EFEM), personal communication, July 15, 2023).

Micro loans of only $50–100 to those living on less than $2 a day, have been found to be an effective poverty reduction tool. Microfinance here refers to micro-credit, micro-savings, micro-insurance, and other approaches that empower entrepreneurs to create businesses and improve financial stability. Micro-credit and micro-savings generally have a positive impact on the health of the poor. This is in relation to the number of days of sickness, nutrition, physical well-being and greater investment in health care and health insurance. Microfinance and micro-savings also generally have positive impacts on food security and nutrition, as well as positive effects on housing, women's empowerment and mental health (The Association des Femmes du Mali pour la Solidarite el le Developpement, personal communication, July 15, 2023; Espoir des Femmes et des Enfants du Mali (EFEM), personal communication, July 15, 2023) [6].

3. Traumatized populations, microfinance and psychoeducation

Microfinance and psychoeducation are powerful, effective interventions that can be applied to uplift and improve the health of many disadvantaged, traumatized groups. Microfinance here referring to small, micro loans with low-income, at-need populations intended to help improve entrepreneurship and economic empowerment capabilities. Psychoeducation here referring to education on mental health concerns for the self and others. Psychoeducation can provide awareness, self-help and group support. The lowest-income populations have higher rates of depression and trauma and need additional support aside from economic empowerment to improve their health, overall circumstances and well-being [7–9]. Trauma here refers to exposure to a traumatic or triggering event. This may be exposure to an actual or threatened death, serious injury, abuse, violence, or sexual violence. Trauma refers to events that cause threats to one's survival or physical existence. It can refer to not only trauma from events that have occurred to individuals, but also to traumatic events such as violence or death to others of familial connection. Traumatic events are different from other stressful life events that create an emotional response. Stressful events do not contain a threat of injury, sexual violation or possible death [10].

Low-income populations are in general, more likely to experience trauma and Post-Traumatic Stress Syndrome (PTSD). They are also more likely to need micro-finance intervention help and support. Many of these populations are living with undiagnosed and untreated PTSD, and often experience discrimination, poverty, and handicaps such as chronic mental or physical illness. Individuals with severe mental illness almost universally have trauma exposure to one or multiple traumas. This trauma and trauma treatment is greatly underdiagnosed and untreated worldwide. Individuals exposed to trauma, often struggle with other issues such as poverty, depression, chronic medical conditions and substance use disorders. These populations are globally underserved and less likely to seek assistance after a traumatic event. Mindfulness, Cognitive Behavior Therapy, mental health first aid, psychoeducation with cognitive restructuring, and exposure therapy are useful interventions for trauma [11].

Trauma psychoeducation is an increasingly popular intervention. However, it is important that it is provided in a human-centered, relationship-focused, culturally-sensitive way that emphasizes compassion, resiliency and strength-building. Psychoeducation on trauma can help someone understand how the trauma they experienced may impact their functioning and how they can manage those negative impacts. This psychoeducation can be used before or after exposure to a traumatic event. Important goals of trauma-focused psychoeducation include an increased understanding of common trauma reactions; building knowledge and skills to help normalize those reactions; and learning healthy mechanisms to reduce those reactions. There is very little research done on the impact of psychoeducation after a traumatic event. Psychoeducation on trauma is much more effective when resilience and recovery is emphasized, not only painful trauma symptoms. This education should help participants not view themselves as broken, or damaged, but to understand their trauma experience is connected to their trauma reactions [10].

Psychoeducation regarding trauma and mental health is more effective when focused on resilience, adaptation, self-care and self-compassion. Another important aspect of psychoeducation is building and maintaining supportive and trusting relationships. Individuals that have experienced threats, sexual assault, neglect and other types of abuse, have great difficulty forming supportive relationships. Positive, supportive, interpersonal relationships can help lessen the effect of stressors, difficult reactions and trauma responses. They can also provide a sense of connection and safety. Another important component of trauma psychoeducation is that it is more impactful when provided soon after the traumatic experience occurs; is provided repeatedly due to the time it may take to process what is being learned; provided in a culturally-sensitive and human-centered way, and to dispel common misunderstandings regarding trauma. Psychoeducation can also integrate practical tools like mindfulness, relaxation training, yoga, emotional support animals, music therapy and other forms of support [10].

4. The value of combined microfinance and psychoeducation interventions

Microfinance and health education programs are more effective than only microfinance or health education alone. This is particularly true if the intervention is longer in duration. Integrated approaches that combine multiple interventions into one, are necessary for achieving Sustainable Development Goals and for income and health equity. Progress was made towards the Millennium Development Goals from 2000 to 2015; however, more than one billion people continue to experience extreme poverty worldwide. In addition to this, the statistics on poverty do not clearly show the variation and inequality within country populations. In general, there is a heavier poverty burden on women, rural populations, and indigenous groups. These groups also have reduced access to income-generating activities and health care services. Microfinance is special in that it is a set of generally-defined financial services to help poor families, and in particular women, improve their economic status, livelihoods and financial security. It can be delivered through microfinance institutions, self-help groups, cooperatives, village banks or savings groups and is adaptable to most circumstances of the poorest [12] (The Association des Femmes du Mali pour la Solidarite el le Developpement, personal communication, July 15, 2023; Espoir des Femmes et des Enfants du Mali (EFEM), personal communication, July 15, 2023).

Structures that provide supportive groups such as self-help groups, microfinance institutions and savings groups, provide an opportunity for financial inclusion. These educational support groups provide opportunities such as health education, psychoeducation, financial or literacy support, and other types of support. These groups also provide platforms for psychoeducation and life-skill support. With these groups, women can also be informally educated, learn positive practices and health behaviors. The group support provides an essential layer of empowerment and an opportunity to increase the level of success beyond just the microfinance loans alone [12] (The Association des Femmes du Mali pour la Solidarite el le Developpement, personal communication, July 15, 2023; Espoir des Femmes et des Enfants du Mali (EFEM), personal communication, July 15, 2023).

Depression is one of the greatest health issues worldwide, and a significant part of depression is not only mindset and belief systems, but also a sense of lack of hope and future possibilities; also, not having power or control over your life and feelings of helplessness. Microfinance groups that support women can help improve depression by alleviating hopelessness and increasing levels of empowerment and support. Micro-finance and self-help groups provide reliable, low-cost and sustainable ways to support impoverished mothers and children. The health benefits of the microfinance groups include neonatal and material mortality reduction, improved child feeding, reduced child malnutrition, reduced child illness, reduced sexually transmitted disease, reduced gender-based violence and improved familial mental health [12] (The Association des Femmes du Mali pour la Solidarite el le Developpement, personal communication, July 15, 2023; Espoir des Femmes et des Enfants du Mali (EFEM), personal communication, July 15, 2023).

Our social, physical and economic environments that individuals live directly impact their level of mental well-being and inform the creation of mental illness. When individuals live in or grow up in poverty they are at much higher risk for mental illness. The World Health Organization (WHO) has been increasing highlighting the importance and interconnection between social determinants of health and global health security. Social determinant interventions make a major positive impact on mental health, physical health and suicide outcomes. Certain groups such as impoverished children, adolescents, women and elderly are at higher risk of mental illness due to poverty [13].

5. Successful global health security approaches

5.1 Inclusion of mental health in microfinance groups

Mental health is currently seen as one of the most important global health and international development issues. It has recently been included in the United Nations Sustainable Development Goals (SDGs) through the identification of how greatly mental illness contributes to the overall disease burden. The Movement for Global Mental Health is a network that has grown from the identification of mental health as being one of the most important issues of our time by the United Nations and the World Health Organization. Mental health and economic development became more highlighted on the global health agenda through the WHO in 2010 with the 'Mental Health and Poverty Project.' This report highlights the association between mental health as a significant health factor and its connection to poverty. Implementing psychoeducation and poverty reduction in a joint venture is addressed as an effective global health security intervention. However, before this report, the first Global Burden of Disease (GBD) studies were provided by the World Bank and the World Health Organization in 1991 and provided the initial foundation to assert mental health and poverty reduction initiatives as a WHO critical priority and part of the Sustainable Development Goals (SDGs) [14].

5.2 Inclusion of health education in microfinance groups

A majority of microfinance initiatives function through cooperative group dynamics that expand health and social well-being through accompanying health education. The phenomenon of combined microfinance and health education initiatives, have been poorly investigated. However, effective interventions that combine public health needs and economic empowerment are essential for progress and development. Microfinance impacts at least 200 million households worldwide through more than 3000 microfinance initiatives. It is a wide-spread mechanism to support the poorest populations with not only micro-loans but also fundamental health and social service needs. This is done through health education, health care, basic education, insurance and other significant concerns. Micro-finance interventions are uniquely suited to addressing complicated social and health issues among the poorest populations because of their already existing wide-spread, global reach. The addition of services into microfinance initiatives also makes them more effective as mechanisms to sustainably lift impoverished families out of poverty and to greater levels of health [15].

Although research is limited on microfinance initiatives that incorporate psychoeducation programs, case studies exist that demonstrate the effectiveness of health education with microfinance. In Mongolia for example, an HIV and sexual risk reduction curriculum combined with a savings-led microfinance program, proved effective in improving participant outcomes. This program was provided for sex workers, and demonstrated consistent positive effects. An intervention in Egypt improved working conditions of children through microfinance loans that provided training on workplace safety for children. In South Africa, a microfinance program implemented a participatory learning and action curriculum called Sisters-For-Life (SFL). The aim was to reduce the level of intimate partner violence and rape. This intervention resulted in reductions in intimate partner violence and sexual violence. An intervention in West Bengal, India with adolescent girls combined a microfinance initiative program with a non-formal education called Learning Games for Girls (LGG). The training provided financial, health and sexual health education to help prevent sexual violence and HIV/AIDS. It also resulted in positive outcomes for participants [15].

Another effective example occurred in Nigeria where a microfinance program integrated education on breastfeeding and maternal health with added songs, drama, and weekly text and voice messages through mobile phones. This intervention found improved maternal and child health outcomes. In Ghana, malaria education was integrated into microfinance initiatives with greater overall results [15]. A qualitative investigation of an agriculture and finance intervention in Kenya found that participants experienced significant improvements in farming practices, food security and nutrition, and protection from unplanned economic and weather-related issues. Food-security knowledge, skills and funding helped to improve overall outcomes [16].

Organizational strategies that combine health education with microfinance initiatives are more successful in improving health behaviors and their associated outcomes. Providing health education during microfinance loan meetings is the most used approach and requires the least number of resources. It is a low-cost, high-impact, sustainable approach to delivering health education. Systems that provide health education or microfinance as only stand-alone interventions are insufficient to address these borrower's needs. However, when these two aspects are combined into one integrated approach, it consistently leads to positive health and social outcomes for poor, at-need communities [15] (The Association des Femmes du Mali pour la Solidarite el le Developpement, personal communication, July 15, 2023; Espoir des Femmes et des Enfants du Mali (EFEM), personal communication, July 15, 2023).

5.3 Inclusion of female borrowers in microfinance groups

Fadikpe et al. [17] examined 735 cases across 105 Microfinance Institutions among 26 countries in Sub-Saharan Africa from 2011 to 2017. This assessment was critical for understanding sustainability and longevity of microfinance programs. This evaluation found that the greater the number of borrowers, the better the financial return. In addition to this, an important component of repayment and sustainability was having a higher number of female borrowers enrolled in the microfinance programs than male borrowers. Female borrowers are essential for the sustainability of microfinance institutions as the female borrowers are much more likely than their male counterparts to repay these loans. The results of this continent-wide study propose that microfinance institutions intentionally increase the number of female borrowers enrolled in these initiatives. In addition to this, governments should increase support to microfinance institutions operating in at-need, impoverished regions. Thirdly, microfinance institutions should be specially trained to work with and support low-income, high need populations (The Association des Femmes du Mali pour la Solidarite el le Developpement, personal communication, July 15, 2023; Espoir des Femmes et des Enfants du Mali (EFEM), personal communication, July 15, 2023) [17].

6. Challenges in implementing sustainable, micro-finance programs for at-need groups

There are other specific challenges and vulnerabilities faced by different groups that receive microfinance loans in different environments throughout the world. These groups include refugees, survivors of violence, individuals living in poverty, minority groups, and particularly women in disempowered circumstances. A significant goal of these programs is to help support women in particular as they experience greater discrimination and poverty due to gender prejudices. The Mudra Yojana is a government-backed microcredit initiative that helps support female entrepreneurs begin a business or expand an existing one with lower interest loans. A study based on 417 female beneficiaries from West Bengal, India assessed the impact of these loans alone on the well-being of these women. This program targeted low-income women that were motivated to create a business or expand a current small business. The results of this quantitative study found that this program encouraged and supported female entrepreneurship, and increased their income, job skills and ability to obtain employment. In addition to this, the women in the study experienced increased financial, social, political and psychological empowerment. These women became active change-makers for themselves, their culture and family. Assisting women with these low-interest, no collateral loans had a multiplying impact that uplifted society [18].

Although there are major positives to targeting low-income, at-need female borrowers, there are also be challenges in this approach. Specifically, successful business endeavors by impoverished, uneducated women (especially those with children) can upset cultural and societal norms. This is due to the increased levels of female empowerment, power, decision-making control and buying power women can gain due to their business success. These positive changes for women can trigger domestic violence dynamics among male family members that feel threatened and disempowered by the female borrower's success. As a result, the female borrowers may experience increased levels of physical, sexual, verbal, emotional or financial abuse from these male family members or male community members. The profits from the female borrowers, or their financial gains to be used for loan repayment, can also be confiscated by male family members due to their perceived loss of power. Another aspect that is problematic in the sustainability and longevity of these microfinance initiatives is political instability, crime, violence, and larger economic problems that disrupt local systems. Some regions have focused on helping support female borrowers with savings groups that have their own bank account which is not accessible by non-group members. These savings groups are meant to help female borrowers manage both wider societal and also destructive, familial destructive dynamics (The Association des Femmes du Mali pour la Solidarite el le Developpement, personal communication, July 15, 2023; Espoir des Femmes et des Enfants du Mali (EFEM), personal communication, July 15, 2023).

7. Important elements of psychoeducation and microfinance for at-need populations and groups

There are helpful tools to implement in psychoeducation for individuals involved in microfinance intervention programs. Some of the psychoeducation that is relevant to integrate with microfinance includes understanding how stress and trauma impacts our mind's ability to function well. It also includes information on abuse, relationships and roles we may be engaging in that we are unaware of. The use of microfinance can interrupt these cycles and shift roles you may not know you are participating in, or to become aware of unhealthy, disempowering roles and dynamics you have been involved in. Additional relevant aspects to incorporate into psychoeducation for vulnerable populations include self-care and grounding exercises for support; education on understanding your window of tolerance for distress and increasing distress tolerance; understanding your triggers and trigger scale; education and understanding of role and re-enactments you may be involved in; and healthy versus unhealthy relationships [19].

Self-care for psychoeducation refers to conducting and participating in activities, mechanisms and strategies that help maintain, repair and develop individual health and well-being. Self-care helps individuals increase awareness of their needs and internal experience of stress and difficulty. Mindful awareness of internal states helps decrease distress, improve emotional regulation, stabilize and reduce trauma symptoms, and improve one's experience of safety, security, competence and well-being. Trauma often occurs because the perpetrator's desires came at the cost of another. Self-care helps with managing stressors, triggers, and emotional regulation so we can function at a higher level. Daily self-care is essential for improving well-being in vulnerable populations. Simple self-care activities such as practiced breathing, journaling, mindfulness practices, self-compassion reflection, exercise, time with friends, taking a walk, time in nature, mindful gentle yoga can all be supportive [19].

Other aspects to incorporate into psychoeducation for microfinance participants include education on what is termed the window of tolerance. The window of tolerance refers to the level of arousal or stimulation an individual can manage for daily stress and challenge. When one experiences trauma, the window of tolerance to stressors diminishes and it becomes much more difficult to manage stressors and everyday needs. Self-care practices can help improve the window of tolerance so that individuals with trauma can handle a greater number of stressors. Self-care is also supportive for managing chronic states of hyperarousal and hypo-arousal. Past trauma tends to easily activate the fight, flight or freeze response, therefore methods to manage these responses are important [19].

Psychoeducation on the existence of the window of tolerance, as well as ways to expand the window of tolerance is supportive as a tool in psychoeducation in conjunction with microfinance interventions. Another important aspect of psychoeducation is discussing the trigger scale. Trigger refers to internal or external phenomenon that remind the individual of their trauma and bring their trauma feelings forward. It is something that occurs in the present and brings up the fight/flight/freeze/or collapse survival response. The trigger scale assists individuals in slowing down, noticing and acknowledging their response to triggers. By mindfully noticing reactions, it creates a space to reduce activation and improve the sense of empowerment and choice regarding reactivity. Other psychoeducational points regarding the Trigger Scale are to ask clients if any symbols, images, ideas or words are associated with the trigger. Also, to ask individuals on a scale of "0" to "10" (with "0" being a state of calm), how triggered they are feeling in relation to certain issues [19].

In the case of microfinance initiatives, it is relevant to have psychoeducation on possible triggers while engaging in selling products or repaying loans. Additional psychoeducation interventions include mindfulness practices to help individuals see they are safe in the here and now and skills to help them notice the present and being calm in their bodies in the moment. Also, exercises to help someone identify that they are in the "there and then," meaning back when they experienced the trauma. *What thoughts, emotions, bodily sensations help to distinguish the present versus the trauma state? Are there any particular triggers that activate past traumas and bring the experience of distress into the present?* [19].

Additional psychoeducational tools are educating individuals on aspects of the brain so they can better understand what they are experiencing in relation to their trauma. Specifically, the understanding that the brain has been hardwired for survival and to keep us alive. This can be useful for understanding and having compassion for survival reactions to past trauma and decrease self-blame and shame. In addition to this, the brain inherently has a negativity bias. This is also tied to survival so that we are aware of potential threats that could hurt us. However, it also means that negative experiences, negative beliefs and negative thoughts may seem more important than positive. Thirdly, the brain is flexible and plastic and can change continuously and heal itself throughout one's lifetime. It is not only during childhood that the brain can be flexible and heal. Through the implementation of continual, conscious, mindful practices, the creation of new neural pathways can be created over time. Also, over time, integrating self-care, and soothing and calming mechanisms can aid in new, positive, neural pathway creation [19].

Other helpful psychoeducational interventions include understanding roles you and others may play such as perpetrator, rescuer, victim, neglectful bystander and what the patterns are in those. Creating your own business and engaging in micro-finance interventions changes your normal role and perception of traits. It can be supportive to understand the roles you were formally playing and the roles you would like to play, as well as others in your life. Engaging in these roles is often tiring and unfulfilling as well as repetitive over time, and can interfere with succeeding in new, empowering endeavors. Therefore, education, awareness and consciously creating an authentic life by behaving as who you want to be, is also important in this process of awareness; also, education on self-esteem and boundaries, what they mean, and how trauma and stress can negatively impact both is valuable to include [19].

There is a difference between internally driven self-esteem and externally driven self-esteem. Internally driven self-esteem comes from inside, and from mindful presence of our own self-worth. Externally driven self-esteem comes from outside and is fragile and changing. Vulnerable populations benefit from education on internally driven self-esteem and focusing on how to make this better. Healthy self-esteem is relevant and important for being a successful entrepreneur or business owner, poor self-esteem of participants can negatively impact microfinance efforts and initiatives. Healthy self-esteem means having kindness for yourself in spite of imperfections, believing you are enough and valuable regardless of outside events. Healthy boundaries mean not allowing harmful people or situations into your life that can hurt your self-esteem, but still allowing connection as much as possible [19].

8. Case study of microfinance and psychoeducation intervention among Malian women

According to the World Health Organization (WHO), the population of Mali is over 18 million and at least 15% of the population is living with disability. However, due to the lack of health and economic empowerment data in Mali it is likely this number is much higher. At this time, there are little, if any, government programs to assist individuals with disabilities [20]. Depression is currently the leading cause of disability in the world and the greatest health burden from a collective perspective. Although data is very limited on impoverished, recovering regions like Mali, it is very likely that depression is also a significant concern in Mali along with economic poverty. Therefore, interventions that address both economic empowerment and group and family-based psychoeducation for trauma and depression are worthwhile and important to explore [20–22].

There are very limited interventions for improving child mental health and mental health in francophone West Africa and areas such as Mali. Interventions that only address behavior and mental health alone are insufficient for families living in absolute poverty and low-income regions. A randomized cluster study of children ages 10–15 years from 12 villages in francophone Africa (N = 360), found that psychosocial intervention that included all family members along with economic empowerment strategies was an innovative, effective approach for improving well-being of families living in extreme poverty. Close to 90% of the world's children are in low and middle-income countries and the disease burden and disability from mental illness is growing in these regions. The 2030 U.N. Sustainable Development Goals included mental health and well-being as a priority concern. Global mental health prevention and poverty are of key global health concern, as well as finding effective interventions to address this. Training on livelihoods, 1–1 mentoring, family coaching that targeted all family members and seed grants were provided to help assist families with both psychoeducation and economic empowerment. These interventions found reductions in symptoms of depression, improved self-esteem and decreased symptoms of trauma. Interventions that conducted only economic empowerment or only psychoeducational initiatives alone, were not as effective in improving mental health and economic outcomes. The combination of the two together through family-based behavioral interventions is a potentially effective, innovative approach to prevent and address mental health concerns in low-income and poverty-stricken situations [20–22].

A case study of an early intervention in central Mali in the Bandiagara region also demonstrates early signs that the combination of psychoeducational group support with microfinance efforts for women living in absolute poverty, can be effective even after violence, trauma and worsening poverty has occurred (Association des Femmes du Mali pour la Solidarite el le Developpement, personal communication, June 16, 2023; Happiness Learned LLC, personal communication, June 16, 2023). On January 18th, 2012, the National Movement for the Liberation of Azawad (MNLA) attacked a small city in Northern Mali and many Malian soldiers at a Mali military camp died, the surviving soldiers were then executed. This began a civil war within Mali that went on for many years afterward and destroyed countless poverty and health intervention efforts that had been conducted previously [21]. However, a group of 43 extremely impoverished women were enrolled in the beginning of April 2023 into a program with combined microfinance and group psychoeducational support. These 43 women all survived by going to the garbage dump and landfill every day to find items within the trash to survive from or hopefully sell. They frequented Le Depot de Lafiabougou and Le Depot D'Ordures de Lafiabougou on a regular basis and survived in abject poverty (Association des Femmes du Mali pour la Solidarite el le Developpement, personal communication, June 16, 2023; Happiness Learned LLC, personal communication, June 16, 2023; Espoir des Femmes et des Enfants du Mali (EFEM), personal communication, July 15, 2023).

However, since the beginning of April, these women each received $100 in micro-loans, group support and psychoeducation on self-esteem, healthy relationships, abuse and strength-building exercises. As of mid-June 2023, all of these women no longer visit the landfill or garbage dump at all. All of these women are also highly engaged and active in the development of their new businesses. They have found psychoeducation to be extremely supportive and helpful in empowering and motivating them to continue the work they are doing. In only 2 months, all the participants express lower levels of depression and trauma symptoms and higher levels of hope, well-being and empowerment since before they received the microfinance and psychoeducational support (Association des Femmes du Mali pour la Solidarite el le Developpement, personal communication, June 16, 2023; Happiness Learned LLC, personal communication, June 16, 2023; Espoir des Femmes et des Enfants du Mali (EFEM), personal communication, July 15, 2023).

Since June 15th, of 2023, a second initiative in the Mopti/Bandiagara area of Mali has begun to assist an additional 75 women with micro-loans. All 75 women are highly motivated, and already have their own individual, small businesses. Through micro-loans of $50 each, group support, and psychoeducation, they are working to increase the viability of their businesses and expand their profit-making margins. This newest initiative is meant to empower and uplift not only themselves but their families, other women and their community. These two projects will continue to grow and be expanded on to include other regions and groups of women that could benefit in the area. The goal is to eventually include at-need women throughout all of Mali by mid-2024 (Association des Femmes du Mali pour la Solidarite el le Developpement, personal communication, June 16, 2023; Happiness Learned LLC, personal communication, June 16, 2023; Espoir des Femmes et des Enfants du Mali (EFEM), personal communication, July 15, 2023).

9. Conclusion

This chapter provides an overview of the relevance of microfinance initiatives for low-income, at-need populations. It also highlights the significant intersection of addressing both the mental health sector and economic empowerment sector synchronously for well-being improvement and development. Mental health or economic empowerment as stand-alone initiatives are not as impactful in helping these populations experience improved outcomes. Depression and trauma are significant worldwide problems, and those living in absolute poverty are at high risk of both. In addition, due to the mental health factors, economic empowerment alone is insufficient to adequately the needs of these populations. Interventions that incorporate multiple initiatives simultaneously are needed in the future to help uplift and improve the health and well-being of the world's most vulnerable.

Acknowledgements

I would like to acknowledge *The Association des Femmes du Mali pour la Solidarite el le Developpement* (AFMSD), Espoir des Femmes et des Enfants du Mali (EFEM) and Happiness Learned, LLC for their invaluable contributions to this chapter.

Conflict of interest

"The authors declare no conflict of interest."

Thanks

Thank you to both *Happiness Learned*, LLC, *Espoir des Femmes et des Enfants du Mali* (EFEM) and *The Association des Femmes du Mali pour la Solidarite et le Developpement* for your invaluable contributions to this chapter.

Author details

Sara Spowart
University of South Florida, St. Petersburg, Tampa, United States

*Address all correspondence to: sspowart@usf.edu; sspowart@mail.usf.edu

References

[1] Wollburg C, Steinert JI, Reeves A, Nye E. Do cash transfers alleviate common mental disorders in low-and middle-income countries? A systematic review and meta-analysis. PLoS One. 2023;**18**(2):e0281283

[2] Chikwira C, Vengesai E, Mandude P. The impact of microfinance institutions on poverty alleviation. Journal of Risk and Financial Management. 2022;**15**(9):393

[3] World Health Organization. Delivering Global Health Security through Sustainable Financing; 26-27 July 2017; Seoul, Republic of Korea (No. WHO/WHE/CPI/2018.38). World Health Organization; 2018

[4] Suicide Worldwide in 2019: Global Health Estimates. Geneva: World Health Organization; 2021. License: CC BY-NC-SA 3.0 IGO

[5] Biswas MP, Rao MRM. Role of NGO in empowering women through microfinance: A conceptual study. Journal of Small Business and Entrepreneurship Development. 2014;**2**(2):141-150

[6] Van Rooyen C, Stewart R, De Wet T. The impact of microfinance in sub-Saharan Africa: A systematic review of the evidence. World Development. 2012;**40**(11):2249-2262

[7] Alesane A. Microfinance, Livelihoods and Poverty Reduction in Ghana. Taylor & Francis; 2022

[8] Charlery A, White S-AR, Majeed I, Phillip T-M. Trauma education and stigma reduction in global settings: An evaluation of the impact of a one-day trauma psychoeducation workshop with community stakeholders in the Caribbean nation of Saint Lucia. International Journal of Environmental Research and Public Health. 2020;**17**(7):2255. DOI: 10.3390/ijerph17072255

[9] Bika, Subalova M, Locke C. Microfinance and small business development in a transitional economy: Insights from borrowers' relations with microfinance Organisations in Kazakhstan. The Journal of Development Studies. 2022;**58**(1):183-203. DOI: 10.1080/00220388.2021.1956472

[10] Whitworth. The role of psychoeducation in trauma recovery: Recommendations for content and delivery. Journal of Evidence-Based Social Work. 2016;**13**(5):442-451. DOI: 10.1080/23761407.2016.1166852

[11] Mueser, Rosenberg SD, Rosenberg HJ. Treatment of Posttraumatic Stress Disorder in Special Population: A Cognitive Restructuring Program. 1st ed. American Psychological Association; 2009

[12] Lorenzetti LM, Leatherman S, Flax VL. Evaluating the effect of integrated microfinance and health interventions: An updated review of the evidence. Health Policy and Planning. 2017;**32**(5):732-756

[13] Wahlbeck C-S, Haaramo P, Parkkonen J. Interventions to mitigate the effects of poverty and inequality on mental health. Social Psychiatry and Psychiatric Epidemiology. 2017;**52**:505-514

[14] Mills C. From 'invisible problem' to global priority: The inclusion of mental health in the sustainable development goals. Development and Change. 2018;**49**(3):843-866

[15] Ruducha J, Jadhav M. A review of organizational arrangements in microfinance and health programs. Journal of Global Health Reports. 2018;**1**

[16] Nicastro TM, Pincus L, Weke E, Hatcher AM, Burger RL, Lemus-Hufstedler E, et al. Perceived impacts of a pilot agricultural livelihood and microfinance intervention on agricultural practices, food security and nutrition for Kenyans living with HIV. PLoS One. 2022;**17**(12):e0278227

[17] Fadikpe AAA, Danquah R, Aidoo M, Chomen DA, Yankey R, Dongmei X. Linkages between social and financial performance: Evidence from sub-Saharan Africa microfinance institutions. PLoS One. 2022;**17**(3):e0261326

[18] Agarwala V, Maity S, Sahu TN. Female entrepreneurship, employability and empowerment: Impact of the mudra loan scheme. Journal of Developmental Entrepreneurship. 2022;**27**(01):2250005

[19] Hershler. In: Hershler, editor. Looking at Trauma: A Tool Kit for Clinicians. The Pennsylvania State University Press; 2021. DOI: 10.1515/9780271092287

[20] Séverin. Mali. African Disability Rights Yearbook2021. p. 7. Available from: https://doi.org/10.29053/2413-7138/2019/v7a8

[21] Bencherif, Campana A, Stockemer D. Lethal violence in civil war: Trends and micro-dynamics of violence in the northern Mali conflict (2012-2015). Studies in Conflict and Terrorism. 2023;**46**(5):659-681. DOI: 10.1080/1057610X.2020.1780028

[22] Ismayilova L, Karimli L, Sanson J, Gaveras E, Nanema R, Tô-Camier A, et al. Improving mental health among ultra-poor children: Two-year outcomes of a cluster-randomized trial in Burkina Faso. Social Science & Medicine. 2018;**208**:180-189

Section 5

Cigarette Uses and Global Health

Chapter 13

Regulatory and Policy-Making of E-Cigarettes Usage

Sharifa Ezat Wan Puteh, Norayuni Ismail and Nur Ismah Izzati Ismail

Abstract

Setting a suitable age limit of e-cigarette user should be established. This requirement considers the need for youth protection against e-cigarette misuse as such childproofing and age limits. Appropriate advertising without aiming for children to curb underage users. Advertisements could be done within sellers' or distributors' compound to keep vigilant control of appropriate or come of age users. Another reason for promoting e-cigarette use are to encourage smoking cessation and give information and incentives to smokers who are unable to stop to transition to less dangerous nicotine delivery methods. Addictive behaviors toward nicotine and complications from smoking e-cigarette should be warned and exposed to the public and users especially on newcomers as health warnings. Safety threshold of constituents should be complied and limit the strength of nicotine in the fluid could be done to reduce harm on users. An e-cigarette aerosol contains a variety of chemicals such as glycols, volatile organic compounds, and metals. The chemicals used have to be monitored for its safety threshold, where potential harm can be demoted. Harm causing effects of public vaping are considered for public vaping ban enforcement. While, many are opposed to the idea of vaping as medicinal treatment.

Keywords: age limit, advertising, health warning, safety threshold, public vaping, medicinal

1. Introduction

The tobacco pandemic is still very much alive and thriving, despite the fact that tobacco use is declining globally as shown statically. Initiatives to minimize the burden of diseases associated to tobacco use have been recognized and put into practise in order to end nicotine addiction. One of the well-recognized projects is the creation of nicotine replacement therapy (NRT), which temporarily replaces much of the nicotine from cigarettes to lessen incentive to use tobacco and nicotine withdrawal symptoms. This technique makes it easier to stop smoking cigarettes completely. Alternative nicotine delivery methods, such as gum, transdermal patches, nasal spray, inhalers, and sublingual tablets or lozenges, are increasingly included in programmes to aid people in quitting smoking [1]. Although long-term nicotine replacement therapy provides smokers an option, research has shown that it has no greater effect on harm reduction or stopping rates [2].

Soon after, it was reportedly intended that the invention of electronic cigarettes would make it possible to turn tobacco harm reduction from a theoretical idea into a practical alternative to smoking. A small percentage of smokers who support tobacco control view harm reduction as an even more crucial supplemental (rather than an alternative) method to conventional tobacco control [3]. According to the Centers for Disease Control and Prevention, "e-cigarettes" include electronic cigarettes, vapes, e-hookahs, vape pens, and other devices that electronically deliver nicotine [4]. While one study on vaping, which included seven countries—South Korea, Russia, Poland, Germany, the United Kingdom, and France—found that the number of vapers increased by up to 85% between 2013 and 2015, from 2.8 million to 5.1 million [5]. Adult vapers in Malaysia increased from 3.2 percent in 2016 to 4.9 percent in 2019 [6].

But there are a lot of concerns about how vaping will impact your health. It's important to realize that vape emissions include more than simply "harmless water vapour" [7]. Metals, glycols, and volatile organic compounds are among the substances in the aerosol that pure vapes emit. According to reports, the amount is normally considerably lower than that of a regular cigarette, but depending on the gadget used, it might still be greater. For instance, a device with an open system may be hotter, which might result in more e-liquid thermal breakdown [8]. Vapes can expose users to large amounts of ultrafine particles, which raise the risk of cardiovascular disease and non-cancerous lung illness similarly to traditional cigarette smoking [8]. Additionally, it could contribute to second-hand aerosol exposure, which is the passive inhalation of vape users' emissions [8], and indoor air pollution [7]. This rapid global uptake of electronic cigarette use, also known as vaping, has created a policy conundrum for public health, with opinions widely divided between those urging caution out of concern for safety and/or the potential for smoking to become more socially acceptable and those emphasizing the potential for harm reduction [8].

2. Childproofing and age limits

Different e-cigarette policies are developing over the world. E-cigarettes can now be regulated as either tobacco products, drugs, consumer goods, or none of the above. The Food and Drug Administration (FDA) in the U.S. has declared that it would extend its authority to regulate tobacco products to include e-cigarettes. To safeguard users and the general public, governments and the majority of public health professionals agree that e-cigarette regulation is necessary. However, how this should be accomplished is still a hotly debated topic. The majority of American smokers and vapers were found to support several of the proposed FDA regulations regarding safety and age, despite not being aware that the FDA does not regulate e-cigarettes. While Australian vapers' views on regulation indicated support for safeguarding those under the age of 18 but against the medical route of regulation, which limits access [9].

Setting a suitable age limit of e-cigarette user should be established. This requirement considers the need for youth protection against e-cigarette misuse. Everyone agreed that childproofing beverages was essential from a safety standpoint. E-liquid bottle opening should be out of the reach of little children. The majority of vapers also concurred that 16–18 age limits were reasonable. The risk of nicotine addiction and having to be the same age as smoking were the main arguments made [9]. Before the FDA's "deeming" rule asserting authority over e-cigarettes was published in May 2016, there was no federal regulation of e-cigarettes in the United States. The law, which came into force in August 2016, requires warning labels on e-cigarettes beginning in August 2018 and created a countrywide minimum age for purchasing of 18 starting immediately [10]. While the United Kingdom and Northern Ireland under the Medicines and Healthcare products Regulatory Agency (MHRA) whom an authority accountable for carrying out most of the requirements of Part 6 of the Tobacco and Related Products Regulations 2016 (TRPR), as amended requiring child-resistant and tamper-evident packaging for nicotine-containing products as well [11].

Between 2011 and 2015, comparisons of teen cigarette and e-cigarette usage in South Korea and the U.S. were observed. Adolescent e-cigarette usage stayed consistent at low levels in South Korea, where they were severely controlled between 2011 and 2015, while it surged in the United States, where they were subject to limited municipal controls but no federal ones. Both nations saw a decline in current cigarette usage, but South Korea had a decline in the combined prevalence of e-cigarette and cigarette use, while the U.S. saw a rise [10]. There are also worries that e-cigarettes might serve as a gateway into smoking among adolescents. A gateway impact has been recorded in certain regions in the U.S. although the data for this is still equivocal [12]. E-cigarettes were immediately controlled in South Korea once they were introduced to the market in 2007. By 2008, South Korea considered e-cigarettes a tobacco product and prohibited sales to minors [10].

3. Appropriate advertising and marketing

Stimson (Gerry Stimson is a sociologist who has been promoting a harm reduction approach to public health since 1987, first related to drug use and later to alcohol and tobacco control) hypothesizes that massive e-cigarette usage may be caused by the product being a consumer-driven factor rather than having its roots in the traditional areas of public health impact, such as medicine [13]. Whatever the cause, regulatory frameworks have lagged behind consumer behavior. For instance, more than 2 million people in the United Kingdom have used e-cigarettes [14]. Between 2010 and 2012, use more than doubled [15]. Although knowledge and use vary between nations, this commercial industry is also global and expanding quickly [16]. Since its inception, the electronically commercialized e-cigarette sector has also gained momentum and grown significantly [17]. Consequently, online purchases allow for the avoidance of national regulatory regimes.

In the United States, the implementation of various e-cigarette policy measures, ranging from restrictive to liberal, has started in certain jurisdictions. Retail access limits, which include legislation requiring a retail license to sell e-cigarettes over the counter, are one of the measures put in place by the United States. Other individual governments that are considering vaping regulations; for instance, Washington State has suggested prohibiting the sale of e-cigarettes online, banning flavors other than menthol/tobacco, and taxing all vaping goods by 95% [9]. Nonetheless, countrywide law enforcement of e-cigarette in the U.S. came into force in 2016. By 2018, there were no limitations on tastes or advertising, and no taxes were implemented under the law [10, 18].

The European Union's Tobacco Products Directive (EU-TPD), which was adopted in 2014 and put into effect in 2016, governs policy in the European Union (EU). This uses a "twin-track system," where goods are generally governed by tobacco laws, but stronger liquids (those containing more than 20 mg) or those with medicinal claims may be governed by laws governing pharmaceuticals. As a result, virtually all advertising is prohibited, and Member States are allowed to determine how to enforce measures like online and cross-border sales and public vaping. Meanwhile. the majority of American smokers and vapers shown reduced support for limits on consumer choice, such as banning advertising and flavoring of e-juice. Internationally, there is also suspicion over the motives of regulators (such as governments eager to boost tax revenues and business entities eager to increase profit) [9].

Appropriate advertising without aiming for children to curb underage users. Advertisements could be done within sellers' or distributors' compound to keep vigilant control of appropriate or come of age users. Another reason for promoting e-cigarette use are to encourage smoking cessation and give information and incentives to smokers who are unable to stop to transition to less dangerous nicotine delivery methods [19]. On the other hand, opinions on a ban on e-cigarette advertising varied significantly. Both for and against limiting e-cigarette ads, several analogies with gambling, alcohol, and tobacco advertisements were made. Few believed that it was appropriate to outlaw commercials on the grounds that the hazards were not yet understood, but the majority said that marketing to adults should be promoted for the sake of the public health [9].

The updated EU-TPD provided the foundation for e-cigarette regulation at the EU level. It contained requirements for the permitted nicotine levels in e-liquids as well as standards for packaging and labelling. In 2016, when the Tobacco Act (TA2016) was updated, Finland incorporated the EU-TPD rules into domestic law. A significant regulatory change for e-cigarettes was included in the renewal of the TA2016 in addition to the implementation of the new EU-TPD standards. In 2014, under the previous regulatory framework (TA2016), 2% of the general population of Finland currently used e-cigarettes. Other Nordic nations, such Denmark (3%) and Sweden (1%), have likewise seen around the same amount of e-cigarette use. It is important to note that although e-cigarettes were rigorously controlled, they were allowed to join the market with licensing. Vaping prohibitions and restrictions on point-of-sale displays were among the rules. Additionally, the selling of e-cigarettes and nicotine liquids over international borders as well as domestically, including online, was prohibited. For example, in Finland, by the end of 2019, a total of 8061 retail sale permits for tobacco products had been awarded, 362 for both tobacco products and nicotine liquids, and 59 for nicotine liquids solely, according to the national registry kept by the National Supervisory Authority for Welfare and Health (Valvira). Therefore, the majority of metropolitan towns across the country have at least one retail location with a nicotine liquids license. The EU-TPD left it up to the Member States to take into consideration in their domestic law any potential regulation of e-liquid flavors. Few nations have laws governing e-liquid flavors, but the TA2016 in Finland includes a restriction on flavors other than tobacco (including menthol) [20].

Although several nations, like Estonia, Hungary, and some U.S. counties, have enacted flavor bans or limitations, these policies are still uncommon internationally [20]. Most nations that ban or limit the sale of e-cigarettes also forbid or restrict sponsorship, marketing, or advertising. The U.K.'s current regulations state that e-cigarette advertisements must explicitly state that the product is not a tobacco product and may not cross-promote tobacco brands or tobacco goods. Additionally, advertisements cannot include actors who are or appear to be under 25 smoking e-cigarettes or otherwise having a key role in the product or service [21]. To add some more, sellers are compelled by MHRA to notify and publish all information about e-cigarettes and e-liquids before they may be sold [11]. In contrast, Southeast Asian nations are attractive targets for the e-cigarette sector due to their high smoking population and underdeveloped e-cigarette marketplaces. For instance, Southeast Asian markets are targets for Juul Labs (is an American electronic cigarette company which once reached its highest peak at $38 billion in market value), partially controlled by Altria Group (formerly Philip Morris). In a 2019 interview, the president of Juul's Asia-Pacific South division referred to Asia as a "high-priority region". Southeast Asian nations have a wide range of e-cigarette policy responses, from outright bans to minimal or no controls. Additionally, the countries' approaches to regulation vary. It also been observed that advertisements showcasing young female models and point-of-sale promos heavily targeted young people in the area with fashionable vape pen designs and a broad range of e-liquid flavors. Given the low frequency of female smoking in Southeast Asia, the targeting of youth, particularly female youth, is at odds with the idea that e-cigarettes are meant to aid current smokers in quitting [12].

In Asia, some nations have legalized e-cigarettes, including the Philippines, South Korea, while others—including the United Arab Emirates, Thailand, and Singapore—have not, including Japan, which only regulates the sale of e-cigarettes that do not contain nicotine. Therefore, public health policy makers in nations where e-cigarettes are still regulated, like Singapore, are faced with a conundrum: legalize e-cigarette use with the goal of enticing smokers of traditional cigarettes to switch to the ostensibly lower risk product despite the potential risk of creating a new generation of e-cigarette users, or keep e-cigarette prohibition in place and work toward an endgame for traditional cigarettes [22]. But now, for Singapore, Singapore has modified its laws to prohibit the sale, possession for sale, import, and distribution of e-cigarettes. Selling, keeping anything for sale, importing, or distributing e-vaporizers and associated parts is illegal. Anyone found guilty might be sentenced to a fine of up to S$10,000 and up to six months in prison. The penalties for using and having a vape is up to S$2000 [23].

In 2008, South Korea has taken the step to prohibit advertisements on television, radio, and billboards. Not to mention, that nation also prohibited sales by Internet and mail, and levied excise taxes. A regulation stating that e-cigarette parts, such as the battery, atomizer, and cartridge, are dangerous to adolescents under the Adolescent Protection Act 14 was published by the Korean Ministry of Gender Equality and Family in November 2011. As a result, the sale, rental, and distribution of the dangerous instruments to adolescents was outlawed. Violators may face fines or imprisonment. Additionally, this rule mandates that sellers of such commodities designate their goods as "hazardous to adolescents" [11].

4. Health warnings and complications

Addictive behaviors toward nicotine should be warned and exposed to the public and users especially on newcomers. Advertising was the subject of two questions: whether commercials ought to be outlawed, and if e-cigarette goods ought to have health warnings. Most people believed that if they linked to addiction, health warnings should be included. Many vapers underlined that warnings ought to be supported by evidence, provided that the evidence is based on science rather than guesswork [9].

Another study revealed nicotine dependence affects cigarette smokers' pulmonary functioning condition [24]. According to one study, adolescent smokers who vape propylene glycol/glycerol aerosol at high wattage with or without nicotine suffer prolonged transcutaneous oxygen tension declines and airway epithelial damage [25]. Additionally, it was shown that vape users had significantly worse lung function characteristics than the control group, which had peripheral obstructive airway impairment [26].

A recent Polish research raised the possibility that vapes are extremely addictive since younger people who use vapes have greater levels of nicotine dependency than those who use traditional cigarettes. Additionally, dual users have been found to have a greater reliance on vapes than regular cigarettes [27]. The use of vapes can expose those who have never used tobacco to nicotine, perhaps predisposing them to nicotine dependency. This would therefore result in the usage of further tobacco products in the future [28].

In addition, particulate matter from second-hand aerosol (SHA), which comes from vapes, includes fine and ultrafine particles, 1,2-propanediol, volatile organic chemicals, certain harmful metals, and nicotine, is a new form of air pollution. It has been demonstrated that SHA contains more metals than second-hand smoke (SHS), such as nickel and chromium. When compared to background air levels, PM 1.0 and PM 2.5 concentrations in SHA are between 14 and 40 times and 6 to 86 times higher, respectively [8].

E-liquids with flavorings and related aerosols include a number of hazardous ingredients and have the potential to be cytotoxic. The flavors of e-cigarettes make them more appealing to young people and are a major factor in the beginning of e-cigarette usage. Young people favor sweet flavors over other flavors, and teenagers are more likely than adults to use flavor-enhanced e-cigarettes. However, flavors make products more appealing to adults as well, and they greatly contribute to prolonged e-cigarette usage. E-cigarettes with a tobacco flavor or without one may be used more frequently by older people and dual users than by younger persons and ex-smokers. The most popular flavor among adult current e-cigarette users in the U.S., Canada, the U.K., and Australia has been fruit flavor, however variety-seeking, flavor transitions, and multiple flavor usage may occur [29].

An exemplary action by South Korea where right after marketization of e-cigarette, the requirement of health warning labels made mandatory. On nicotine cartridges, written health warnings started to appear in 2015 nation widely. The South Korean's Fair Trade Commission issued an order in October 2012 requiring two e-cigarette producers to retract their fraudulent health claims in accordance with the Act on Fair Labeling and Advertising, which forbade e-cigarette manufacturers from making such claims about their products [10].

5. Safety threshold of constituents

Limit the strength of nicotine in the fluid could be done to reduce harm on users. An e-cigarette aerosol contains a variety of chemicals such as glycols, volatile organic compounds, and metals. The chemicals used have to be monitored for its safety threshold, where potential harm can be demoted. The idea that vaping should be confined to certain flavors in order to avoid tempting minors was contested by several vapers from the U.S. and the E.U. as well. A restriction of nicotine to 20 mg for sale in normal stores in accordance with the EU Tobacco Products Directive (EU-TPD) was another topic of discussion. Some vapers expressed agreement or ambivalence. Many vapers were worried that this would not completely satiate the nicotine needs of heavy smokers. Regulation to increase safety, both for batteries and chargers as well as the components of liquids, was, nevertheless, welcomed [9]. Meanwhile, the MHRA has restrict the use of certain compounds, such as colorings, caffeine, and taurine for U.K. and Northern Ireland [11].

In the United States in 2019, 68 e-cigarette users died and over 2800 were hospitalized with e-cigarette or vaping product use associated lung injury (EVALI), a condition that resembles acute pneumonia. These events were due to vaping e-liquids in combination with a fatal constituent namely marijuana oil, which is frequently obtained informally, has the potential to be deadly. Stringent control in constituents used to produce e-liquids needs to be monitored to avoid these kind of incidence [12].

6. Ban on public vaping

Harm causing effects of public vaping should be measured to consider public vaping ban enforcement. For example, in Farrimond's study that in terms of public usage, the participants of the study advocated against a blanket prohibition due to a perceived lack of scientific proof of damage. The participants did, however, accept the autonomy principle, which states that people and organizations have the authority to limit vaping. In keeping with current smoking regulations, some of the participants advised prohibiting vaping in locations like schools, hospitals, and around food [9]. It is also found that e-cigarettes also expose users to high levels of ultrafine particles that pose disease risks similar to exposure with conventional cigarettes [29]. It can also be a source of indoor air pollution [7] and second-hand aerosol exposure to emissions from e-cigarette users [8]. There is minimal proof that secondhand exposure to e-cigarette vapor or aerosol is harmful to their health. There is evidence to support the claim that using e-cigarettes raises the level of fine particulate matter dispersed in the air. However, the particulate matter's makeup is different from that of cigarette smoke, its concentrations are far lower than those brought on by cigarette smoke, and sometimes it can be difficult to tell them apart from airborne particles in non-smoking and non-vaping surroundings [21].

Furthermore, a limited number of nations outlaw the use of e-cigarettes entirely, while others just forbid its use in particular types of enclosed public venues or on public transit. Policies might differ even between nations. Similar to how different a nation's states have different legislation from each other [21]. However, in Farimond's study, total banning of vaping has vapers claimed that it would simply benefit tobacco businesses as regular cigarettes are currently not outlawed. They also pointed out the danger that switching from smoking to e-cigarettes posed. A few people also mentioned "stealth vaping," which refers to using a vape device in places where it is illegal or where the rules are hazy. Vaping was believed to make this simpler because there is no scent, which improves discretion. Several European nations have considered banning public vaping, and some study has looked into opinions regarding these proposals (for example, France and Wales). Approximately half of the Spanish people disapproved of vaping in public, whereas slightly over half approved of it in the workplace. They also noted that the least support for public usage was seen in health care facilities, hospitals, and schools. Support for prohibitions on using e-cigarettes inside closed spaces has also been connected to perceptions of high danger [9].

Both conventional and social media have been used to discuss the public health conundrum around e-cigarette legislation and regulation. They may be discovered online, in blogs, vape forums, and on websites like Twitter as well as in newspapers.

A "right to vape" is the focus of a revived social advocacy movement. Even vapers who have no interest in politics are probably aware of the political agenda. There might be regional variations in this political drive. Given that e-cigarette usage is rather substantial due to their ubiquitous availability, the policy agenda may be especially obvious in the United Kingdom. Public controversy has also been sparked by the adoption of Article 20 of the EU-TPD in 2016 and suggested restrictions on vaping in public. The views of vapers toward law and policy may be viewed not just as a question of politics but also as an issue of identity. It has been noted that smoking has become moralized as a social sin as opposed to a personal lifestyle decision. Similar to what was discovered in Australia, the majority of vapers opposed the licensing of medical devices, and some even rejected the idea of a medicalized conception of vaping. This resemblance to other contemporary works leads one to believe that the transnational nature of the 21st-century vaper's policy position. Through social media (such as forums), vapers communicate with one another across international borders to exchange information on goods and technology as well as, for some, to serve as political activists for the "right to vape" [9].

The situation of the modern vaper with regard to regulation is both political and psychological. Insistence on their "right to vape" at the cost of others was not common among vapers. The concept of autonomy—which states that groups and people have the freedom to decide for themselves whether to permit vaping—was used to handle the conflict between the "right to vape" and "the rights of others." Additionally, several participants recommended refraining from vaping in public in places where smoking norms or restrictions already exist, such as around children, food, or hospitals. This might be seen as a strategy to lessen social stigma, similar to that associated with smoking, by positioning oneself as a "pro-social," "considerate," and socially conscious vaper. Participants also accomplished this by highlighting the value of "protecting youngsters," since "damage to innocents" is a significant factor in the stigma associated with smoking. The vapers in this group were actively concerned about preventing nicotine addiction in the next generation and supported a number of regulations (childproofing, age restrictions on sale, advertising restrictions, health warnings, etc.) to achieve this. It is important to note that this is not just a rhetorical device [9].

7. Medicinal regulation

Whether e-cigarettes should be controlled "as medications (like nicotine gum/patches) rather than consumer items" was the question put to the vapers in Farrimond study. Most participants opposed such restriction. Because they did not view their vaping as a medicinal treatment, several participants opposed medical regulation. Others expressed worry about the lack of variety and product availability if supplied solely via medical practitioners. Some people had more favorable opinions of the advantages of medical regulation [9].

8. Comparative table of legislative actions between countries mentioned

Based on the subjects mentioned above, a comparative table of legislative actions taken between the countries is shown the **Table 1**.

Subject	Country involved	Actions taken	References
Childproofing and age limit	United States	Countrywide minimum age for purchasing of 18	[10]
	United Kingdoms & Northern Ireland	Child-resistant and tamper-evident packaging for nicotine-containing products	[11]
	South Korea	• Prohibited sales to minors • Prohibit advertisements on television, radio, and billboards • Prohibited sales by Internet and mail, and levied excise taxes	[10]
Appropriate advertising and marketing	United States	• Retail access limits, which include legislation requiring a retail license to sell e-cigarettes over the counter	[9, 10, 18]
	European Union	• Requirements for the permitted nicotine levels in e-liquids • Were allowed to join the market with licensing • Vaping prohibitions and restrictions on point-of-sale displays • Prohibit selling of e-cigarettes and nicotine liquids over international borders as well as domestically • Including virtual advertising prohibition	[9, 20]
	United Kingdoms & Northern Ireland	• Advertisements must explicitly state that product is not a tobacco product, no cross-promote tobacco brands or tobacco goods • Advertisements cannot include actors who are or appear to be under 25 • Sellers to notify and publish all information about e-cigarettes and e-liquids before sold	[11, 25]
	South Korea	Stating that e-cigarette parts are dangerous to adolescents	[11]
Health warnings and complications	United States	Warning labels on e-cigarettes	[10]
	European Union	Standards for packaging and labelling	[11]
	South Korea	• Health warning labels made mandatory • Forbade fraudulent health claims	[10]
Safety threshold of constituents	European Union	Restriction of nicotine to 20 mg for sale in normal stores	[11]
	United Kingdoms & Northern Ireland	Restrict the use of certain compounds, such as colorings, caffeine, and taurine	[11]
Ban on public vaping	Still debated in e-cigarettes legalized countries		
Medicinal regulation	Still debated in e-cigarettes legalized countries		

Table 1.
Comparative table of legislative actions taken between the countries.

9. Conclusions

Similar to smoking, reduced e-cigarette usage may be predicted by more stringent e-cigarette legislation. It is conceivable that stringent laws against smoking and using e-cigarettes, such as taxes, marketing restrictions, use limits, prohibitions on remote sales and point-of-sale transactions, and flavor limitations, will make e-cigarette use less common. Increased regulations on flavoring tobacco products can reduce teen cigarette and e-cigarette usage. E-cigarettes may have distinct smoking cessation effects when used as consumer and therapeutic goods, underscoring the importance of the regulatory framework in outcomes associated with nicotine and tobacco use. It is recommended that countries with lax rules, big populations, and high smoking rates control e-cigarettes before their usage becomes established in their cultures, especially among the younger generation.

Conflict of interest

The authors declare no conflict of interest.

Author details

Sharifa Ezat Wan Puteh*, Norayuni Ismail and Nur Ismah Izzati Ismail
Faculty of Medicine, National University of Malaysia, Kuala Lumpur, Malaysia

*Address all correspondence to: shaezat@gmail.com

References

[1] Wadgave U, Nagesh L. Nicotine replacement therapy: An overview. International Journal of Health Sciences. 2016;**10**(3):425-435

[2] Ellerbeck EF, Nollen N, Hutcheson TD, Phadnis M, Fitzgerald SA, Vacek J, et al. Effect of long-term nicotine replacement therapy vs standard smoking cessation for smokers with chronic lung disease: A randomized clinical trial. JAMA Network Open. 2018;**1**(5):e181843. DOI: 10.1001/jamanetworkopen.2018.1843

[3] Britton J, McNeill A. Nicotine regulation and tobacco harm reduction in the UK. The Lancet. 2013;**381**:1879-1880

[4] Centers for Disease Control and Prevention (CDC). 2019. Outbreak of Severe Pulmonary Disease Associated with Using E-Cigarette Products: Investigation Notice. Available from: https://www.cdc.gov/tobacco/basic_information/e-cigarettes/severe-lung-disease.html [Accessed: September 7, 2019]

[5] Ernst & Young LLP. E-Cigarettes: An Emerging Category. London, UK: Ernst & Young LLP; 2016

[6] Institute for Public Health (IPH) Malaysia. Tobacco & E-Cigarette Survey among Malaysian Adolescents (TECMA). Kuala Lumpur: Institute for Public Health, National Institutes of Health, Ministry of Health Malaysia; 2016

[7] Grana R, Benowitz N, Glantz SA. E-cigarettes: A scientific review. Circulation. 2014;**129**(19):1972-1986

[8] World Health Organization (WHO) FCTC. Electronic Nicotine Delivery Systems and Electronic Non-Nicotine Delivery Systems (ENDS/ENNDS). Moscow, Russian Federation. 13-18 October 2014

[9] Farrimond H. E-cigarette regulation and policy: UK vapers' perspectives. Addiction. 2016;**111**(6):1077-1083. DOI: 10.1111/add.13322

[10] Lee S, Kimm H, Yun JE, Jee SH. Public health challenges of electronic cigarettes in South Korea. Journal of Preventive Medicine and Public Health. 2011;**44**(6):235-241

[11] Medicines and Healthcare products Regulatory Agency (MHRA). Guidance – E-cigarettes: regulations for consumer products [internet]. 2016. Available from: https://www.gov.uk/guidance/e-cigarettes-regulations-for-consumer-products#:~:text=The%20requirements%3A,no%20more%20than%2020mg%2Fml [Accessed: August 18, 2022]

[12] Van der Eijk Y, Ping GTP, Ong SE, et al. E-cigarette markets and policy responses in Southeast Asia: A scoping review. International Journal of Health Policy and Management. 2021;**11**(9):1616-1624. DOI: 10.34172/ijhpm.2021.25

[13] Stimson G, Costall P. UK Public Health doctors and e-cigarettes — why this matters [internet]. 2014. Available from: http://nicotinepolicy.net/gerry-stimson/673-uk-public-health-doctors-and-e-cigarettes-why-this-matters [Accessed: May 11, 2015]

[14] Action for Smoking on Health (ASH). Use of Electronic Cigarettes in Great Britain: ASH Factsheet. London, UK: ASH; 2015

[15] Dockrell M, Morison R, Bauld L, McNeill A. E-cigarettes: Prevalence and attitudes in Great Britain. Nicotine & Tobacco Research. 2013;**15**:1737-1744

[16] Gravely S, Fong GT, Cummings KM, Yan M, Quah ACK, Borland R, et al. Awareness, trial, and current use of electronic cigarettes in 10 countries: Findings from the ITC project. International Journal of Environmental Research and Public Health. 2014;**11**:691-704

[17] Yamin CK, Bitton A, Bates D. E-cigarettes: A rapidly growing internet phenomenon. Annals of Internal Medicine. 2010;**153**:607-609

[18] US Food and Drug Administration (FDA). Deeming tobacco products to be subject to the federal food, drug, and cosmetic act, as amended by the family smoking prevention and tobacco control act; restrictions on the sale and distribution of tobacco products and required warning statements for tobacco products. USA: US Food and Drug Administration. Federal Register. 2016;**81**(90):28973-29106. PMID: 27192730

[19] SCOHRE. Evaluation of the Legislative Framework for Tobacco Control: Call for Evidence. European Union (EU): International Association of Smoking Control and Harm Reduction; 2022

[20] Ruokolainen O, Ollila H, Karjalainen K. Correlates of e-cigarette use before and after comprehensive regulatory changes and e-liquid flavour ban among general population. Drug and Alcohol Review. 2022;**41**:1174-1183

[21] Brose LS, Partos TR, Hitchman SC, et al. Tobacco Control. 2017;**26**:e7-e15

[22] Doan TTT, Tan KW, Dickens BSL, et al. Tobacco Control. 2020;**29**:522-530

[23] Abu Baker J. Significant increase in vape cases in Singapore; HSA steps up enforcement [internet]. 2022. Available from: https://www.channelnewsasia.com/singapore/significant-increase-vape-cases-recent-years-hsa-steps-enforcement-2718246#:~:text=In%20Singapore%2C%20it%20is%20an,of%20up%20to%20S%242%2C000 [Accessed: August 25, 2022]

[24] Mohesh G, Sembulingam PA. The impact of cigarette smoking on lung function in smokers with differences in their nicotine dependency. International Journal of Medical Research and Health Sciences. 2016;**5**:36-41

[25] Chaumont M, Borne P, Bernard A, Muylem A, Deprez G, Ullmo J, et al. Fourth generation E-cigarette vaping induces transient lung inflammation and gas exchange disturbances: Results from two randomized clinical trials. American Journal of Physiology-Lung Cellular and Molecular Physiology. 2019;**316**(5):L705-L719

[26] Meo SA, Ansary MA, Barayan FR, Almusallam AS, Almehaid AM, Alarifi NS, et al. Electronic cigarettes: Impact on lung function and fractional exhaled nitric oxide among healthy adults. American Journal of Men's Health. 2019;**13**(1)

[27] Jankowski M, Krzystanek Z, Majek L, Lawson & Brozek G. E-cigarettes are more addictive than traditional cigarettes—A study in highly educated young people. International Journal of Environmental Research and Public Health. 2019;**16**:2279

[28] Jaber RM, Mirbolouk M, DeFilippis AP, Maziak W, Keith R, Payne T, et al. Electronic cigarette use prevalence, associated factors, and pattern by cigarette smoking status in the United States from Nhanes (National Health and nutrition

examination survey), 2013; 2014. Journal of the American Heart Association. 2018;**7**(14):e008178

[29] Glantz SA, Bareham DW. E-cigarettes: Use, effects on smoking, risks, and policy implications. Annual Review of Public Health. 2018;**39**:215-235

Chapter 14

Global Regulatory Approaches towards E-Cigarettes, Key Arguments, and Approaches Pursued

Marissa Smith and Shona Hilton

Abstract

A range of regulatory approaches are being applied to e-cigarettes globally. This chapter examines the reasons for this and what this means for broader tobacco control efforts. The chapter starts with a discussion of tobacco control and how evidence has influenced the development of international tobacco control policies. The chapter then explores the development and emergence of e-cigarettes. It identifies and discusses the arguments and evidence used in the e-cigarette regulatory debates. The chapter concludes by suggesting that research in this domain could improve our understanding of what factors influence the regulatory environment, thus why different regulatory approaches as pursued.

Keywords: electronic cigarettes, e-cigarettes, regulation, harm reduction, precautionary

1. Introduction

A key challenge for regulation of electronic cigarettes (e-cigarettes) has been keeping pace with the speed at which the e-cigarette market has emerged. But before examining regulation, it is worth considering the broader public health context in which e-cigarettes emerged and tobacco control efforts to reduce the morbidity and mortality associated with tobacco use. The health effects associated with smoking emerged in the 1950s and 1960s [1, 2]. By the 1990s, passive or environmental smoke was also found to have carcinogenic properties [3]. Since then, the tobacco control community (including public health experts, clinicians, and decision-makers) has worked together to reduce tobacco use and has been successful in supporting the implementation of various policies and frameworks such as the World Health Organisation (WHO) Framework Convention on Tobacco Control (FCTC). To address the global tobacco epidemic, the WHO developed the world's first public health treaty, the FCTC [4]. It was adopted by the World Health Assembly in 2003 and legally entered into force in 2005. The international treaty provides a comprehensive strategy for member Parties to address and combat the tobacco epidemic. It details a range of evidence-based measures to reduce tobacco demand (Articles 6–14) and supply (Articles 15–17) [4]. Between 2007 and 2014, it is estimated that nearly 22 million future premature smoking-attributable deaths were prevented as a result of the strong implementation of the FCTC [5]. Similarly, Dubray et al. [6] found that overall, countries with higher levels of implementation of the FCTC experienced greater decreases in current tobacco smoking between 2006 and 2009.

To assist parties to meet their commitment to the treaty and implement appropriate policies, in 2008, the WHO developed the MPOWER framework for tobacco control. This framework corresponds to WHO FCTC articles: Article 20 (Monitoring tobacco use and prevention policies); Article 8 (Protect people from tobacco smoke); Article 14 (Offer help to quit tobacco use); Articles 11 and 12 (Warn about the dangers of tobacco); Article 13 (Enforce bans on tobacco advertising, promotion, and sponsorship); and Article 6 (Raise taxes on tobacco) [4, 7].

Ngo et al. [8] reported a reduction in smoking prevalence and cigarette consumption during 2007–2014 as a result of the implementation of the MPOWER framework. The FCTC has served as a powerful tool to initiate, support, and advance national and global tobacco control policies. Evidence suggests that strong implementation of the FCTC and MPOWER framework can lead to significant reductions in tobacco use [6, 8, 9].

Unlike tobacco products, where most countries have coalesced around a series of regulatory approaches meant to shrink the market for the products over time, the development of alternative nicotine products, for example, e-cigarettes, has polarised the tobacco control debate. Their rapid proliferation, the limited evidence base on the long-term health effects, and their patterns of use among different population groups have led to controversial political and public health debates, with public health policymakers and researchers finding themselves with divergent views. As a result, a variety of regulatory approaches have been pursued. Before discussing the regulatory approaches pursued, it is pertinent to discuss the emergence of e-cigarettes.

2. The rapid emergence of e-cigarettes as a regulatory challenge

Across the world, policy debates about tobacco control have been markedly altered by the rapid proliferation of e-cigarettes which have been readily available to global markets since 2004. This has meant that regulation has often lagged behind and been unable to keep pace with their increasing popularity, use, and availability. In addition to the rapid emergence of e-cigarettes, debates about them have led to a breakdown of old public health alliances, resulting in the polarisation of tobacco control arguments and debates about regulation.

Developing regulation has also been challenged by the speed at which a variety of models or 'generations' became available. First-generation e-cigarettes (sometimes referred to as 'cigalikes') were designed to mimic the look and feel of combustible cigarettes [10]. They are not rechargeable or refillable. Second-generation e-cigarettes are larger and are generally refillable using e-liquids [11]. E-liquids are nicotine-containing liquid solutions that are consumed in e-cigarettes. However, some solutions may contain no nicotine. Third-generation e-cigarettes (tanks or mods) are much larger than the previous generations and are refillable and rechargeable [10, 12]. They are modifiable devices ('mods'), meaning the user can customise the substances in the device [13]. The fourth generation of e-cigarettes is called 'Pod Mod'. They contain a prefilled or refillable 'pod' or pod cartridge with a modifiable 'mod' system ('Pod-Mod') [12]. Pod Mods are available in many shapes, sizes, and colours, and the most common brands worldwide include JUUL and Suroin. **Figure 1** illustrates the four generations of e-cigarette products available on the market.

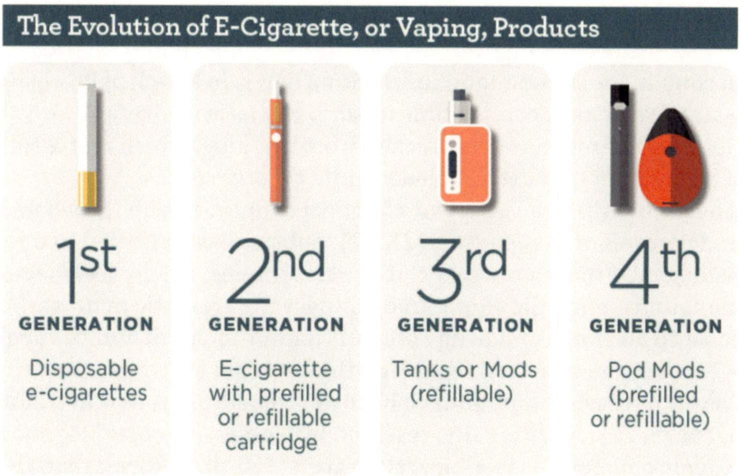

Figure 1.
Illustration of the four generations of e-cigarette or vaping products. Texas department of state health services. 2020. What is Vaping? [Online]. Texas Department of State Health Services, Tobacco Prevention and Control Bureau. Available: https://www.dshs.state.tx.us/Vaping/WhatisVaping/ [Accessed 27 January 2021]., reproduced with permission from Texas Department of State Health Service.

This rapid emergence of e-cigarettes and the numerous generations and flavourings available has led to various concerns being raised including the risks, benefits and safety of these products. Policymakers find it hard to keep up with the rapid evolution of e-cigarettes, meaning regulations often have to be amended to include the next generation of e-cigarette. The next section will review some of the current arguments and evidence in e-cigarette debates, including the toxicology of e-cigarettes and the arguments about the use of e-cigarettes as a harm reduction tool, which have been used as evidence for pursuing a particular regulatory approach.

3. Arguments and evidence in the e-cigarette regulatory debate

The development and population exposure to e-cigarettes have created a 'moral quandary' [14]. The tobacco control community remains divided on the evidence base and the appropriate approach for regulation. This section will examine some of the arguments and evidence used by different sides of the e-cigarette policy debate.

3.1 Should regulation take account of evidence on the health risks associated with e-cigarette use?

Regulation could be warranted if there are health risks associated with e-cigarettes. Research on the health effects of e-cigarettes is increasing. The toxicology of e-cigarettes is an area that has been extensively studied by various scientific bodies. E-cigarette operation does not involve combustion, therefore no smoke or other harmful combustion products, such as tar and carbon monoxide, are formed [15, 16]. However, the content of e-cigarettes is a key concern for those considering whether further regulation is warranted. The variations in product design and e-liquid compositions among the variety of brands available affect the toxicants and chemicals released in the aerosol and delivered to the user [17]. E-liquids are available in a variety of nicotine concentrations, with levels ranging from 0 mg/mL (i.e., no nicotine) to over 59 mg/mL [18, 19], and a single e-liquid cartridge for some devices can contain the same amount of nicotine that is in a pack of 20 cigarettes [20]. For general reference, combustible tobacco cigarette smokers absorb about 1 mg (range = 0.3–2 mg) of nicotine systemically from smoking, which represents about 80–90% of the amount of nicotine inhaled [13].

Research has identified a variety of chemical components in the cartridges, e-liquids and aerosols of e-cigarettes [21, 22]. Substances identified in e-liquids and aerosols include nicotine, tobacco-specific nitrosamines, aldehydes, metals, volatile organic compounds, phenolic compounds, polycyclic aromatic hydrocarbons, flavours, tobacco alkaloids and drugs (such as amino-tadalafil and rimonabant) [17, 18, 23–28]. Despite concerns regarding the contents of e-cigarettes, research has found the levels of these compounds to be lower than those found in traditional cigarettes [18, 24, 25, 28]. Additionally, research by Goniewicz et al. [24] showed that the carcinogenic compounds in e-cigarettes are 9–450 times lower than the levels found in traditional cigarettes and are comparable to the levels found in currently licenced nicotine-containing products. This could suggest that regulation does not need to mirror the regulation of tobacco cigarettes. However, there have also been concerns about the effects of flavoured substances administered by inhalation. For instance, there are some chemicals that, although approved for ingestion, have adverse health effects when inhaled including diacetyl, acetylpropionyl, acetoin, cinnamaldehydes and benzaldehyde [13]. There is also the issue of passive exposure although current research largely shows that second-hand vapour from e-cigarettes exposes bystanders to nicotine and other chemicals, is much less than from cigarette smoke [24, 29, 30].

Other health risks also muted in regulatory debates are about the risk of nicotine intoxication and fatal poisoning, particularly in young children if a high nicotine-content solution is ingested [31, 32]. There have been incidents of children ingesting e-liquids used by parents/families to fill their e-cigarettes, leading to a large number of calls to poison centres and several cases of fatal nicotine ingestion [33]. Data from published case reports state that the ingestion of 4 mL of a 12 mg/mL nicotine-containing solution would be lethal for an adult [34]. It is argued that the risk of accidental poisoning in children due to e-cigarettes is not different from household devices and chemicals [35].

Although existing research does not provide a definitive conclusion on the safety of e-cigarettes, research suggests that they are less harmful than tobacco products and are comparable in toxicity to approved nicotine replacement therapies (NRT) [15, 30]. Concerning the long-term health effects, the United Kingdom's (UK) National Centre for Smoking Cessation and Training stated that although they do not know the long-term risks, the "magnitude of any risks that may emerge from long-term e-cigarette use is likely to be small" [30, p.34]. However, some researchers and public health bodies and organisations argue that much is unknown about the long-term health effects of e-cigarette use, and we need focused research to study this [36–38].

3.2 Should regulation take account of evidence on whether e-cigarettes are associated with lung injury?

In 2019, the United States of America (USA) reported a rise in people, particularly those under 30, being admitted to hospital suffering from pneumonia-like lung injuries; none were traceable to a microbial source, but all reported recently using e-cigarettes [39, 40]. The Centers for Disease Control and Prevention (CDC) referred to the outbreak of severe lung illness as e-cigarette or vaping product use-associated lung injury (EVALI). All individuals with EVALI reported using e-cigarette products, most of whom reported using their e-cigarette devices to ingest tetrahydrocannabinol (THC), the primary psychoactive compound in cannabis [41, 42]. Vitamin E acetate is strongly associated with EVALI, and it has been added to THC cartridges by cost-cutting manufacturers who would claim that their products contained more THC than they did, as Vitamin E acetate increased the viscosity of the THC [40]. It is important to note that not all EVALI cases have been associated with THC-containing products and that in certain individuals, nicotine-containing or flavoured e-cigarettes may also cause acute lung inflammation and injury [40, 43, 44]. King et al. [40] argue that the use of e-cigarette products by youths is unsafe, regardless of whether they contain nicotine or THC, and the risks posed by these products are further heightened by the EVALI outbreak.

Other countries such as the UK, Australia, Canada and New Zealand were on alert for lung injuries caused by e-cigarette use after the outbreak in the USA. As of January 2020, in the UK there have been two potential cases of EVALI [45], occurring during a similar time period to the USA outbreak. UK public health experts argue that the EVALI outbreak could damage the reputation of e-cigarettes. In Australia, where there are no confirmed reports of EVALI, public health experts argued that the EVALI outbreak in the USA further entrenched the negative perception of e-cigarettes and therefore supported their regulatory approach [46]. In Canada, 20 EVALI cases were reported; eight were classified as confirmed and 12 as probable [47]. In New Zealand, where no cases were reported, public health experts and policymakers understood EVALI was not caused by nicotine-containing e-cigarettes and that precautionary policies towards that market were unlikely to solve that public problem.

3.3 Should regulation consider that e-cigarettes are a useful harm reduction tool?

Regulation needs to consider harm reduction as a strategy for reducing health risks. Harm reduction has been a pillar of public health practices, an example is the use of methadone and needle exchanges rather than eliminating intravenous drug use. However, harm reduction approaches are often controversial (including the example above) because it has been argued that they accommodate rather than eliminate risky behaviours [48]. Since the development of e-cigarettes, public health experts and tobacco control advocates have debated the role of e-cigarettes as a harm reduction tool. Several public health experts believe e-cigarettes can play a role in eliminating smoking-related diseases and consider them to be a breakthrough in harm reduction development [49–52]. Whereas other public health experts argue that caution should be taken when endorsing e-cigarette products until crucial evidence becomes available [53]. E-cigarettes are popular among smokers due to their ability to replicate the behavioural and physical aspects of smoking [54, 55]. E-cigarettes are often termed a short-term tobacco harm reduction tool, as they do not contain tobacco or tar, which are known to cause numerous smoking-related diseases, including cardiovascular disease. As there is no long-term evidence yet available, the debate about using them as a long-term tobacco harm reduction tool will continue, but this raises the question of what regulation should be in place until we have long-term evidence?

3.4 Is regulation needed to prevent e-cigarettes from becoming a gateway to youth smoking?

One of the main concerns and important aspects in debates concerning the regulation of e-cigarettes is whether e-cigarettes increase tobacco smoking among youths, a gateway effect. Some in the tobacco control community argue that research has shown that youths who use e-cigarettes are more likely to start smoking compared with those who do not [56–61].

Another issue that has been raised relates to the increasing number of e-liquid flavours now available. In 2014, it was estimated there were 7764 unique flavours, with an average of 242 new flavours being added per month [62, 63]. The vast majority of flavours are related to confectionery (e.g., candyfloss, marshmallow, vanilla, cola, bubble-gum), and in 2020, it was estimated that there were over 15,000 different flavours available on the market [64, 65]. The question being asked is if this variety of e-liquid flavours is attracting youths to try e-cigarettes. Research has shown that the variety of available flavours is one of the top reasons for experimentation with e-cigarettes among youths, in addition to peer influence and curiosity [66–70]. Compared with adults, youths are more likely to use sweet e-liquid flavoured e-cigarettes, and their popularity among youths and the rates of prevalence have significantly increased in recent years [71, 72]. Research shows that youths perceived fruit and sweet flavoured e-cigarettes to be less harmful compared with tobacco flavour e-cigarettes [73–75]. Harrell et al. [72] argue that the elimination or restriction of flavoured e-liquids (particularly sweet and fruit flavours) could potentially aid youth and young adult prevention efforts. Already, Finland and several states in the USA (including Chicago and New York City) have brought in legislation to prohibit the sale of flavoured e-cigarettes [76, 77].

Several public health experts have disputed the gateway effect, arguing that the youths smoking prevalence continues to decline; therefore, e-cigarettes cannot be causing smoking among youths [78, 79]. It has also been argued that research has found that smoking more often preceded vaping rather than vice versa (i.e., most youths who had tried e-cigarettes are already smoking or have previously experimented with cigarette smoking) [80–82].

3.5 Is regulation needed to prevent e-cigarettes renormalising smoking?

Concerns over the renormalisation of smoking have been raised by numerous researchers and tobacco control advocates (including [83–85]). The renormalisation hypothesis suggests the growing prevalence and visibility of e-cigarette use could undo 'decades of work' in tobacco control regulation and shift social norms surrounding the extent to that smoking is once again seen as 'normal' behaviour [86–88].

Sæbø and Scheffels [87] and Hallingberg et al. [89] argue that the renormalisation hypothesis assumes cigarettes and e-cigarettes are viewed as similar to one another. E-cigarette products are evolving over time and as discussed previously, new models no longer resemble traditional cigarettes compared with earlier generations. Therefore, this needs to be considered when evaluating the renormalisation debate [87, 89] and considering the need for the regulation of e-cigarettes.

By contrast, some researchers argue that e-cigarettes may denormalise smoking through the social display of an alternative behaviour and cause some youth to not smoke who would otherwise have become smokers [89]. From this perspective, aligning e-cigarettes and tobacco regulation could result in the perception that the products are equal and potentially cause the renormalisation of smoking [89].

3.6 Is regulation needed to reduce the risk of dual use?

The issue of dual use relates to whether e-cigarette users will continue to use both tobacco cigarettes and e-cigarettes for an extended period of time [90]. Some researchers argue that from a population-level public health perspective, dual use could provide an opportunity to reduce the burden of tobacco use if it represents a temporary stage before smokers switch to solely e-cigarette use or quit tobacco products completely [90–92].

Nayak et al. [91] found that higher proportions of dual users have a stronger intention to quit compared with cigarette smokers. Similarly, research by Nabi-Burza et al. [93] showed that dual users may have higher rates of contemplating smoking cessation than individuals who only smoke cigarettes, suggesting that dual users may be using e-cigarettes for harm reduction or as a step towards cessation. However, it is possible that dual use could prolong nicotine addiction and consequently inhibit smoking cessation among smokers who might otherwise quit smoking [90, 94–96]. Concerns about the dual use of hazardous and reduced hazard products add another layer of complexity to the e-cigarette regulatory debate.

3.7 Do e-cigarettes lead to smoking cessation and if so, what does this mean for regulation?

Since the development of e-cigarettes, there has been an increase in the number of smokers who use and enquire about e-cigarettes when attempting to quit smoking [97, 98]. Currently, available medications include NRT, Varenicline (Champix) and Bupropion (Zyban) [99]. There are severeal published randomised controlled trials (RCTs) evaluating whether nicotine-containing e-cigarettes increase smoking cessation compared with placebos, financial incentives and behavioural therapy or NRT (including [97, 100–106]).

A 2016 Cochrane review [102] found that data from research by Caponnetto et al. [100] and Bullen et al. [101] support an effect of nicotine e-cigarettes on cessation when compared with placebo e-cigarettes, but has low certainty in the evidence due to the small number of trials (n=2), low event rates and wide confidence intervals [102]. The study by Bullen et al. [101] compares e-cigarettes to standard NRT, which is the most relevant comparator for clinicians. Unfortunately, the trial design placed the NRT group at a disadvantage compared with the e-cigarette group, as the NRT group was given vouchers for purchasing patches while the e-cigarette group was provided with e-cigarettes [101]. The authors of the review [102] were unable to determine if e-cigarettes were better than a nicotine patch for smoking cessation due to the low number of participants in the study. Furthermore, the review indicated that none of the studies, included in the review, found that smokers who used e-cigarettes short- to mid-term (for 2 years or less) had an increased health risk compared with smokers who did not use e-cigarettes [102].

Since the 2016 Cochrane review, three RCTs have been completed [103–105]. Hajek et al. [103] conducted the largest RCT of e-cigarettes compared with NRT to date, finding that nearly twice as many participants quit smoking at 1 year in the vaping group (18.0%) compared with the NRT group (9.9%). Participants in the NRT groups were allowed to choose the NRT product they use, this included using combination NRT (i.e., using two forms of NRT together, which is the most effective way to use NRT [107]) [103]. All three RCTs have found nicotine-containing e-cigarettes to be at least as effective as NRT, and some found that vaping was more effective [103–105].

The 2014 and 2016 Cochrane reviews both demonstrated low certainty in the evidence regarding the efficacy of e-cigarettes as a smoking cessation tool [97, 102]. A 2021 Cochrane review [106] found that nicotine e-cigarettes were superior to placebo e-cigarettes and at least as effective as NRT for smoking cessation, which is consistent with findings from other RCTs [103–105]. In addition, the review stated that there is moderate certainty in the evidence that nicotine-containing e-cigarettes increase the quit rate compared with NRT and non-nicotine-containing e-cigarettes [106]. As with the previous Cochrane reviews, there is imprecision due to the small number of trials, often with low event rates [97, 102, 106]. More evidence is required about the effects of e-cigarettes concerning smoking cessation, particularly due to the development of newer types of e-cigarette devices that have better nicotine delivery compared with older generations of e-cigarettes [108, 109].

This evidence is against a backdrop of the fact that e-cigarette use continues to increase globally despite uncertainty regarding their long-term health impacts and their effectiveness for tobacco smoking. This uncertainty creates unique challenges for governments and policymakers as they attempt to optimally regulate these products in a way that maximises the public's health. The next section will discuss current e-cigarette regulatory approaches and the variation across jurisdictions.

4. Regulation of e-cigarettes

Current approaches to e-cigarette regulation appear to fall within a spectrum of options ranging from a singular focus on health protection, whereby policies intend to prevent the dangers of e-cigarettes, to a singular focus on using e-cigarettes for harm reduction, whereby policies intend to reduce the more harmful effects of smoking tobacco. Regulation options include prohibition, regulation as medicinal products, poisons, tobacco products, consumer products and/or unique products.

4.1 Regulatory spectrum

A simplified view suggests that approaches to e-cigarette regulation fall within a spectrum of options. The spectrum ranges from a singular focus on a 'harm reduction' approach at one end to a singular focus on a 'precautionary' approach at the other end [110–113] (**Figure 2**). The main difference between the two ends of the spectrum is the population on which the recommendations are focused. The 'harm reduction' approach focused on the potentially positive health effects e-cigarettes pose to conventional smokers. In contrast, the 'precautionary' approach generally focuses on the health effects e-cigarettes pose to non-smokers, particularly youths and young people.

Both the 'harm reduction' and 'precautionary' approaches apply restrictions on e-cigarettes and tobacco products; however, in different ways. Adopting a 'harm reduction' approach does not require weak regulation of e-cigarette products; instead, it ensures that e-cigarette products are available as a smoking cessation tool for smokers who are unwilling or unable to quit smoking, meaning that the negative health effects caused by smoking can be reduced while minimising any exposure (resulting

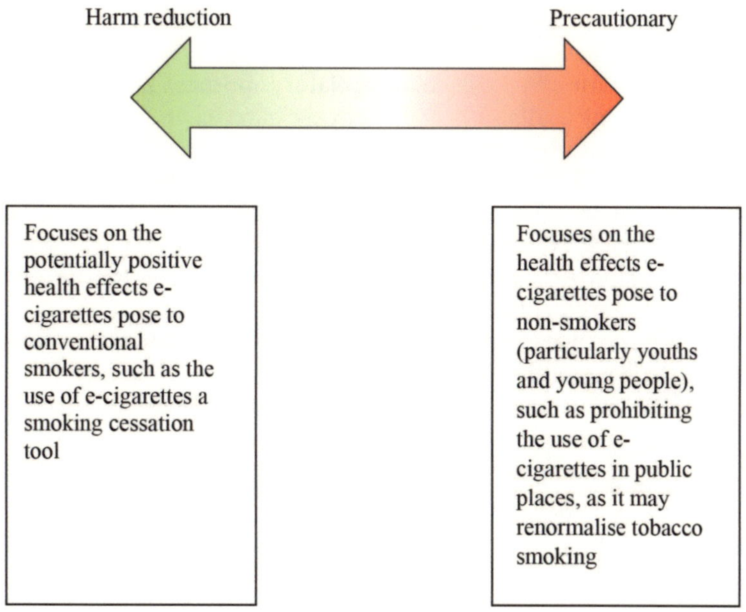

Figure 2.
A representation of the regulatory spectrum towards e-cigarette regulation.

in potentially positive health effects) among non-smokers and youths. While the 'precautionary approach' adopts stronger e-cigarette regulations to prevent initiation and use of e-cigarettes among non-smokers and youths.

4.1.1 Harm reduction approach

Harm reduction can be described as a way to reduce the negative health effects or health behaviours by making less harmful products available for use as a substitute for more harmful products [114]. The harm reduction approach acknowledges that cigarette users become addicted to nicotine and cannot easily stop smoking; it is, therefore, desirable to reduce the harms associated with the use of combustible cigarettes, by encouraging users to switch to a less harmful product (e.g., e-cigarettes) [115]. However, advocates of harm reduction do not always share the same views regarding the ultimate goals of e-cigarette use; some advocates argue that the goal should be to quit these harmful products entirely, whereas others believe risk minimisation is sufficient [116, 117].

4.1.2 Precautionary approach

Countries that are concerned about preventing the initiation of new users may choose to pursue prohibitive regulations that restrict the supply and demand (e.g., increasing taxes) of e-cigarette products. Numerous public health experts often argue that e-cigarettes are harmful, normalise smoking behaviour [83, 85] and serve as a gateway to nicotine addiction and even more harmful tobacco consumption for non-smokers and youth [56, 60, 61]. Rather than aiding in smoking cessation, they may believe the sale of e-cigarettes will encourage continued use of conventional cigarettes resulting in the dual use of both products, consequently inhibiting complete cessation [90, 96, 118, 119].

4.2 Current regulatory approaches

There is much variation in the current regulatory approaches adopted by countries, and this affects the availability and use of e-cigarettes and the perceived harms of e-cigarettes by the country's citizens. The perceived harmfulness of e-cigarettes among policymakers and citizens may affect the choice of regulatory framework adopted in a given country. The ways in which policymakers perceive and classify e-cigarettes will influence the regulatory approach pursued and will affect decisions about whether e-cigarettes should be included under existing legislation or whether new legislation is required [120].

Table 1 provides an overview of the variation between countries showing what approach countries have adopted.

Approach	Number of countries	Countries
Prohibition	30	Argentina, Brazil, Brunei Darussalam, Cambodia, Colombia, Egypt, The Gambia, India, Iran, Kuwait, Lao People's Democratic Republic, Lebanon, Mauritius, Mexico, Nepal, Nicaragua, Oman, Panama, Qatar, Seychelles, Singapore, Sri Lanka, Suriname, Syria, Thailand, Timor-Leste, Turkey, Turkmenistan, Uganda, Uruguay
Medicinal Products	20	Austria, Belgium, Canada, Chile, Denmark, Estonia, Finland, France, Iceland, Ireland, Jamaica, Japan, Norway, Philippines, South Africa, Sweden, Thailand, United Kingdom, United States, Venezuela
Poisons or Hazardous Substances	4	Australia, Belgium, Malaysia, Brunei Darussalam
Tobacco Products	54	Argentina, Austria, Azerbaijan, Bahrain, Brazil, Brunei Darussalam, Bulgaria, Colombia, Costa Rica, Croatia, Ecuador, Estonia, Finland, Georgia, Germany, Greece, Honduras, Indonesia, Iran, Italy, Latvia, Lithuania, Maldives, Malta, Mauritius, Mexico, Moldova, Nepal, The Netherlands, New Zealand, Nicaragua, Norway, Palau, Panama, Paraguay, Poland, Romania, Senegal, Seychelles, Singapore, Slovakia, Slovenia, South Korea, Spain, Sweden, Tajikistan, Thailand, Togo, Turkey, Turkmenistan, United Kingdom, United States, Venezuela, Vietnam
Consumer Products	15	Australia, Canada, France, Germany, Greece, Hungary, Iceland, Indonesia, Ireland, Moldova, South Korea, Switzerland, United Kingdom, United States, Venezuela
Unique Products	68	Argentina, Austria, Azerbaijan, Bahrain, Barbados, Belgium, Brazil, Bulgaria, Cambodia, Canada, Costa Rica, Croatia, Cyprus, Czech Republic, Denmark, Ecuador, El Salvador, Estonia, Fiji, Finland, France, The Gambia, Georgia, Germany, Greece, Ireland, Israel, Italy, Jamaica, Jordan, Kuwait, Lao People's Democratic Republic, Latvia, Lebanon, Lithuania, Luxembourg, Malta, Moldova, Nepal, The Netherlands, Norway, Oman, Panama, Paraguay, Poland, Portugal, Qatar, Romania, Saudi Arabia, Serbia, Slovakia, Slovenia, Spain, Sri Lanka, Suriname, Sweden, Switzerland, Syria, Tajikistan, Thailand, Timor-Leste, Turkey, Turkmenistan, Uganda, Ukraine, United Arab Emirates, United Kingdom, Uruguay

Table 1.
Countries' regulatory approaches towards e-cigarettes [121].

4.2.1 Prohibition

Prohibiting all legal access to e-cigarettes is often motivated by the precautionary approach and the desire to avoid all possible risks, whether or not those risks are scientifically authenticated [122]. This approach typically prohibits the manufacture, import and export, sale and/or possession of e-cigarettes. Thirty countries around the world (including Argentina, Egypt, Lebanon and Singapore) have prohibited all legal access to e-cigarettes, regardless of nicotine concentration [121]. For example, Singapore's Tobacco Control Act prohibits the sale, possession, distribution and importation of e-cigarettes in the country [121, 123]. The prohibition of e-cigarettes falls within the precautionary approach end of the regulatory spectrum. Prohibiting legal access to e-cigarette products discourages e-cigarette initiation (particularly among non-smokers and youths), prevents the renormalisation of smoking [124] and prevents the health risks associated with dual use. However, several concerns have been raised. Firstly, by prioritising non-smokers and youths, the approach may prevent tobacco smokers from accessing a less harmful product [119, 122], as it removes e-cigarettes from the market. Secondly, prohibiting legal access to e-cigarettes may cause consumers to purchase e-cigarettes from illegal sources, and these products may not be quality-assured, thus more harmful [110]. Regulatory approaches need to consider these.

4.2.2 Regulation as medicinal products

Regulating e-cigarettes as medicinal products is motivated by a desire to strictly limit e-cigarettes to those who will use them as a smoking cessation tool [103]. This approach prohibits legal access to e-cigarettes except when used as a smoking cessation tool. Regulatory mechanisms under this classification include restricting sales to accredited pharmacies, applying strict regulation of internet sales in order to ensure pharmaceutical standards are being met and requiring a medical prescription for purchase [125]. Most countries that have pursued this regulatory approach also pursue other approaches in conjunction. For example, Norway regulates e-cigarettes as medicinal products, tobacco products and as unique products [121]. Pursuing a combined approach increases accessibility to e-cigarettes by creating an additional pathway for accessing these products.

Twenty countries around the world (including Austria, Iceland and the Philippines), regulate e-cigarettes as medicinal products [121]. For example, the Philippines classifies e-cigarettes as medicinal products and medical devices [121], meaning they must pass assurance checks (including all quality, efficacy and safety evaluations) conducted by the Food and Drug Authority of the Philippines before they can be sold [126].

This approach addresses several of the key health concerns at both ends of the regulatory spectrum. By preventing non-smokers from legally accessing e-cigarettes prevents initiation, while simultaneously allowing current smokers to access e-cigarettes and reduce the harms associated with conventional tobacco smoking and eventually quit smoking. Caponnetto et al. [125] state that there is a major advantage to this approach; most countries already have well-established regulations for medicinal products. In addition, Campus et al. [110] explains if e-cigarette products were regulated and prescribed as medicinal products, they could potentially be provided or reimbursed by health insurance plans. This coverage could serve as a financial incentive for smokers to completely switch from conventional cigarettes to e-cigarettes, as it would ideally decrease or eliminate the cost of e-cigarettes for users of the product. While there are advantages, several limitations have also been raised. Lengthy pharmaceutical approval processes could create an interim black market for unregulated e-cigarette purchases [119]. Many e-cigarette manufacturers may lack the necessary expertise or resources to register their products or comply with stringent medicinal regulatory standards [125, 127]. Therefore, companies may choose to never go through the approval process and the black market may consequently become permanent [110, 119].

Applying medicinal regulations to e-cigarettes also creates unique challenges [125] regarding access to these products. Requiring a prescription to use e-cigarettes will limit accessibility and may encourage potential users to continue using conventional tobacco products.

4.2.3 Regulation as poisons or hazardous substances

Regulating e-cigarettes as a poison or hazardous substance is based upon the poisonous and potentially fatal nature of high nicotine concentrations [118]. With the focus on preventing nicotine overdose, possible regulatory mechanisms include banning nicotine-containing e-cigarettes or placing restrictions on nicotine concentrations in e-liquids [110]. Four countries have adopted this regulatory approach: Australia, Belgium, Malaysia and Brunei Darussalam [121]. In Australia, nicotine is classified as a dangerous poison; therefore, it is illegal to possess or use nicotine as a non-therapeutic good [128, 129]. However, there are currently two ways that Australians can legally purchase nicotine-contain e-cigarettes: through the personal importation scheme, or through a compounded pharmacy [129]. The personal import scheme enables Australians to ask a medical doctor to apply to the Therapeutics Goods Administration to allow the importation of up to a 3-month supply of nicotine for use in e-cigarettes for therapeutic purposes [119, 130]. Non-nicotine e-cigarettes are currently not regulated as a therapeutic good; therefore, they can be sold and used legally [130, 131]. In Brunei Darussalam, e-cigarette regulation focuses specifically on nicotine concentration. E-liquids with a nicotine concentration above 7.5% are classified as a poison, whereas those with a nicotine concentration under this amount are classified as tobacco products [121, 132]. Prohibiting nicotine-containing e-liquids would help address and potentially achieve the goal of preventing current non-smokers from developing an addiction to nicotine. However, this approach does not pay attention to or address the potential risks associated with non-nicotine e-liquids [110] and may complicate and/or impede the achievement of smoking cessation goals [122]. Similar to the approach pursued by Brunei Darussalam, countries that wish this regulatory approach may consider limiting the nicotine concentration in e-liquids.

4.2.4 Regulation as tobacco products

Fifty-four countries regulate e-cigarettes as tobacco products (including Finland, the USA and Vietnam) [121]. For example, the United States (U.S.) Food and Drug Administration (FDA) has regulatory authority over all tobacco products, including e-cigarettes [133], except when e-cigarettes are marketed as drugs or combination products (i.e., to use as a smoking cessation tool) [121].

The U.S. FDA defines tobacco products as 'any product made or derived from tobacco that is intended for human consumption, including any component, part, or accessory of a tobacco product' [134]. Based on this definition, it has been argued that the classification of e-cigarettes as tobacco products is legally justified by the fact that nicotine is derived from tobacco [116, 127]. Many policymakers argue that e-cigarettes should be classified as tobacco products to include them in already well-established tobacco legislation [125, 130]. Under this approach, e-cigarettes would be legally available for purchase, similar to conventional tobacco products [123], and they would be subject to regulatory requirements, such as product labelling requirements, restrictions on advertising and minimum age requirements for purchase [116, 123, 125].

Tobacco control legislation is mostly well established, therefore classifying e-cigarettes as tobacco products would allow current legislation to apply to e-cigarette products. While this would be advantageous, it is worth considering the potential limitations of pursuing this approach. Campus et al. [110] argue that from a harm reduction perspective, regulating e-cigarettes solely as tobacco products may discourage people from switching completely to a less harmful alternative. Furthermore, e-cigarettes do not always contain nicotine, meaning they do not fit with the previous definition [122]. In terms of the precautionary approach, the same arguments motivating the strict regulation of tobacco products can be applied to e-cigarettes, in that the latter are also highly addictive products that cause harm and may serve as a gateway to even more harmful behaviours [79, 82, 119].

4.2.5 Regulation as consumer products

Similar to regulating e-cigarettes as tobacco products, countries can regulate e-cigarettes as consumer products, meaning they can be included in existing legislation relating to consumer protection [110]. If pursuing this regulatory approach, e-cigarettes would be subject to the same regulations as other consumer products and would be available to purchase in convenience shops, speciality shops (i.e., vape shops) and on the internet [122]. Countries that choose to pursue this regulatory approach could create quality control standards for e-cigarette products [125] such as child-resistant packaging, labelling regulations regarding nicotine concentrations [122], as well as post-market surveillance and product recall systems [110]. In doing so, this would help protect consumers from unsafe or faulty devices and e-liquids [125]. Campus et al. [110] highlight that it is important to consider that consumer protections vary substantially across countries; therefore, regulation as a consumer product will inevitably have different meanings in different countries.

Fifteen countries currently regulate e-cigarettes as consumer products [121]. In Hungary, e-cigarettes are regulated primarily as consumer products [121] and are subject to Article 20 of the European Union (EU) Tobacco Products Directive (TPD) [135]. The directive establishes safety and quality requirements for e-cigarettes, packaging and labelling rules, as well as monitoring and reporting requirements for manufacturers and importers [135]. By regulating the sale of e-cigarettes as consumer products, Hungary aims to achieve multiple competing goals. Firstly, introducing warning labels on e-cigarettes will warn non-smokers and non-users not to use the products. Secondly, prohibiting e-cigarette advertising will help prevent non-smokers and non-users, particularly youths, from pursuing smoking-related behaviours, while still allowing current smokers to access e-cigarette products to assist in their quit attempts.

Farsalinos and Le Houezec [122] argue that this regulatory approach fails to address the issues surrounding nicotine concentrations and may potentially give the impression that e-cigarettes are safe for anyone to use. Several countries (including Australia, France, Moldova and Switzerland) have opted to regulate non-nicotine e-cigarettes as consumer products while implementing stricter approaches for nicotine-containing e-cigarettes including prohibition or regulating them as poisons or hazardous substances [121].

4.2.6 Regulation as unique products

Policymakers may choose to classify e-cigarettes as a unique product, therefore creating new legislation that relates specifically to e-cigarette products. Sixty-eight countries currently regulate e-cigarettes as a unique product, including Canada, Denmark, Saudi Arabia and Uganda [121]. In Canada, e-cigarettes are regulated under several Acts [121]; Tobacco & Vaping Products Act (TVPA), the Canada Consumer Product Safety Act, the Food & Drugs Act and the Non-Smokers' Health Act [136]. The TVP aims to prevent youth from using tobacco and e-cigarettes (i.e., precautionary) while allowing adult smokers to access e-cigarettes as a less harmful smoking alternative (i.e., harm reduction) [137]. The TVPA prohibits the sale of e-cigarettes to those under 18, as well as the sale of e-cigarettes that may be appealing to youth in the way that they look or function (i.e., certain flavours) [136, 137]. In addition, Canada has banned lifestyle advertising, advertising that is appealing to youth and the use of testimonials and endorsements [121]. While Canada has taken a relatively moderate approach to regulating e-cigarettes, other countries have pursued more restrictive approaches, while still regulating e-cigarettes as a unique product. For example, Cambodia, which has also classified e-cigarettes as a unique product, prohibits the sale, importation and use of e-cigarettes in the country [138]. This example constitutes a precautionary approach.

Regulating e-cigarettes as a unique product acknowledges that no existing regulatory classification may be suitable. This approach enables policymakers to tailor and modify e-cigarette regulations to the unique goals of their country. Therefore, this regulatory approach can draw upon aspects from both ends of the regulatory spectrum. As mentioned previously, Canada is an example whereby regulating e-cigarettes as a unique product, and policymakers have been able to pursue both a precautionary and harm reduction approach. Whereas, if countries view e-cigarettes as entirely harmful, regulating them as a unique product allows the pursuit of a precautionary approach. However, pursuing this approach requires countries to develop and adopt new legislation and considerable resources must be dedicated to the process.

How countries choose to regulate e-cigarettes will also depend on contextual factors including, epidemiological features of smoking and/or vaping and the need to be consistent with previous tobacco control policies. Policymakers might want to consider developing policy approaches and solutions that facilitate harm reduction for certain population groups (e.g., smokers), while simultaneously protecting the health of other population groups (e.g., non-smoking adults and youths). Tailoring regulation of e-cigarette policies for each jurisdiction might allow for the achievement of certain policy goals and objectives. Policymakers would need to determine which goals and objectives to prioritise and which ones cannot be optimally achieved. While this is a difficult balance to achieve, the situation is further complicated by the fact that the long-term health impacts of e-cigarettes are currently unknown [134, 139–141]. Unfortunately, there is no one-size-fits-all solution, and it is not possible to achieve all competing objectives, meaning some competing objectives cannot be met. E-cigarettes are a relatively new product to the market and globally, countries are still in the process of determining the most effective policies. Policymakers should consider learning from other countries policies and from international organisations such as the WHO to facilitate cross-country learning related to e-cigarettes [110].

5. Conclusions

E-cigarette regulation poses a real challenge for public health in determining which regulatory approach is most likely to improve population health and protect people from the damaging effects of tobacco smoking. This is evident from the variation of different approaches adopted across countries in taking a more 'harm reduction' or 'precautionary' approach. As the regulatory debate continues to evolve, it is likely a new 'middle ground' will emerge in the regulation of e-cigarettes as public health experts and tobacco control advocates alter their position on e-cigarette regulations in response to new evidence. In this chapter, we have summarised the global regulatory approaches towards e-cigarettes and debated some of the key arguments and approaches pursued by different countries. Despite various regulatory approaches being pursued, public health experts and tobacco control advocates are all focusing on the same goals—to reduce tobacco use and related harms.

Conflict of interest

The authors declare no conflict of interest.

Author details

Marissa Smith* and Shona Hilton
MRC/CSO Social and Public Health Sciences Unit, University of Glasgow, Glasgow, UK

*Address all correspondence to: marissa.smith@glasgow.ac.uk

References

[1] Doll R. Evolution of knowledge of the smoking epidemic. In: Boyle P, Gray N, Henningfield J, Seffrin J, Witold Z, editors. Tobacco: Science, Policy and Public Health. Oxford, UK: Oxford University Press; 2010. pp. 3-16

[2] Berridge V. The policy response to the smoking and lung cancer connection in the 1950s and 1960s. The Historical Journal. 2006;**49**(4):1185-1209

[3] Scientific Committee on Tobacco and Health. Report of the Scientific Committee on Tobacco and Health. London, UK: The Stationary Office; 1998. pp. 1-118

[4] World Health Organisation. WHO Framework Convention on Tobacco Control. Geneva, Switzerland: World Health Organisation; 2003

[5] Levy DT, Borland R, Lindblom EN, Goniewicz ML, Meza R, Holford TR, et al. Potential deaths averted in USA by replacing cigarettes with e-cigarettes. Tobacco Control. 2018;**27**(1):18-25

[6] Dubray J, Schwartz R, Chaiton M, O'Connor S, Cohen JE. The effect of MPOWER on smoking prevalence. Tobacco Control. 2015;**24**(6):540-542

[7] World Health Organisation. MPOWER in Action. Geneva, Switzerland: World Health Organisation; 2013

[8] Ngo A, Cheng K-W, Chaloupka FJ, Shang C. The effect of MPOWER scores on cigarette smoking prevalence and consumption. Preventive Medicine. 2017;**105**(1):10-14

[9] Gravely S, Giovino GA, Craig L, Commar A, D'Espaignet ET, Schotte K, et al. Implementation of key demand-reduction measures of the WHO framework convention on tobacco control and change in smoking prevalence in 126 countries: An association study. The Lancet Public Health. 2017;**2**(4):166-174

[10] Williams M, Talbot P. Design features in multiple generations of electronic cigarette atomizers. International Journal of Environmental Research and Public Health. 2019;**16**(16):2904-2919

[11] Grana R, Benowitz N, Glantz S. E-cigarettes: A scientific review. Circulation. 2014;**129**(19):1972-1986

[12] Centers for Disease Control and Prevention. E-Cigarette, or Vaping, Products Visual Dictionary. Atlanta, Georgia: Centers for Disease Control and Prevention; 2020

[13] National Academies of Sciences Engineering and Medicine. Public Health Consequences of E-Cigarettes. Washington, D.C., USA: The National Academies Press; 2018. Report No.: 978-0-309-46834-3

[14] Loddenkemper R, Kreuter M. The tobacco epidemic. Progress in Respiratory Research. 2015;**42**(2):258-267

[15] Farsalinos KE, Polosa R. Safety evaluation and risk assessment of electronic cigarettes as tobacco cigarette substitutes: A systematic review. Therapeutic Advances in Drug Safety. 2014;**5**(2):67-86

[16] Action on Smoking and Health. Briefing: Electronic Cigarettes. London, UK: Action on Smoking on Health; 2018

[17] Wang G, Liu W, Song W. Toxicity assessment of electronic cigarettes. Inhalation Toxicology. 2019;**31**(7): 259-273

[18] Cheng T. Chemical evaluation of electronic cigarettes. Tobacco Control. 2014;**23**(2):11-17

[19] Erythropel HC, Anastas PT, Krishnan-Sarin S, Malley SS, Jordt SE, Zimmerman JB. Differences in flavourant levels and synthetic coolant use between USA, EU and Canadian Juul products. Tobacco Control. 2021;**30**(4):453-455

[20] Willett JG, Bennett M, Hair EC, Xiao H, Greenberg MS, Harvey E, et al. Recognition, use and perceptions of JUUL among youth and young adults. Tobacco Control. 2019;**28**(1):115-116

[21] Herrington JS, Myers C. Electronic cigarette solutions and resultant aerosol profiles. Journal of Chromatography A. 2015;**1418**(1):192-199

[22] Kucharska M, Wesołowski W, Czerczak S, Soćko R. Testing of the composition of e-cigarette liquids—Manufacturer declared vs. true contents in a selected series of products. Medycyna Pracy. 2016;**67**(2):239-253

[23] Hadwiger ME, Trehy ML, Ye W, Moore T, Allgire J, Westenberger B. Identification of amino-tadalafil and rimonabant in electronic cigarette products using high pressure liquid chromatography with diode array and tandem mass spectrometric detection. Journal of Chromatography A. 2010;**1217**(48):7547-7555

[24] Goniewicz ML, Knysak J, Gawron M, Kosmider L, Sobczak A, Kurek J, et al. Levels of selected carcinogens and toxicants in vapour from electronic cigarettes. Tobacco Control. 2014;**23**(2): 133-139

[25] Orr MS. Electronic cigarettes in the USA: A summary of available toxicology data and suggestions for the future. Tobacco Control. 2014;**23**(2):18-22

[26] Margham J, McAdam K, Forster M, Liu C, Wright C, Mariner D, et al. Chemical composition of aerosol from an E-cigarette: A quantitative comparison with cigarette smoke. Chemical Research in Toxicology. 2016;**29**(10):1662-1678

[27] Flora JW, Wilkinson CT, Sink KM, McKinney DL, Miller JH. Nicotine-related impurities in e-cigarette cartridges and refill e-liquids. Journal of Liquid Chromatography & Related Technologies. 2016;**39**(17-18):821-829

[28] Takahashi Y, Kanemaru Y, Fukushima T, Eguchi K, Yoshida S, Miller-Holt J, et al. Chemical analysis and in vitro toxicological evaluation of aerosol from a novel tobacco vapor product: A comparison with cigarette smoke. Regulatory Toxicology and Pharmacology. 2018;**92**(1):94-103

[29] Czogala J, Goniewicz ML, Fidelus B, Zielinska-Danch W, Travers MJ, Sobczak A. Secondhand exposure to vapors from electronic cigarettes. Nicotine & Tobacco Research. 2014;**16**(6):655-662

[30] McEwen A, McRobbie H. Electronic Cigarettes: A Briefing for Stop Smoking Services. London, UK: National Centre for Smoking Cessation and Training; 2016

[31] Gupta S, Gandhi A, Manikonda R. Accidental nicotine liquid ingestion: Emerging paediatric problem. Archives of Disease in Childhood. 2014;**99**(12):1149

[32] Bartschat S, Mercer-Chalmers-Bender K, Beike J, Rothschild MA, Jübner M. Not only smoking is deadly:

Fatal ingestion of e-juice-a case report. International Journal of Legal Medicine. 2015;**129**(3):481-486

[33] Quail MT. Nicotine toxicity: Protecting children from e-cigarette exposure. Nursing. 2020;**50**(1):44-48

[34] Mayer B. How much nicotine kills a human? Tracing back the generally accepted lethal dose to dubious self-experiments in the nineteenth century. Archives of Toxicology. 2014;**88**(1):5-7

[35] Wagener TL, Siegel M, Borrelli B. Electronic cigarettes: Achieving a balanced perspective. Addiction. 2012;**107**(9):1545-1548

[36] Rigotti NA. Balancing the benefits and harms of E-cigarettes: A National Academies of Science, Engineering, and Medicine report. Annals of Internal Medicine. 2018;**168**(9):666-667

[37] Darville A, Hahn EJ. E-cigarettes and atherosclerotic cardiovascular disease: What clinicians and researchers need to know. Current Atherosclerosis Reports. 2019;**21**(5):15-23

[38] Sapru S, Vardhan M, Li Q, Guo Y, Li X, Saxena D. E-cigarettes use in the United States: Reasons for use, perceptions, and effects on health. BMC Public Health. 2020;**20**(1):1518-1538

[39] Centers for Disease Control and Prevention. 2019 Lung Injury Surveillance Primary Case Definitions: Centre for Disease Control and Prevention. Atlanta, Georgia; 2019. Available from: https://www.cdc.gov/tobacco/basic_information/e-cigarettes/assets/2019-Lung-Injury-Surveillance-Case-Definition-508.pdf

[40] King BA, Jones CM, Baldwin GT, Briss PA. The EVALI and youth vaping epidemics—Implications for public health. New England Journal of Medicine. 2020;**382**(8):689-691

[41] U.S. Department of Health and Human Services. E-Cigarette Use among Youth and Young Adults: A Report of the Surgeon General. Maryland, USA: U.S. Department of Health and Human Services; 2016

[42] Koslow M, Petrache I. A finale on EVALI?: The abated but not forgotten outbreak of acute respiratory illness in individuals who vape. Journal of the American Medical Association Network Open. 2020;**3**(11):e2019366

[43] Schweitzer KS, Chen SX, Law S, Van Demark M, Poirier C, Justice MJ, et al. Endothelial disruptive proinflammatory effects of nicotine and e-cigarette vapor exposures. American Journal of Physiology-Lung Cellular and Molecular Physiology. 2015;**309**(2):175-187

[44] Layden JE, Ghinai I, Pray I, Kimball A, Layer M, Tenforde MW, et al. Pulmonary illness related to E-cigarette use in Illinois and Wisconsin—Final report. New England Journal of Medicine. 2020;**382**(10):903-916

[45] UK Government. E-cigarette use or vaping: Reporting suspected adverse reactions, including lung injury. 2020. Available from: https://www.gov.uk/drug-safety-update/e-cigarette-use-or-vaping-reporting-suspected-adverse-reactions-including-lung-injury

[46] Munsif M, Hew M, Dabscheck E. E-cigarette or vaping product use-associated lung injury (EVALI): A cautionary tale. Medical Journal of Australia. 2020;**213**(3):109-110

[47] Baker MM, Procter TD, Belzak L, Ogunnaike-Cooke S. Vaping-associated lung illness (VALI) in Canada: A descriptive analysis of VALI cases

reported from September 2019 to December 2020. Health Promotion and Chronic Disease Prevention in Canada. 2022;**42**(1):37-44

[48] Thomas R, Parker LS, Shiffman S. The ethics of tobacco harm reduction: An analysis of E-cigarette availability from the perspectives of utilitarianism, bioethics, and public health ethics. Nicotine & Tobacco Research. 2020;**23**(1):3-8

[49] Cahn Z, Siegel M. Electronic cigarettes as a harm reduction strategy for tobacco control: A step forward or a repeat of past mistakes? Journal of Public Health Policy. 2011;**32**(1):16-31

[50] Britton J, McNeill A. Nicotine regulation and tobacco harm reduction in the UK. The Lancet. 2013;**381**(9881):1879-1880

[51] Hajek P. Electronic cigarettes have a potential for huge public health benefit. BMC Medicine. 2014;**12**(1):225-228

[52] Cox S, Dawkins L. Global and local perspectives on tobacco harm reduction: What are the issues and where do we go from here? Harm Reduction Journal. 2018;**15**(1):32-33

[53] Chapman S. E-cigarettes: Does the new emperor of tobacco harm reduction have any clothes? European Journal of Public Health. 2014;**24**(4):535-536

[54] Rahman MA, Hann N, Wilson A, Mnatzaganian G, Worrall-Carter L. E-cigarettes and smoking cessation: Evidence from a systematic review and meta-analysis. PLoS One. 2015;**10**(3):e0122544

[55] Green LW, Fielding JE, Brownson RC. The debate about electronic cigarettes: Harm minimization or the precautionary principle. Annual Review of Public Health. 2018;**39**(1):189-191

[56] Dutra LM, Glantz SA. Electronic cigarettes and conventional cigarette use among us adolescents: A cross-sectional study. Journal of the American Medical Association Pediatrics. 2014;**168**(7):610-617

[57] Moore GF, Littlecott HJ, Moore L, Ahmed N, Holliday J. E-cigarette use and intentions to smoke among 10-11-year-old never-smokers in Wales. Tobacco Control. 2014;**25**(2):147-152

[58] Barrington-Trimis JL, Berhane K, Unger JB, Cruz TB, Huh J, Leventhal AM, et al. Psychosocial factors associated with adolescent electronic cigarette and cigarette use. Pediatrics. 2015;**136**(2):308-317

[59] Bunnell RE, Agaku IT, Arrazola RA, Apelberg BJ, Caraballo RS, Corey CG, et al. Intentions to smoke cigarettes among never-smoking US middle and high school electronic cigarette users: National Youth Tobacco Survey, 2011-2013. Nicotine & Tobacco Research. 2015;**17**(2):228-235

[60] East K, Hitchman SC, Bakolis I, Williams S, Cheeseman H, Arnott D, et al. The association between smoking and electronic cigarette use in a cohort of young people. Journal of Adolescent Health. 2018;**62**(5):539-547

[61] Khouja JN, Suddell SF, Peters SE, Taylor AE, Munafò MR. Is e-cigarette use in non-smoking young adults associated with later smoking? A systematic review and meta-analysis. Tobacco Control. 2020;**30**(1):8-15

[62] Zhu S, Sun J, Binnevie E, Cummins S, Gamst A, Yin L, et al. Four hundred and sixty brands of e-cigarettes and counting: Implications for product regulation. Tobacco Control. 2014;**23**(3):3-9

[63] Tierney PA, Karpinski CD, Brown JE, Luo W, Pankow JF. Flavour chemicals

in electronic cigarette fluids. Tobacco Control. 2016;**25**(1):10-15

[64] Henry TS, Kligerman SJ, Raptis CA, Mann H, Sechrist JW, Kanne JP. Imaging findings of vaping-associated lung injury. American Journal of Roentgenology. 2020;**214**(3):498-505

[65] Campaign for Tobacco-Free Kids. E-cigarettes: Flavored Products Fuel a Youth Epidemic Campaign for Tobacco-Free Kids. 2020. Available from: https://www.tobaccofreekids.org/what-we-do/industry-watch/e-cigarettes

[66] Kong G, Morean ME, Cavallo DA, Camenga DR, Krishnan-Sarin S. Reasons for electronic cigarette experimentation and discontinuation among adolescents and young adults. Nicotine & Tobacco Research. 2015;**17**(7):847-854

[67] Bold K, Kong G, Cavallo D, Camenga D, Krishnan-Sarin S. Reasons for trying E-cigarettes and risk of continued use. Pediatrics. 2016;**138**(3):e20160895

[68] Audrain-McGovern J, Strasser AA, Wileyto EP. The impact of flavoring on the rewarding and reinforcing value of e-cigarettes with nicotine among young adult smokers. Drug and Alcohol Dependence. 2016;**166**(1):263-267

[69] Czoli CD, Goniewicz M, Islam T, Kotnowski K, Hammond D. Consumer preferences for electronic cigarettes: Results from a discrete choice experiment. Tobacco Control. 2016;**25**(1):30-36

[70] Zare S, Nemati M, Zheng Y. A systematic review of consumer preference for e-cigarette attributes: Flavor, nicotine strength, and type. PLoS One. 2018;**13**(3):e0194145

[71] Stanton CA, Villanti AC, Watson C, Delnevo CD. Flavoured tobacco products in the USA: Synthesis of recent multidiscipline studies with implications for advancing tobacco regulatory science. Tobacco Control. 2016;**25**(1):1-3

[72] Harrell MB, Weaver SR, Loukas A, Creamer M, Marti CN, Jackson CD, et al. Flavored e-cigarette use: Characterizing youth, young adult, and adult users. Preventive Medicine. 2017;**5**(1):33-40

[73] Ford A, MacKintosh AM, Bauld L, Moodie C, Hastings G. Adolescents' responses to the promotion and flavouring of e-cigarettes. International Journal of Public Health. 2016;**61**(2):215-224

[74] Pepper JK, Ribisl KM, Brewer NT. Adolescents' interest in trying flavoured e-cigarettes. Tobacco Control. 2016;**25**(1):62-66

[75] Cooper M, Harrell MB, Pérez A, Delk J, Perry CL. Flavorings and perceived harm and addictiveness of E-cigarettes among youth. Tobacco Regulatory Science. 2016;**2**(3):278-289

[76] Amendment of chapter 4-64 of municipal code by adding new section 4-64-098 regarding flavored tobacco products and amending section 4-64-180. 2013

[77] Ollila E. See you in court: Obstacles to enforcing the ban on electronic cigarette flavours and marketing in Finland. Tobacco Control. 2020;**29**(1):175-180

[78] Bauld L, MacKintosh AM, Eastwood B, Ford A, Moore G, Dockrell M, et al. Young People's use of E-cigarettes across the United Kingdom: Findings from five surveys 2015-2017. International Journal of Environmental Research and Public Health. 2017;**14**(9):973-985

[79] Chapman S, Bareham D, Maziak W. The gateway effect of E-cigarettes:

Reflections on Main criticisms. Nicotine & Tobacco Research. 2019;**21**(5):695-698

[80] de Lacy E, Fletcher A, Hewitt G, Murphy S, Moore G. Cross-sectional study examining the prevalence, correlates and sequencing of electronic cigarette and tobacco use among 11-16-year olds in schools in Wales. BMJ Open. 2017;**7**(2):e012784

[81] Berry KM, Reynolds LM, Collins JM, Siegel MB, Fetterman JL, Hamburg NM, et al. E-cigarette initiation and associated changes in smoking cessation and reduction: The population assessment of tobacco and health study, 2013-2015. Tobacco Control. 2019;**28**(1):42-49

[82] Mendelsohn CP, Hall W. Does the gateway theory justify a ban on nicotine vaping in Australia? The International Journal on Drug Policy. 2020;**78**:102712

[83] Fairchild AL, Bayer R, Colgrove J. The renormalization of smoking? E-cigarettes and the tobacco "endgame". New England Journal of Medicine. 2013;**370**(4):293-295

[84] World Health Organisation. Electronic Nicotine Delivery Systems. Geneva, Switzerland: World Health Organisation; 2014

[85] Voigt K. Smoking norms and the regulation of E-cigarettes. American Journal of Public Health. 2015;**105**(10):1967-1972

[86] Hsu R, Myers AE, Ribisl KM, Marteau TM. An observational study of retail availability and in-store marketing of e-cigarettes in London: Potential to undermine recent tobacco control gains? BMJ Open. 2013;**3**(12):e004085

[87] Sæbø G, Scheffels J. Assessing notions of denormalization and renormalization of smoking in light of e-cigarette regulation. The International Journal on Drug Policy. 2017;**49**:58-64

[88] Aleyan S, Cole A, Qian W, Leatherdale ST. Risky business: A longitudinal study examining cigarette smoking initiation among susceptible and non-susceptible e-cigarette users in Canada. BMJ Open. 2018;**8**(5):e021080

[89] Hallingberg B, Maynard OM, Bauld L, Brown R, Gray L, Lowthian E, et al. Have e-cigarettes renormalised or displaced youth smoking? Results of a segmented regression analysis of repeated cross sectional survey data in England, Scotland and Wales. Tobacco Control. 2020;**29**(2):207-216

[90] Wills TA, Knight R, Williams RJ, Pagano I, Sargent JD. Risk factors for exclusive e-cigarette use and dual e-cigarette use and tobacco use in adolescents. Pediatrics. 2015;**135**(1):43-51

[91] Nayak P, Pechacek TF, Weaver SR, Eriksen MP. Electronic nicotine delivery system dual use and intention to quit smoking: Will the socioeconomic gap in smoking get greater? Addictive Behaviors. 2016;**61**(1):112-116

[92] Owusu D, Huang J, Weaver SR, Pechacek TF, Ashley DL, Nayak P, et al. Patterns and trends of dual use of e-cigarettes and cigarettes among U.S. adults, 2015-2018. Preventive Medicine. 2019;**16**:101009

[93] Nabi-Burza E, Regan S, Walters BH, Drehmer JE, Rigotti NA, Ossip DJ, et al. Parental dual use of e-cigarettes and traditional cigarettes. Academic Pediatrics. 2019;**19**(7):842-848

[94] Jha P, Ramasundarahettige C, Landsman V, Rostron B, Thun M, Anderson RN, et al. 21st-century hazards of smoking and benefits of cessation in

the United States. New England Journal of Medicine. 2013;**368**(4):341-350

[95] U.S. Department of Health and Human Services. The Health Consequences of Smoking—50 Years of Progress. Maryland, USA: U.S. Department of Health and Human Services; 2014

[96] Hilton S, Weishaar H, Sweeting H, Trevisan F, Katikireddi SV. E-cigarettes, a safer alternative for teenagers? A UK focus group study of teenagers' views. BMJ Open. 2016;**6**(11):e013271

[97] McRobbie H, Bullen C, Hartmann-Boyce J, Hajek P. Electronic cigarettes for smoking cessation and reduction. Cochrane Database of Systematic Reviews. 2014;(9):CD010216. DOI: 10.1002/14651858.CD010216.pub2

[98] NHS. Using E-cigarettes to Stop Smoking. NHS; 2019. Available from: https://www.nhs.uk/live-well/quit-smoking/using-e-cigarettes-to-stop-smoking/

[99] NHS. Stop Smoking Treatments. NHS; 2019. Available from: https://www.nhs.uk/conditions/stop-smoking-treatments/

[100] Caponnetto P, Campagna D, Cibella F, Morjaria JB, Caruso M, Russo C, et al. EffiCiency and safety of an eLectronic cigAreTte (ECLAT) as tobacco cigarettes substitute: A prospective 12-month randomized control design study. PLoS One. 2013;**8**(6):e66317

[101] Bullen C, Howe C, Laugesen M, McRobbie H, Parag V, Williman J, et al. Electronic cigarettes for smoking cessation: A randomised controlled trial. The Lancet. 2013;**382**(9905):1629-1637

[102] Hartmann-Boyce J, McRobbie H, Bullen C, Begh R, Stead LF, Hajek P. Electronic cigarettes for smoking cessation. Cochrane Database of Systematic Reviews. 2016;(9):CD010216. DOI: 10.1002/14651858.CD010216.pub3

[103] Hajek P, Phillips-Waller A, Przulj D, Pesola F, Myers Smith K, Bisal N, et al. A randomized trial of E-cigarettes versus nicotine-replacement therapy. New England Journal of Medicine. 2019;**380**(7):629-637

[104] Lee SH, Ahn SH, Cheong YS. Effect of electronic cigarettes on smoking reduction and cessation in Korean male smokers: A randomized controlled study. Journal of the American Board of Family Medicine. 2019;**32**(4):567-574

[105] Walker N, Parag V, Verbiest M, Laking G, Laugesen M, Bullen C. Nicotine patches used in combination with e-cigarettes (with and without nicotine) for smoking cessation: A pragmatic, randomised trial. The Lancet Respiratory Medicine. 2020;**8**(1):54-64

[106] Hartmann-Boyce J, McRobbie H, Butler AR, Lindson N, Bullen C, Begh R, et al. Electronic cigarettes for smoking cessation. Cochrane Database of Systematic Reviews. 2021;(9):CD010216. DOI: 10.1002/14651858.CD010216.pub6

[107] U.S. Department of Health and Human Services. Smoking Cessation: A Report of the Surgeon General. Washington D.C., USA: U.S. Department of Health and Human Services; 2020. Contract No.: 10 November

[108] Farsalinos KE, Spyrou A, Tsimopoulou K, Stefopoulos C, Romagna G, Voudris V. Nicotine absorption from electronic cigarette use: Comparison between first and new-generation devices. Scientific Reports. 2014;**4**(1):4133-4140

[109] Tattan-Birch H, Brown J, Shahab L, Jackson SE. Trends in use of e-cigarette

device types and heated tobacco products from 2016 to 2020 in England. Scientific Reports. 2021;**11**(1):13203-13214

[110] Campus B, Fafard P, St Pierre J, Hoffman SJ. Comparing the regulation and incentivization of e-cigarettes across 97 countries. Social Science & Medicine. 2021

[111] Hawkins B, Ettelt S. The strategic uses of evidence in UK e-cigarettes policy debates. Evidence & Policy. 2019;**15**(4):579-596

[112] Smith KE, Ikegwuonu T, Weishaar H, Hilton S. Evidence use in E-cigarettes debates: Scientific showdowns in a 'wild west' of research. BMC Public Health. 2021;**21**(1): 362-378

[113] Smith MJ, Skivington K, Hilton S, Katikireddi SV. Exploring e-cigarette public health recommedations: A compartive document analysis of four jurisdictions [manuscript submitted for publication]. 2022

[114] Hawk M, Coulter RWS, Egan JE, Fisk S, Reuel Friedman M, Tula M, et al. Harm reduction principles for healthcare settings. Harm Reduction Journal. 2017;**14**(1):70-78

[115] Buckell J, Fucito LM, Krishnan-Sarin S, Malley S, Sindelar JL. Harm reduction for smokers with little to no quit interest: Can tobacco policies encourage switching to e-cigarettes? Tobacco Control. 2022:tobaccocontrol-2021-057024

[116] Fairchild AL, Bayer R. Smoke and fire over e-cigarettes. Science. 2015;**347**(6220):375-376

[117] Fairchild A, Colgrove J. Out of the ashes: The life, death, and rebirth of the "safer" cigarette in the United States. American Journal of Public Health. 2004;**94**(2):192-204

[118] Kenkel DS. Healthy innovation: Vaping, smoking and, public policy. Journal of Policy Analysis and Management. 2016;**35**(2):473-479

[119] Hall W, Gartner C, Forlini C. Ethical issues raised by a ban on the sale of electronic nicotine devices. Addiction. 2015;**110**(7):1061-1067

[120] Kennedy RD, Awopegba A, De León E, Cohen JE. Global approaches to regulating electronic cigarettes. Tobacco Control. 2017;**26**(4):440-445

[121] Institute for Global Tobacco Control. Country Laws Regulating E-cigarettes: A Policy Scan. Baltimore, MD: Johns Hopkins Bloomberg School of Public Health; 2020. Available from: https://www.globaltobaccocontrol.org/e-cigarette_policyscan

[122] Farsalinos KE, Le Houezec J. Regulation in the face of uncertainty: The evidence on electronic nicotine delivery systems (e-cigarettes). Risk Manag Healthc Policy. 2015;**8**:157-167

[123] Campaign for Tobacco-Free Kids. Tobacco Control Laws 2021. Available from: https://www.tobaccocontrollaws.org/legislation/country/singapore/ec-policies#:~:text=Analysis-,The%20law%20bans%20the%20import%2C%20distribution%2C%20sale%2C%20offer%20for,this%20policy%20is%20not%20applicable

[124] Kaufman N, Mahoney M. E-cigarettes: Policy options and legal issues amidst uncertainty. The Journal of Law, Medicine & Ethics. 2015;**43**(1_suppl):23-26

[125] Caponnetto P, Saitta D, Sweanor D, Polosa R. What to consider when

regulating electronic cigarettes: Pros, cons and unintended consequences. The International Journal on Drug Policy. 2015;**26**(6):554-559

[126] Rules and Regulations on Electronic Nicotine Delivery System (ENDS) or Electronic Cigarettes 2014-0008. 2014

[127] Hajek P, Foulds J, Houezec JL, Sweanor D, Yach D. Should e-cigarettes be regulated as a medicinal device? The Lancet Respiratory Medicine. 2013;**1**(6):429-431

[128] Douglas H, Hall W, Gartner C. E-cigarettes and the law in Australia. Australian Family Physician. 2015;**44**(6):415-418

[129] Berridge V, Hall W, Taylor S, Gartner C, Morphett K. A first pass, using pre-history and contemporary history, at understanding why Australia and England have such different policies towards electronic nicotine delivery systems, 1970s–c. 2018. Addiction. 2021;**116**(9):2577-2585

[130] Klein DE, Chaiton M, Kundu A, Schwartz R. A literature review on international E-cigarette regulatory policies. Current Addiction Reports. 2020;**7**(4):509-519

[131] Yong H-H, Borland R, Balmford J, McNeill A, Hitchman S, Driezen P, et al. Trends in E-cigarette awareness, trial, and use under the different regulatory environments of Australia and the United Kingdom. Nicotine & Tobacco Research. 2015;**17**(10):1203-1211

[132] Jin P, Jiang JY. E-cigarettes in ten southeast Asian countries: A comparison of national regulations. Global Health Journal. 2017;**1**(3):1-10

[133] U.S. Food and Drug Administration. Deeming Tobacco Products to be Subject to the Federal Food, Drug, and Cosmetic Act, as Amended by the Family Smoking Prevention and Tobacco Control Act; Restrictions on the Sale and Distribution of Tobacco Products and Required Warning Statements for Tobacco Products. Washington D.C., USA: U.S. Food and Drug Administration; 2016

[134] Callahan-Lyon P. Electronic cigarettes: Human health effects. Tobacco Control. 2014;**23**(2):36-40

[135] European Commission. Tobacco Products Directive (2014/40/EU). Brussels, Belgium: European Commission; 2014. p. 1-38

[136] Government of Canada. Vaping Product Regulations. 2019. Available from: https://www.canada.ca/en/health-canada/services/smoking-tobacco/vaping/product-safety-regulation.html#a1

[137] Government of Canada. Tobacco and Vaping Products Act 2018. Available from: https://www.canada.ca/en/health-canada/services/health-concerns/tobacco/legislation/federal-laws/tobacco-act.html

[138] Circular on Measures to Prevent and Terminate Consumptions, Sales, and Imports of SHISHA and E-Cigarette in the Kingdom of Cambodia, No. 001/14. 2014

[139] Kaisar MA, Prasad S, Liles T, Cucullo L. A decade of e-cigarettes: Limited research & unresolved safety concerns. Toxicology. 2016;**365**(1):67-75

[140] Chaffee BW. Electronic cigarettes: Trends, health effects and advising patients amid uncertainty. Journal of the California Dental Association. 2019;**47**(2):85-92

[141] Erku DA, Kisely S, Morphett K, Steadman KJ, Gartner CE. Framing and scientific uncertainty in nicotine vaping product regulation: An examination of competing narratives among health and medical organisations in the UK, Australia and New Zealand. International Journal of Drug Policy. 2020;**78**:102699. DOI: 10.1016/j.drugpo.2020.102699

Chapter 15

The Electronic Cigarette Use in Canada – Local and Global Considerations

Rudra Dahal

Abstract

Since its invention in 2003, electronic cigarettes' (EC) users have been growing worldwide. ECs were first introduced in the market in Canada in 2004, and they remained illegal until 2018. ECs were initially marketed as a safer and cleaner alternative for the traditional combustible smoking and smoking cessation measures. Statistics show that EC use prevalence is the highest among the youths (15–19) and adolescents (20–24) years of age. EC has to promote cessation as it supplies nicotine to smokers prevent nicotine withdrawal syndrome and reduce motivation to continue smoking. EC use becomes a gateway to tobacco use and nicotine addiction. Nicotine exposure to youth and adolescents can damage the developing brain. EC use is also associated with an increased heart attack rate and other health problems. There are various reasons for using ECs, such as curiosity, quitting combustible smoking, or cutting down the number of cigarette use. Many people start ECs use before the age of 19 years. Majority of vapers like fruit flavor. Dual combustible cigarette smoking and EC use is a burning issue globally, including in Canada.

Keywords: electronic cigarette, Canada, dual smokers, smoking cessation, electronic cigarette flavors

1. Introduction

Cigarette smoking is the primary cause of preventable deaths in Canada [1]. From 1960 to 2015, traditional combustible cigarette smoking prevalence has reduced from 50 to 13% in Canada [2] which is a good sign for public health. Even though, electronic cigarette (EC) is emerging in the Canadian general population which is a public health threat in this generation. The majority of Canadian EC users start smoking during their adolescence period.

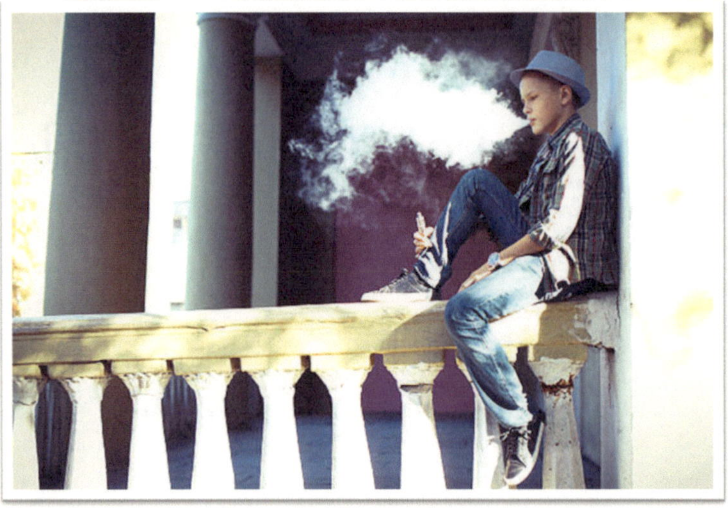

Image credit: Pixabay.

EC also known as e-cigarettes or "vape," is vaporized nicotine, cannabis, or only flavored products contained in a battery-powered electronic nicotine delivery device. EC use has increased in recent times globally, which has also been used as an alternative to combustible cigarette smoking. Since the invention of EC in 2003, its availability, popularity, and use have been widely growing [3]. ECs were first introduced in the Canadian market in 2004 and became legal in 2018. They were initially marketed as a safer and cleaner alternative to traditional combustible cigarettes and are used extensively for smoking cessation and relapse prevention [4]. ECs are typically considered a harm reduction strategy as they involve vapor that contains a smaller amount of toxic chemicals than the traditional combustible cigarettes [3, 5]. However, this impression is misleading, erroneous, and meant for marketing purposes.

The prevalence of EC use is varied and increasing globally, specifically in high-income countries, including Canada. The prevalence is reportedly higher in adolescents (15–19 years) and youths (20–24 years) [2, 3, 6–8]. For instance, in the US, current EC use was 11.7% in 2017 and reached 27.5% in 2019 [9]. In the UK, EC use was 1.7% in 2012, arose to 7.1% in 2019 [10]. Similarly, in Eastern Europe- EC use in Russia was 33.4%, Slovakia 34.4%, and Lithuania 55.6% [11]. In the middle East, studies in the University students in Saudi Arabia found the prevalence of EC use between 10 and 27.2% [12]. According to the European Commission, EC use prevalence in European Union countries ranges between more than 0.2% to less than 7% [13].

According to the Canadian Tobacco, Alcohol, and Drugs Survey, in the general Canadian population aged 15 years or older, the prevalence of past-30-days EC use was 3%, it was 2% in 2013, and that of ever tried EC was 15%, which was 9% in 2013. The prevalence was higher among youths and young adults over the period [6–8]. In the US, the past 30 days EC use was 11.7% in 2017 and reached 27.5% in 2019 [9].

The public health impact of EC use is attached to its effects on conventional smoking and health risks. ECs are recommended in harm reduction programs for cigarette smokers as an alternative to traditional tobacco or a cigarette smoking cessation measure [14]. EC can promote smoking cessation as it supplies nicotine to cigarette users and prevents nicotine withdrawal syndromes, which reduces motivation for conventional cigarette smoking. However, its effectiveness for smoking cessation is controversial, given the range of smoking outcomes reported by research- some smokers quit smoking by switching to EC, some become dual users, and remaining smokers quit tobacco and discontinue EC use [2, 15]. Furthermore, EC use as a measure of smoking cessation seems relevant to adult smokers as most youths and young adults who use ECs are non-smokers. Although the evidence around the health benefits and risks of EC use is unclear, the use of EC by smokers as a harm reduction or smoking cessation measure may gain health benefits. However, EC use may increase among non-smokers, former smokers, and dual users [16]. Alternatively, EC use may serve as a gateway for cigarette smoking initiation [2, 6, 15].

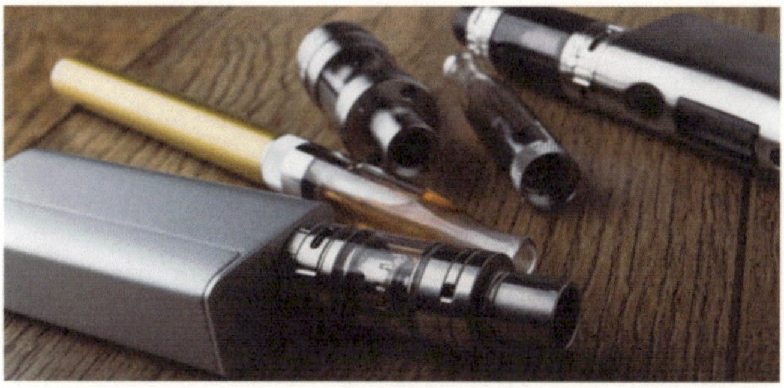

Image credit: Pixabay.

The prevalence of past-30 days of EC use was 14% among non-smoker youths and 11% among non-smoker young adults in Canada [6]. Various systematic reviews and longitudinal studies reported strong associations between EC use and the subsequent smoking behavior, whereby youths and adolescents who use EC have more than two times increased intention to cigarette smoking in the future than those who do not use EC [2, 17]. Therefore, the increased prevalence of EC use is a critical public health concern because, in addition to its health risks, it may interrupt the declining trends of cigarette smoking over the past decades and may add to the future population-level burden of cigarette smoking.

2. Some facts about ECs

Fact # 1. ECs are battery-operated devices that mimic the smoking experience using an inhalation and heating process, which vaporizes the e-liquid within the device. The e-solution differs in composition, but mostly propylene or vegetable glycol or can contain other ingredients and flavors. It may or may not contain nicotine.

Fact # 2. ECs containing nicotine are legal for adults 18 years and older in the Canadian market.

Fact # 3. Evidence shows that ECs are less harmful than conventional tobacco smoking [18].

Fact # 4. The previous study demonstrated few potential benefits to ECs as a smoking cessation device, but current research remains inconclusive. The body of evidence is fast-growing and shifting in this area of research [19, 20].

Fact # 5. Evidence shows that it would be less harmful to cease smoking entirely rather than dual-use.

Fact # 6. Individual who has tried other cessation methods and have not had success try ECs. Individuals who failed to quit smoking would be better off using ECs over the long term rather than continuing to be smoking a combustible cigarette.

Fact # 7. Health concerns such as long-term inhaling propylene or vegetable glycol and the effects of exposing second-hand smoking are not established yet.

Fact # 8. EC use is associated with an increased risk of heart attack, and both conventional cigarettes and ECs are associated with multiple threats of heart attack to the individual [6].

Fact # 9. There is evidence of child poisoning and accidental exposure, and consumption of e-liquid is on the rise [21].

Fact # 10. Evidence shows that nicotine exposure to youth and adolescents can damage the developing brain [22, 23].

Fact # 11. Emerging evidence proved the potential for ECs to be a gateway to tobacco use and nicotine addiction [24, 25].

Fact # 12. Marketing and promoting ECs are common; primarily, youths are targeted with attractive flavors.

Fact # 13. Research showed that ECs could renormalize and undermine tobacco control and smoking cessation efforts [26].

Fact # 14. ECs are appealing to youth. 23% of students in Canada reported having ever tried ECs. More teens are using ECs [8].

Fact # 15. Various jurisdictions in Canada address EC use in public places to support tobacco control and support clean air initiatives.

Fact # 16. The most common type of EC use in Canada is dual use-where an individual both vapes and smokes combustible tobacco [7].

Fact # 17. 38.6 million EC users live in the countries where EC sales are allowed, 9.5 million in those places where EC use is completely banned, and 10 million live in those areas where EC use has no specific laws [27].

3. Global estimation of EC use

ECs are potentially disruptive innovations for human health. According to the Global Adult Tobacco Survey, which was last conducted in 2017 from 49 countries around the globe found, the number of EC users was 40.3 million [27]. It was estimated that the remaining 152 countries belong to 17.8 million EC users, which gives a total of 58.1 million people who used ECs in 2018. As Jerzyński et al. (2021) projected that among EC users, 2.1 million belong to low-income countries, 7.7 million belong to lower-middle-income countries, 19 million belong to upper-middle-income countries, and 29.3 million belong to higher-income countries. Looking at the above global statistics, it is seen that more than half of EC users live in high-income countries. Likewise, let us compare these numbers region-wise. 4.1 million EC users reside in the African region, 4.2 million in the Eastern Mediterranean region, 4.6 million in the South-East Asian continent, 11.2 million in the Western Pacific area, 15.3 million in the European region, and 18.7 million in the Americas region [27].

4. EC use and legal status in Canada

ECs with or without nicotine are legal in the Canadian market now. In May 2018, Bills S-5: An Act to amend the Tobacco Act and Non-Smokers' Health Act received Royal Assent, which established a new legislative framework to regulate the manufacturing, sale, labeling, and promotions of vaping products in Canada. Sales of vaping products containing nicotine are permitted to adults 18 years and older in Canada. A Canadian study found that more teens use ECs as they see them as fun [28].

5. Age at initiation of EC

According to the Canadian Tobacco and Nicotine Survey (CTNS) [8], 30.57% of males and 31.54% of females initiate EC before 19 years in Canada. From the age group of 20–24 years, male numbers are higher than females. Interestingly, after 45 years of age, more females started EC use than males, which is 21.34% and 17.08%, respectively [8].

6. Causes of EC use

There are numerous reasons for using ECs in Canada. Many Canadians use ECs than prescription medications to quit smoking and nicotine replacement therapy. According to CTNS [8], among Canadians aged 15 years and over who used EC in the past 30 days, the most commonly reported causes were smoking cessation (27%), curiosity (20%), and enjoyment (20%). The generally reported reasons among youth aged 15 to 19 years who used ECs past 30 days were curiosity (29%), enjoyment (29%), and reducing stress (21%). In the young adults who used ECs in the past 30 days, the most common reasons were curiosity (27%) and smoking cessation (20%), while among adults aged 25 years and above, the most common causes were smoking cessation (41%) and avoiding returning to smoking (15%). After looking at the above statistics, we can conclude the following reasons for EC use in Canada:

- Curiosity, just wanted to try it,
- For enjoyment/pleasure,
- To reduce stress or self-calm down,
- To quit combustible smoking,
- To cut down on smoking cigarettes,
- To use where cigarettes are not allowed or permitted,
- To avoid returning to cigarette smoking
- Peer pressure

7. EC and its flavors

When people visit vape stores or websites, they will find a wide variety of colorful pods, cartridges, and bottles (Picture below) filled with various flavored e-liquid. The vape juice is heated in EC devices, and then it creates an aerosol that vapers inhale and enjoy. Vape juices are available in different forms, such as bubble gums, tobacco, candy, and many more.

These flavors are available in the Canadian vape market [8].

- Fruit flavor 42.0%
- Mint or Menthol 17.8%
- Tobacco 13.5%
- No usual taste 9.7%
- Candy 5.6%

Some other flavors are also available in the market, such as dessert, kid's cereals, and flavorless.

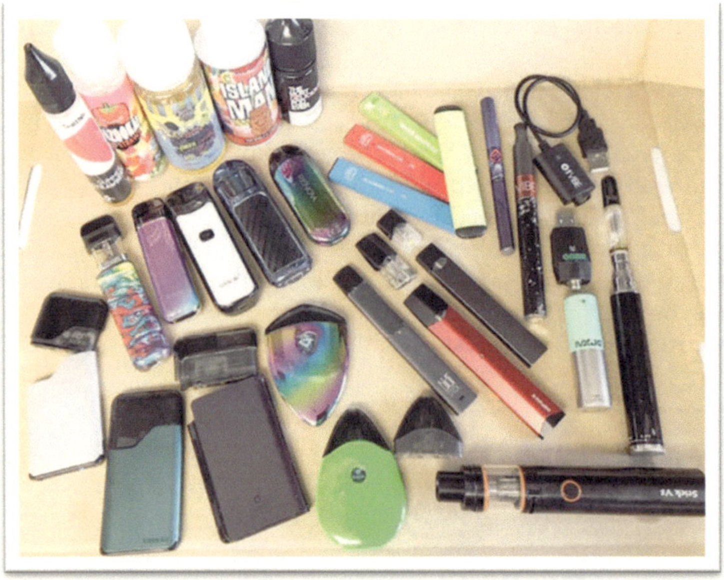

Picture credit: Google.

8. Patterns of ECs use in Canada

13% of Canadian people reported trying an EC in 2015 [2, 6, 7]. Youth (15–19 years of age) and young adults (20–24 years of age) were found to have the highest rate of trying ECs at a rate of 6.3% [8]. EC use dramatically increased between 2013 and 2015 [29]. Dual-use of combustible tobacco and ECs is a burning topic in Canada as it is the most common pattern of EC use among smokers [28].

9. EC use and health risks

There are insufficient studies to establish long-term health risks of ECs [11]. Nevertheless, there are various health risks and side effects of ECs recognized as follows:

- Nicotine addiction [30]
- Hypertension
- Acute inflammatory distress [31]
- Asthma [32]
- Lung Injury [33]
- Atherosclerosis [34]
- Cardiovascular disease [34]
- Headache
- Cough
- Dizziness
- Irritation of mouth and throat
- Nausea and vomiting

10. Sales and marketing of ECs

Legally the manufacturer cannot make a health claim regarding an EC product's ability to aid in smoking cessation or suggest a safer alternative to smoking traditional combustible tobacco unless Health Canada approves the statements. Bill S-5 has prohibited the promotion of flavors too. The legislation also gave the regulatory authority to Health Canada to mandate the application of consumer information, including health warning messages on vaping products. Similarly, the marketing of vaping product has been prohibited in Canada through bill S-5. Nevertheless, it is not that difficult to find online and using other social media platforms. Smokers think that it is their right to smoke in public places, thinking ECs are socially accepted products free of stigmatization and guilt. This positioning is concerning as ECs are being marketed to undermine the hard-fought change in social norms related to tobacco use, thus undermining the progress in tobacco control.

Moreover, there are no location-based restrictions for vaping product advertisements. Though banned in Canada, celebrity ECs endorsements are common, and celebrities often use ECs in entertainment programs, which act as an indirect endorsement. Increasing globalization and the advancement of the digital era means that Canadians can be exposed to EC marketing from countries where regulations are nonexistent or less comprehensive. ECs are rapidly growing in the Canadian market [20, 29].

11. Conclusion

EC use has emerged in present days all around the globe. EC was first introduced in the Canadian market in 2004, becoming legal after 14 years. Initially, it was marketed as a safer and cleaner alternative to the traditional tobacco smoking and relapse prevention tool. The prevalence of EC use is rising in high-income countries, including Canada, and most users are adolescents and youths. The increased prevalence of EC use is a critical public health issue because it may interrupt the declining trend of cigarette smoking; as a result, it may increase the future population-level burden.

EC with or without nicotine is legal in Canada; however, it is illegal for a manufacturer to make a health claim regarding EC product's ability to aid in smoking cessation or suggest a safer alternative to traditional tobacco smoking. Many Canadians initiate EC use before 19 years of age. Canadians use EC for various reasons, such as curiosity, enjoyment and cutdown, and traditional smoking. There are a wide variety of tastes of ECs available in the Canadian market. There are not enough scientific studies to establish the long-term health risks of EC use. Nevertheless, several health risks are documented, including nicotine addiction, cardiovascular diseases, and lung injuries.

Author details

Rudra Dahal
University of Lethbridge, Lethbridge, AB, Canada

*Address all correspondence to: karsdahal@gmail.com

References

[1] Shiplo S, Czoli CD, Hammond D. E-cigarette use in Canada: Prevalence and patterns of use in a regulated market. BMJ Open. 2015;**5**:e007971. DOI: 10.1136/BMJ open-2015-007971

[2] Hammond D, Reid JL, Cole AD, Leatherdale ST. Electronic cigarette use and smoking initiation among youth: A longitudinal cohort study. CMA. 2017;**2017**(189):E1328-E1336. DOI: 10.1503/cmaj.161002

[3] Mehra VM, Keethakumar A, Bohr YM, Abdullah P, Tamim H. The association between alcohol, marijuana, illegal drug use and current use of E-cigarette among youth and young adults in Canada: Results from Canadian tobacco, alcohol and drugs survey 2017. BMC Public Health. 2019;**19**(1):1208. DOI: 10.1186/s12889-019-7546-y

[4] Patten SB, Williams J, Wiens K, Lukmanji A, Dores AK, Isherwood LJ, et al. Emerging patterns of E-cigarette use in the general population. Canadian Journal of Psychiatry. 2021;**66**(5):503-505. DOI: 10.1177/0706743720975591

[5] Carroll Chapman SL, Wu LT. E-cigarette prevalence and correlates of use among adolescents versus adults: A review and comparison. Journal of Psychiatric Research. 2014;**54**:43-54. DOI: 10.1016/j.jpsychires.2014.03.005

[6] Czoli CD, Reid JL, Rynard VL, Hammond D. E-Cigarettes in Canada-Tobacco Use in Canada: Patterns and Trends, 2015 Edition, Special Supplement. Waterloo, ON: Propel Centre for Population Health Impact, University of Waterloo; 2015

[7] Reid JL, Rynard VL, Czoli C, Hammond D. Who is using e-cigarettes in Canada? Nationally representative data on the prevalence of e-cigarette use among Canadians. Preventive Medicine. 2015;**2015**(81):180-183. DOI: 10.1016/j.ypmed.2015.08.019

[8] Statistics Canada. Canadian Tobacco, Alcohol and Drugs Survey (CTADS). 2017. https://www23.statcan.gc.ca/imdb/p2SVFunction+getSurvey&SDD.pl?Function=getSurvey&SDDS

[9] Moritz ED, Zapata LB, Lekiachvili A, Glidden E, Annor FB, Werner AK, et al. Lung injury response epidemiology/surveillance task force (2019). Update: Characteristics of patients in a National Outbreak of E-cigarette, or vaping, product use-associated lung injuries - United States, October 2019. MMWR. Morbidity and Mortality Weekly Report. 2019;**68**(43):985-989. https://doi.org/10.15585/mmwr.mm6843e1

[10] McNeill A, Brose LS, Calder R, Simonavicius E, Robson D. Vaping in England: An Evidence Update Including Vaping for Smoking Cessation, February 2021: A Report Commissioned by Public Health England. London: Public Health England; 2021

[11] Brożek GM, Jankowski M, Lawson JA, Shpakou A, Poznański M, Zielonka TM, et al. The prevalence of cigarette and E-cigarette smoking among students in central and Eastern Europe-results of the YUPESS study. International Journal of Environmental Research and Public Health. 2019;**16**(13):2297. DOI: 10.3390/ijerph16132297

[12] Almutham A, Altami M, Sharaf F, AlAraj A. E-cigarette use among medical students at Qassim university: Knowledge, perception, and prevalence. Journal of Family Medical Primers Care.

2019;**8**:2921-2926. DOI: 10.4103/jfmpc.jfmpc_567_19

[13] European Commission. Special Eurobarometer 458: Attitudes of Europeans Towards Tobacco and Electronic Cigarettes. 2017. Available from: https://data.europa.eu/euodp/en/data/dataset/S2146_87_1_458_ENG

[14] Wang RJ, Bhadriraju S, Glantz SA. E-cigarette use and adult cigarette smoking cessation: A meta-analysis. American Journal of Public Health. 2021;**111**(2):230-246. DOI: 10.2105/AJPH.2020.305999

[15] McMillen RC, Gottlieb MA, Shaefer RM, Winickoff JP, Klein JD. Trends in electronic cigarette use among U.S. adults: Use is increasing in both smokers and non-smokers. Nicotine & Tobacco Research: Official Journal of the Society for Research on Nicotine and Tobacco. 2015;**17**(10):1195-1202. DOI: 10.1093/ntr/ntu213

[16] Hua M, Talbot P. Potential health effects of electronic cigarettes: A systematic review of case reports. Preventive Medicine Reports. 2016;**4**:169-178. DOI: 10.1016/j.pmedr.2016.06.002

[17] Zhong J, Cao S, Gong W, Fei F, Wang M. Electronic cigarettes use and intention to cigarette smoking among never-smoking adolescents and young adults: A meta-analysis. International Journal of Environmental Research and Public Health. 2016;**13**(5):465. DOI: 10.3390/ijerph13050465

[18] National Academies of Science and Engineering. Public Health Consequences of E-cigarettes. 2018 [Cited 2018 Sep 28]. Available from: http://nationalacademies.org/hmd/Reports/2018/public-healthconsequences-of-e-cigarettes.aspx

[19] Grana R, Benowitz N, Glantz SA. E-cigarettes: a scientific review. Circulation. 2014;**129**(19):1972-1986

[20] Journals BMJ. Tobacco control – FDA E-cigarettes: Impact on individual and population. Health. 2014;**23**(2)

[21] Kamboj A, Spiller HA, Casavant MJ, Chounthirath T, Smith GA. Pediatric exposure to e-cigarettes, nicotine, and tobacco products in the United States. Pediatrics. 2016:e20160041

[22] Yuan M, Cross SJ, Loughlin SE, Leslie FM. Nicotine, and the adolescent brain. The Journal of Physiology. 2015;**593**(16):3397-3412

[23] England LJ, Bunnell RE, Pechacek TF, Tong VT, McAfee TA. Nicotine and the developing human: A neglected element in the electronic cigarette debate. American Journal of Preventive Medicine. 2015;**49**(2):286-293

[24] Kandel D, Kandel E. The gateway hypothesis of substance abuse: Developmental, biological, and societal perspectives. Acta Paediatrica. 2015;**104**(2):130-137

[25] Grana RA. Electronic cigarettes: A new nicotine gateway? Journal of Adolescent Health. 2013;**52**(2):135-136

[26] Kumetz EA, Hurst ND, Cudnik RJ, Rudinsky SL. Electronic cigarette explosion injuries. The American Journal of Emergency Medicine. 2016;**34**(11):2252-22e1

[27] Jerzyński T, Stimson GV, Shapiro HL. Estimation of the global number of e-cigarette users. Harm Reduction Journal. 2021;**18**:109. DOI: 10.1186/s12954-021-00556-7

[28] Khoury M, Manlhiot C, Fan CP, Gibson D, Stearne K, Chahal N, et al.

Reported electronic cigarette use among adolescents in the Niagara region of Ontario. Canadian Medical Association Journal. 2016:cmaj-151169

[29] Tozzi J, Bachman J. Big Tobacco Keeps Pushing into e-Cigarettes. Bloomberg Business Week; 2014 [cited 2018 Sep 27]. Available from: http://www.businessweek.com/articles/2014-06-17/big-tobacco-keeps-pushing-into-e-cigarettes

[30] Qanash S, Alemam S, Mahdi E, Softah J, Touman AA, Alsulami A. Electronic cigarette among health science students in Saudi Arabia. Annals of Thoracic Medicine. 2019;**14**:56-62. DOI: 10.4103/atm.ATM_76_18

[31] Farsalinos KE, Polosa R. Safety evaluation and risk assessment of electronic cigarettes as tobacco cigarette substitutes: A systematic review. Therapeutic Advances in Drug Safety. 2014;**5**:67-86. DOI: 10.1177/2042098614524430

[32] Cho JH, Paik SY. Association between electronic cigarette use and asthma among high school students in South Korea. PLoS One. 2016;**11**:e0151022. DOI: 10.1371/journal.pone.0151022

[33] Siegel DA, Jatlaoui TC, Koumans EH, Kiernan EA, Layer M, Cates JE, et al. Update: Interim guidance for health care providers evaluating and caring for patients with a suspected e-cigarette, or vaping, product use associated lung injury - United States, October 2019. MMWR. Morbidity and Mortality Weekly Report. 2019;**68**:919-927. DOI: 10.15585/mmwr.mm6841e3

[34] MacDonald A, Middlekauff HR. Electronic cigarettes, and cardiovascular health: What do we know so far? Vascular Health and Risk Management. 2019;**5**:159-174. DOI: 10.2147/VHRM.S175970